14. MAGNIFICATION:

$$\frac{\textbf{(SID) source-to-image distance}}{\textbf{(SOD) source-to-object distance}} = \text{Magnification factor}$$

15. PENUMBRA FORMULA (Geometric Unsharpness):

$$\frac{\textbf{(FSS) focal spot size} \times \textbf{(OID) object-to-image distance}}{\textbf{(SOD) source-to-object distance}} = \text{Penumbra}$$

16. GRID RADIO:

$$\frac{\textbf{H} \text{ (height)}}{\textbf{D} \text{ (distance)}} = \text{Grid ratio}$$

H = The height of the opaque material, usually lead

D = The distance of the interspace, radiolucent material, between the lead strips

17. AUTOMATIC BRIGHTNESS CONTROL:

Total brightness gain =
Flux gain × minification gain

Minification gain =

$$\frac{(\text{Input screen diameter})^2}{(\text{Output screen diameter})^2}$$

18. TECHNICAL CHANGES FOR PART THICKNESS:

Increase part thickness by 5 cm =
Double (× 2) the mAs
Decrease part thickness by 5 cm = 50%
decrease in mAs

or

kVp = 2 kVp per cm

Casts

Fiberglass: Same as part thickness
(above)

Plaster:

Wet: 15 kVp, or 3 × mAs

Dry: 10 kVp, or 2 × mAs

19. SOURCE-TO-SKIN DISTANCE (SSD):

Fixed radiographic unit: 15" minimum
Portable radiographic unit: 12" minimum
This includes image intensification and
C-arm machines.

20. FAHRENHEIT TO CELSIUS CONVERSION:

9/5 (C) + 32 = Degrees Fahrenheit
5/9 (F) − 32 = Degrees Celsius

21. RADIATION UNITS:

Traditional Units	SI Units
1 rad	0.01 gray
1 rem	0.01 sievert
1 curie	3.7×10^{10} becquerel
1 roentgen	2.58×10^{-4} C/kg of air
100 rad	1 gray
100 rem	1 sievert

Radiography
Study Guide and
Registry Review

Radiography
Study Guide and
Registry Review

Ruth S. Widmer, AAS, RT(R)
Assistant Administrative Director, Radiology
St. Joseph's Hospital and Medical Center
Paterson, New Jersey

Kenneth W. Van Soelen, AAS, RT(R) (MR)
MRI Technologist
The Valley Hospital
Ridgewood, New Jersey

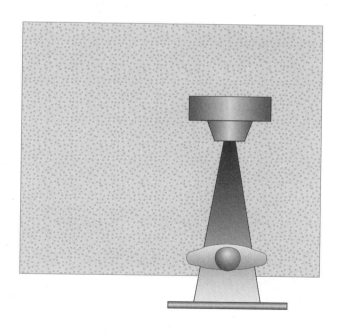

W.B. SAUNDERS COMPANY
A Division of Harcourt Brace & Company
Philadelphia London Toronto Montreal Sydney Tokyo

W.B. SAUNDERS COMPANY
A Division of Harcourt Brace & Company

The Curtis Center
Independence Square West
Philadelphia, Pennsylvania 19106

Library of Congress Cataloging-in-Publication Data

Widmer, Ruth S.

Radiography study guide and registry review / Ruth S. Widmer, Kenneth W.
Van Soelen.—1st ed.

p.   cm.

ISBN 0–7216–7289–2

1. Radiology, Medical—Examinations, questions, etc.   I. Van Soelen, Kenneth W.
II. Title.   [DNLM: 1. Radiography examination questions.   2. Technology,
radiologic examination questions.   WN 18.2 W641r 1999]

R896.W54   1999   616.07′572′076—dc21

DNLM/DLC   98–13364

RADIOGRAPHY STUDY GUIDE AND REGISTRY REVIEW   ISBN 0–7216–7289–2

Printed in the United States of America.

Last digit is the print number: 9   8   7   6   5   4   3   2   1

In memory of Michael Jon Smith, BS, RT(R)
(1955–1997)

To Constance S. Whittemore, BS, RT(R). You are a first-class educator, mentor, and technologist. May this dedication honor you on behalf of all of us whose lives you have touched. Thank you, Connie.

To Ken. For being the initiator of this project as well as my confidant and co-author supreme. You are my true and faithful friend.

To Nora and Kara. To my bright and beautiful daughters, with love and gratitude, for your patience, love, humor, and understanding during the past three years. May this endeavor inspire you both to realize your dreams!

RSW

To Ryan Mitchell, my son. You are my inspiration and motivation. You have given me a new perspective on life—there are no limits. You will always be my best friend. I love you.

To Ingrid, my wife. Thank you for believing in me and giving me the courage to believe in myself. You are a beautiful, caring woman and a wonderful mother. I'll always love you.

To Ruth, my co-author. Without your honesty, encouragement, and support, this project never would have happened. You are a dear friend. I admire and respect you both personally and professionally. Thank you, Ruth.

KVS

To Samy Ayoub, RPh, MS, Pharm D, and Frances Manelis, RN. With special appreciation.

To Marian Spied, RN, JD. Thank you for reviewing specific chapters for professional content accuracy. Your time and suggestions were invaluable.

To Richard Green who photographed our selected radiographs so beautifully.

To Jacquie Ricker who saved us from just one more weekend of keying in questions.

To Lisa Biello who knew a good thing when she saw it.

To Rachael Kelly, our developmental editor, thanks for the day in Philadelphia, for listening to our concerns, and for tying together all the loose ends at a moment's notice.

To Andrew Allen, our editor, for supporting our belief that software is a viable publishing medium.

To all the W.B. Saunders Company staff for their professional expertise, patience, and guidance. Thank you!

RSW and KVS

PREFACE

Our main objective in creating the *Radiography Study Guide and Registry Review* is to ease the burden of studying for the Registry. We hope to provide you with more than you need for the Registry Review in a format that encourages you to read, learn, review, and share. After completing a radiography program, too many students are still bewildered about what material is important. We have included what we believe the ARRT deems important by utilizing their content specifications as our table of contents. In addition, we include all that our dual experiences define as important based on the fact that health care is changing on a daily basis and requires more knowledge and responsibility from every medical professional and paraprofessional. We have included topics that, although they are not yet necessary for Registry requirements, are still needed by radiologic technologists in their everyday knowledge base and/or job performance. These involve increased nursing-related concerns, new pharmaceuticals, oxygen formulas, patient monitoring and performance improvement standards, and future considerations.

Our experience is gained from two different perspectives. One vision encompasses almost 30 years in the medical field of radiography, as student, technologist, educator, and administrator. The second view is from a relatively recent graduate who continued with his education to become multiregistered. He currently performs magnetic resonance imaging. Our common philosophy is that information must be shared. An explanation that requires a synthesis of didactic and clinical experience is most effective. Rather than isolate specific subject material, we have blended multiple subjects, incorporating our own experience, when necessary, to provide you with "holistic" explanations that will help you understand how it all works together. A solution that can be applied in the real-world environment is essential. We believe that we have succeeded in accomplishing that for you.

If you are a confident student or instructor, this book will provide you with a challenging review of standard subject material and updated issues and a wealth of questions and answers. If you are hazy about what your own learning requirements are, this book will quickly define them and provide supporting reference information. As a student, an instructor, or a technologist re-entering the profession: all of you will find benefit in the use of *Radiography Study Guide and Registry Review.*

Our hope is that our endeavor clarifies problematic subject material for you, supports you in the information you already possess, inspires you to always learn more than you really need to know, and most of all helps you to share your knowledge with others.

RSW
KVS

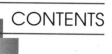

CONTENTS

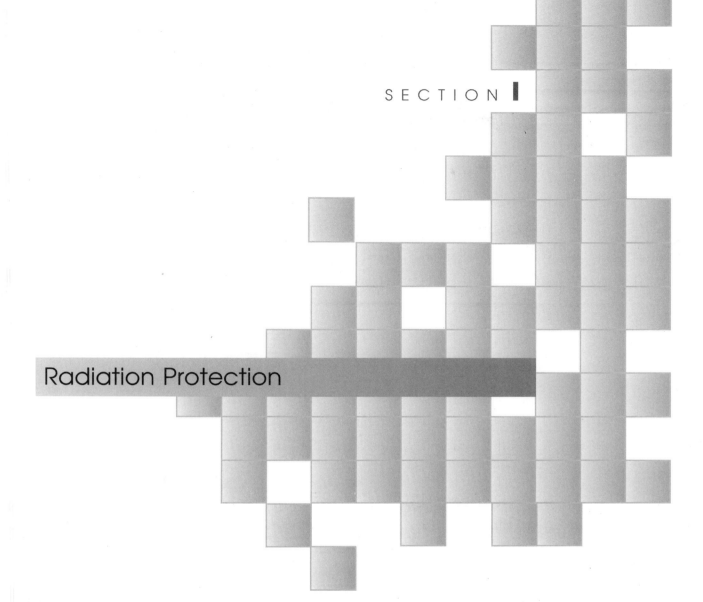

Radiation Protection

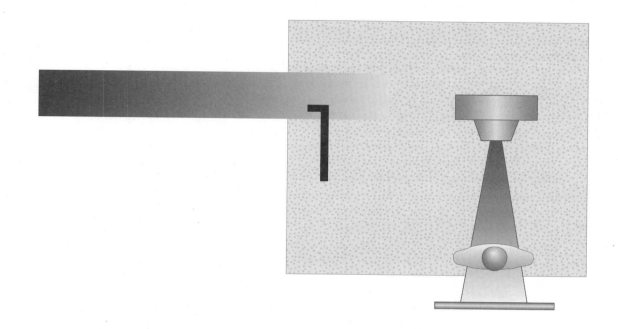

PATIENT
PROTECTION

Glossary

1. **Half-value layer–** The amount of a material necessary to reduce the intensity of radiation to one half of its original intensity.

Example:
A diagnostic unit has a half-value layer of 2.5 mm Al (aluminum). An exposure is measured at 40″ SID (source-to-image distance) and reads 3 mr (milliroentgen)/mAs (milliampere-second). What would be the new exposure reading if 2.5 of Al was placed within the path of the beam? The additional 2.5 Al will reduce the beam's intensity by half, 1.5 mr/mAs.

2. **Half-life–** The time required for a radioactive material to decay to half of its original intensity.

Example:
A dose of iodine-131 measured at 100 mr has a half-life of 6 hours. How long would it take for the isotope to decay completely? The isotope decreases in half for every 6 hours that passes:

100 mr/2	= 50 mr at 6 hours
50 mr/2	= 25 mr at 12 hours
25 mr/2	= 12.5 mr at 18 hours
12.5 mr/2	= 6.25 mr at 24 hours
6.25 mr/2	= 3.125 mr at 30 hours
3.125 mr/2	= 1.5625 mr at 42 hours
1.5625 mr/2	= 0.78125 mr at 48 hours

3. **Relative biological effectiveness (RBE)–** The capability of radiations with different energy transfer rates to produce particular reactions when compared with a reference radiation, usually an x-ray photon of 250 kVp. This helps determine the possible effects of alpha-radiation when compared with the same quantity of x-radiation.

4. **Quality factor (QF)–** A modification factor used in the calculation of the dose that is equivalent to the ability of a dose of any kind of radiation to cause biological damage. These factors are different depending upon the ionizing ability of the radiation. X-radiation and gamma- and beta-radiation have a quality factor of 1, whereas alpha-radiation with fast neutrons has a quality factor of 20. This means that 10 mr of alpha-radiation equals 200 mr of x-radiation.

5. **Linear energy transfer (LET)–** The average energy deposited per unit of path length to a medium by ionizing radiation as it passes through that medium. This means that radiation, such as particle radiation, has a higher LET and has the capability of depositing more energy per unit of tract length; therefore, it has the potential to cause more damage.

6. **Primary radiation–** Radiation that is exiting from the tube port before it interacts with matter (Fig. 1–1).

7. **Remnant radiation–** Radiation that exits from the patient as it travels toward the image receptor. This is the primary radiation minus the radiation that is attenuated by the patient as it travels through the body. This type of radiation is also referred to as exit radiation, or image-forming radiation (Fig. 1–1).

8. **Radiosensitivity–** Refers to structures that are easily affected by ionizing radiation, such as gonads, skin, and lining of the gastrointestinal tract.

9. **Radioresistant–** Refers to structures that are not easily affected by ionizing radiation,

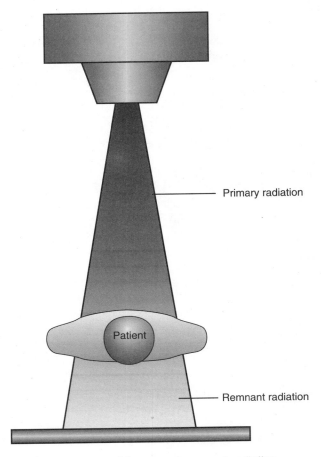

Figure 1-1 ■ Primary and remnant radiation.

Primary radiation

Patient

Remnant radiation

such as brain, nerve tissue, and muscle tissue.

10. **Acute dosage–** A large dosage of radiation delivered over a short period of time, within 24 hours. This type of dosage is delivered by a radiation leakage or meltdown.
11. **Chronic dosage–** A large amount of radiation delivered in small amounts over a long period of time. This type of dosage is delivered by small radiation leakages or excessive diagnostic examinations.
12. **Short-term effects–** Effects of ionizing radiation evident in the exposed individual within 30 days after the exposure. Epilation and erythema are examples of a short-term effect. Onset is sudden after the exposure but effects usually are not permanent.
13. **Long-term effects–** Effects of ionizing radiation in the exposed individual evident 30 days postexposure. Cataracts and cancer are examples of long-term effects; these begin slowly and progress over time and usually are permanent.

REGULATORY AGENCIES

Four agencies perform radiation research and determine limits for radiation exposure and its possible effects. These agencies do not make or enforce laws.

1. **ICRP**—International Council on Radiation Protection
2. **UNSCEAR**—United Nations Scientific Community on the Effects of Atomic Radiation
3. **NAS BEIR**—National Academy of Science, Advisory Committee, Biological Effects of Ionizing Radiation
4. **NCRP**—National Council on Radiation Protection

The Nuclear Regulatory Commission (NRC) reviews the recommendations made by the other agencies listed and enforces them as law. The NRC may be influenced by any of the four agencies.

RADIATION EXPOSURE

Studying the effects of ionizing radiation is very difficult because there is no disease unique to radiation, only radiation syndromes. Therefore, any disease may originate from another cause. To depict accurately the results of radiation exposure, a study must be made over many years and must include a large group of people. Studies have utilized World War II atomic bomb survi-

vors, uranium miners, and the people exposed to the Chernobyl reactor meltdown in the Ukraine.

The number one radiation protection rule is the ALARA concept: *As Low as Reasonably Achievable.* This means that any dose of radiation should yield the lowest amount possible with the highest degree of radiation protection available. And the relative risk of the radiation exposure must not outweigh the potential benefit of the exposure.

BIOLOGICAL EFFECTS OF RADIATION

Radiation interaction is a random process that increases as the amount of energy transferred increases. The energy is deposited very rapidly and is randomly distributed over the exposed area. It cannot be attracted or repelled in one area more than another. The interaction may or may not cause biological or chemical changes; this is also a random process, increasing with the quantity of energy. If biological or chemical changes do occur, they will present only after a latent (delayed) period, in the form of another disease. The damage becomes apparent on the cellular level.

Basic Cellular Anatomy (Macromolecules)

1. **Cytoplasm–** The liquid contained within the cell that bathes all the cellular components. The cytoplasm is composed mostly of water.
2. **Cell membrane–** Gives structure and form to the cell. It serves to contain all the cellular components and provides protection from the surrounding environment.
3. **Endoplasmic reticulum (ER)–** Provides a transport network within the cell. It serves to transport cellular substances from one area to another within the cell. There are two varieties:

   Rough ER—Endoplasmic reticulum with ribosomes
   Smooth ER—Endoplasmic reticulum without ribosomes

4. **Ribosomes–** These organelles are found attached to the endoplasmic reticulum. They receive encoded messages from the nucleus in the form of RNA and use this information to manufacture proteins.
5. **Golgi apparatus–** This component serves as a transport for substances to be transported outside the cell. This organelle acquires proteins and other substances,

packages them, and transports them to the cell membrane.

6. **Mitochondria–** These organelles break down certain substances to create high-energy chemical bonds to be used in the cell for energy. Without these organelles the cell would not be able to carry out its basic life functions. The more energy required by the cell, the more mitochondria will be found in the cell.

7. **Lysosome–** Contains digestive enzymes that are used to detoxify the cell and protect it from invading organisms.

8. **Centrosome–** A spindle-shaped organelle used in cell division.

9. **Nucleus–** Usually located in the center of the cell. It contains all the genetic material, called DNA, and serves as the cellular brain directing all the other organelles in their functions. It is surrounded by a selectively permeable membrane called the nuclear envelope, which serves to contain and protect the genetic material of the cell.

10. **Deoxyribonucleic acid (DNA)–** A highly complex macromolecule controlling all cellular activity. DNA consists of

   1. Deoxyribose
   2. Phosphoric acid
   3. Four bases:
      a. Two purine: adenine and guanine
      b. Two pyrimidine: thymine and cytosine

Mitosis Cell Division (Somatic Cells)
(Fig. 1–2)

Prophase. During this phase, the chromatids condense into chromosomes, and the nuclear envelope begins to disappear. Centrosomes begin to migrate to the opposite side of the cell and form the spindle fibers.

Metaphase. Chromosomes migrate to the middle of the spindle fibers. The chromosomes duplicate, forming kinetochores, which attach to the spindle fibers.

Anaphase. The spindle fibers begin to retract. The kinetochores split and migrate to opposite ends of the spindle.

Telophase. The spindle fibers finish retracting, and the duplicated chromosomes are now located at each end of the cell. The nuclear envelope reappears and the chromosomes change back into chromatids. The cell membrane splits off, and the organelles are randomly divided between the two new daughter cells. Each of the daughter cells has the exact genetic information that the parent cell contained.

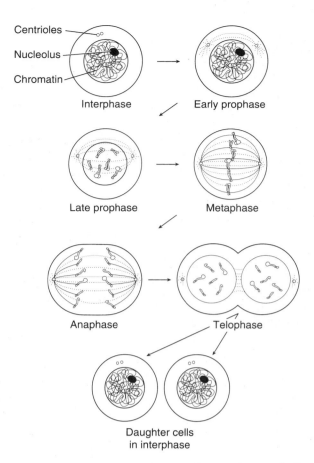

Figure 1-2 ■ Mitosis, shown as occurring in a cell of a hypothetical animal with a diploid chromosome number of six (haploid number three); one pair of chromosomes is short, one pair is long and hooked, and one pair is long and knobbed. (From Dorland's Illustrated Medical Dictionary. 28th ed. Philadelphia, WB Saunders, 1994.)

Meiosis Cell Division (Germ Cells)
(Fig. 1–3)

Germ cells undergo cell division exactly as do somatic cells, through the four phases (P, M, A, T) just described. Once this process is complete, germ cells undergo an additional division without duplicating the genetic material. Therefore the parent cell (46 chromosomes) yields two daughters, each with 46 chromosomes, and two granddaughter cells, each with 23 chromosomes. The granddaughter cells are now ready for procreation.

Cellular Radiation Effects

Direct Effect. This type of interaction occurs when an incoming photon ionizes a macromolecule within a cell. This may cause the macromolecule to dysfunction resulting in structural or chemical changes within the cell. The macromolecule may die or the entire cell may die.

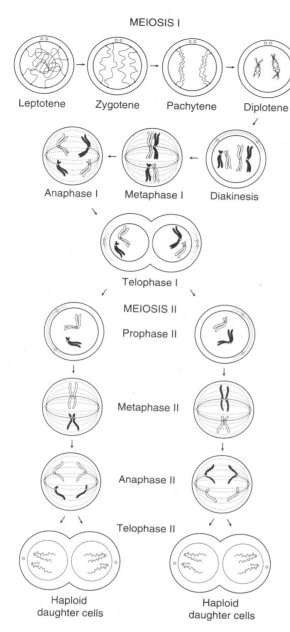

MEIOSIS I

Leptotene   Zygotene   Pachytene   Diplotene

Anaphase I   Metaphase I   Diakinesis

Telophase I

MEIOSIS II

Prophase II

Metaphase II

Anaphase II

Telophase II

Haploid daughter cells   Haploid daughter cells

Figure 1-3 ■ Meiosis. Only 2 of the 23 human chromosome pairs are shown, the chromosomes from one parent in black, those from the other parent in outline. (From Dorland's Illustrated Medical Dictionary. 28th ed. Philadelphia, WB Saunders, 1994.)

Indirect Effect. This type of interaction occurs when the water within the cell (80% to 90% of the cell) becomes irritated by an incoming photon. When water is ionized, it produces a free electron (e^-) and a positively charged water molecule (HOH^+). HOH^+ and e^- may recombine and cause no damage to the cell at all. But, if e^- and HOH^+ do not recombine and e^- rejoins with another water molecule, an unstable water molecule will be created ($e^- + H_2O = HOH^-$). The result is two unstable water molecules, HOH^+

and HOH^-. These water molecules can break apart very easily and form free radicals: HOH^+ = H^+ and *OH (free radical)* and HOH^- = OH^- + *H (free radical)*. The H^+ and the OH^- rejoin and reform a stable water molecule. The free radicals *(OH and H)* are highly energetic but carry no charge. They can cause many reactions to occur within the cell. They may cause damaging chemicals or interfere with the function of the cellular macromolecules. This may result in cellular death or may alter cellular activity (Fig. 1–4).

Dose-Effect Relationships

These relationships may be defined by any of the following examples, which are graphic representations of exposure and response.

The first consideration for dose-response curves:

Threshold. This response requires a minimum amount of exposure before any effect is noted (Figs. 1–5, 1–7).

Nonthreshold. This is a response to any amount of radiation regardless of how small the exposure (Figs. 1–6, 1–8).

The second consideration for dose-response curves:

Linear. The curve or line increases proportional to the exposure (Figs. 1–5, 1–6).

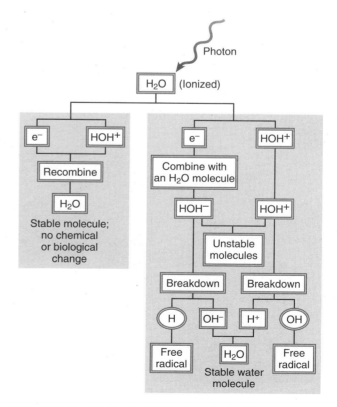

Figure 1-4 ■ Indirect effect of an ionized water molecule.

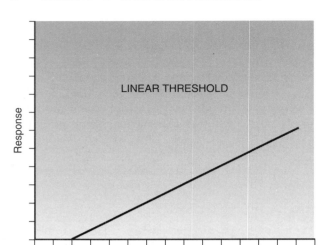

Figure 1-5 ■ Graphic representation of a linear threshold dose response curve.

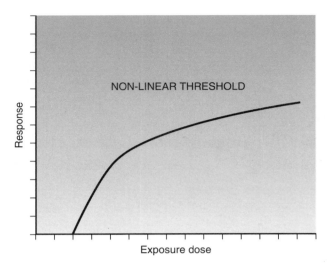

Figure 1-7 ■ Graphic representation of a non-linear threshold dose response curve.

Nonlinear. The curve or line increases but not in proportion to the exposure. This type of response usually is referred to as *curvilinear* or *quadratic*. When applying these dose-response relationships to radiation protection, a non-threshold model is used, even though a threshold model may depict the actual response more accurately (Figs. 1–7, 1–8).

STOCHASTIC EFFECT

This effect is classified as a random response in which the response increases with the dose delivered, but the severity of the response does not necessarily increase. This would be noted in a nonthreshold linear or curvilinear graph. An example of a stochastic effect is cancer.

NONSTOCHASTIC EFFECT

This type of dose response relationship demonstrates a threshold. As the dosage increases, the severity of the response also increases. Therefore, a disease-specific minimum exposure is necessary for a response to occur. An example of a nonstochastic effect is cataracts.

Long-Term Effects

A long-term effect has an extended latent period, with no response for weeks, months, or even years. These radiation exposures are usually chronic, but long-term effects may occur with acute exposures as well. Some long-term effects are discussed next in relation to the various types of radiation.

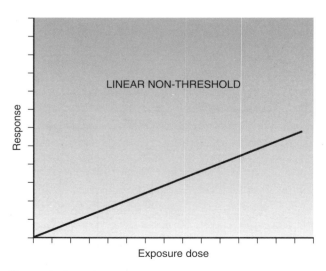

Figure 1-6 ■ Graphic representation of a linear non-threshold dose response curve.

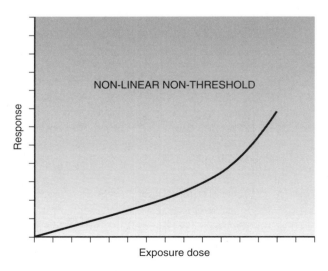

Figure 1-8 ■ Graphic representation of a non-linear non-threshold dose response curve.

Cancer

The carcinogenic effect of radiation has been studied in events such as medical exposure, occupational exposure, and disasters. Using varying types of radiation exposure, scientists are able to demonstrate a correlation between exposure and cancer as a result of the exposure. Exposure dependency results in a stochastic effect and is described by a linear nonthreshold dose-response curve. This is because it is not known how much radiation is needed for carcinogenesis. The important aspect of this research is that the cancer, regardless of type, is no different from cancer that may have occurred without radiation exposure.

Cataracts

Opacification of the lens of the eye denotes a cataract. This is usually caused by an increased amount of epithelial cells—the cells that make up the lens—being sloughed off and accumulating on the lens. A relationship has been identified between radiation exposure to the eyes and the production of cataracts. This is a nonstochastic effect and is described by a threshold nonlinear response curve. Minimum exposure may result in cataract formation. Cataracts may be produced with exposures as low as 200 rad, but are usually from a cumulative chronic exposure.

Life Span Shortening

Shortening of the natural life span due to radiation exposure has been demonstrated through studies of early radiologists. Radiation may accelerate the natural aging process and cause tissue degeneration and disease. The diseases are prematurely induced and are not unique to radiation exposure. Occupational exposure doses for the radiographic technologist do not seem to be a problem in modern radiology departments because of technical advancements and precautions taken by workers. Nuclear medicine technologists appear to receive the largest occupational exposure dose.

LETHAL DOSE

The term *LD 50/30* means that a large dose of radiation delivered over a short period of time will cause 50% of the population to die within 30 days of the exposure. The precise LD 50/30 for humans is not known. Investigators have studied many groups that received large doses of radiation and have quantified an approximate LD 50/ 30 for humans at about 250 to 450 rad, depending upon how the radiation is delivered.

ACUTE RADIATION SYNDROME

This is caused by a large dose of radiation delivered to the whole body over a short period of time: less than 24 hours. Radiation syndromes usually result in death and are characterized by three periods:

Prodromal Period. This phase does not last more than 24 hours after the exposure. It is characterized by nausea, vomiting, anorexia, and apathy.

Latent Period. This phase is characterized by an absence of all symptoms. The body is assessing the damage caused by the radiation but has not responded to it yet. The body undergoes depletion of cells without being able to replenish them. This period lasts until the body is able to recognize the disturbance in homeostasis.

Manifest Period. This phase immediately following the latency period is the actual response to the radiation, radiation sickness. It is divided into three major categories: hematopoietic syndrome, gastrointestinal syndrome, and central nervous system syndrome.

Hematopoietic Syndrome. This syndrome occurs at exposures of between 100 and 1000 rad. The hematopoietic (blood-forming) system is the most radiosensitive system in the body. The onset of this syndrome includes:

- decrease in red blood cells
- decrease in white blood cells
- decrease in thrombocytes (clotting cells)

resulting in a major decrease in immunity and the body's ability to clot. The decrease in bone marrow (blood-forming) cells enables opportunistic pathogens to cause infections or possible hemorrhage. This level of exposure will cause death within 30 days. The latent period is about 2 to 3 weeks. Those affected usually die of infections and/or hemorrhage.

Gastrointestinal Syndrome. This syndrome occurs with exposure doses of between 600 and 1000 rad. It is characterized by damage to the epithelial lining of the gastrointestinal system. This inhibits the normal function of the GI tract and leads to dehydration, nausea, vomiting, ulcerations, and hemorrhage. This syndrome includes many symptoms of the hematopoietic syndrome, allowing for widespread infection from abnormally high levels of the body's own bacterial flora. With an exposure of this magnitude, the latent period lasts only 3 to 5 days and death occurs within 10 to 14 days.

Central Nervous System Syndrome. This syndrome is characterized by exposure doses of between 2000 and 5000 rad. Confusion, disorientation, ataxia, and an increase in intracranial pressure are symptoms. The exposed individual may also experience seizures, periods of agitation, and shock, which usually lead to coma and eventual death. The latent period may range from 15 minutes to 12 hours, with death occurring within 14 to 36 hours.

Somatic Effects

These effects are seen in irradiated individuals. They may be *early* or *late* effects. An early effect is evident in about 30 to 60 days and usually involves an imbalance of the body's natural homeostasis; a late effect may take months or even years to become evident.

Embryonic and Fetal Effects

Genetic effects are congenital and occur only in utero. The magnitude of these effects is proportional to the gestational time that the developing fetus received the radiation exposure, because this is a major factor in determining the radiosensitivity of the fetus. These may be reviewed in the three gestational periods:

First Trimester. This embryonic stage is highly radiosensitive because many cells are undifferentiated and dividing rapidly. Within this stage the implantation period, up to 9 days postconception, is the most radiosensitive. An exposure that elicits a response during this stage usually results in embryonic death.

Second Trimester. Usually this period is a little less radiosensitive because organogenesis has begun, and most cells are differentiated into the rudiments of the organs they are going to form. During this period the embryonic cells divide rapidly and have a high oxygen content, increasing the radiosensitivity according to the Bergonié-Tribondeau law. Exposures during this time probably will not result in embryonic death but may lead to severe fetal malformations.

Third Trimester. Even though the fetus is still considered radiosensitive, this period is the most radioresistant. The effects of an exposure during this time are usually not fatal. They are generally related to the central nervous system. Exposed individuals may later present with low IQs or neurologic problems.

Bone Marrow

Bone marrow contains the blood-forming stem cells. The red blood-forming marrow is more radiosensitive than the fatty yellow marrow. Children have more red bone marrow than do adults, which makes them more radiosensitive. Bone marrow may be affected by a chronic or acute dose of as low as 200 rad, which can disturb the hematopoietic (blood-forming) system. Exposure doses that are delivered to red bone marrow are termed mean marrow dose, or MMD.

Thyroid

This gland is located very superficially in the neck. It is composed mainly of epithelial tissue, which raises its radiosensitivity. It is documented that tumors of the thyroid may occur with doses as low as 50 rad.

Genetic Effects

These effects are caused by irradiation of germ cells (egg and sperm). They do not show in the individuals who are irradiated but rather in their children. Irradiated gonads may interfere with an individual's fertility. With a dose of 200 rad, temporary sterility may occur in both men and women. A dose of 500 to 600 rad may cause permanent sterility. If sterility does not occur and the damaged cell is part of procreation, the effect will become evident in following generations.

A point mutation results from a change in a single base pair in the DNA molecule. In a chromosomal mutation, large regions of a chromosome are affected. Chromosomal aberrations are more common (90%) than point mutations and are discussed later.

Genetically Significant Dose

This is defined as a dose of radiation that, if given to the entire population, would cause significant genetic effects. For humans, such a dose is estimated at about 20 rad. This figure is determined by computing the average dose received by the population with the greatest chance of procreating.

Doubling Dose. A doubling dose is the quantity of radiation that is required to double the amount of mutation that occurs naturally. For example, if Down's syndrome were found in 5% of all living births, the addition of the doubling dose of radiation would increase the occurrence of Down's to 10% in all live births. In humans, the doubling dose is estimated to be about 50 to 250 rad of x-ray or gamma radiation.

Genetic Effect

Genetic effects will occur only if the macromolecule DNA is damaged in the irradiated individual, following which it is used in procreation. The types of DNA mutations caused by ionizing radiation are as follows:

Single Strand, One Break. One break in the chromosome. There are three types of single strand breaks:

1. Terminal deletion—the end of the chromosome is broken off and does not reattach.
2. Inversion—the end is broken and reattached upside down.
3. Duplication—the end of one chromosome is broken and reattaches to the end of another chromosome.

Single Strand, Double Break. Two breaks on the same chromosome. There are four types of double strand breaks:

1. Interstitial deletion—two breaks occur on the same end of the same chromosome.
2. Inversion—two breaks on the same chromosome; the middle free segment inverts and reattaches with the chromosome.
3. Duplication—two breaks on the same chromosome; one or both of the free segments reattach to another chromosome.
4. Translocation—two different chromosomes receive breaks, with the segments of each attaching to the other chromosome.

Acentric and Decentric Formations
Acentric. Two breaks occur to the same chromosome. The smaller fragments join to form the acentric portion of the model while the chromosome forms a ring with its ends joining.

Decentric. Two breaks occur to two different chromosomes. The fragments join and form the acentric portion of the model. The larger parts of the chromosomes join at their broken ends and form the decentric portion of the model.

Relative Tissue Radiosensitivity

Relative tissue radiosensitivity is determined by cellular or tissue composition. This is best described by the *Bergonié-Tribondeau law,* which has three basic principles that determine tissue radiosensitivity:

1. The more mitotic activity occurring, the more radiosensitive the cell or tissue.
2. The less differentiated the cell or tissue, the more radiosensitive the cell or tissue.
3. The higher the oxygen content at the time of irradiation, the more radiosensitive the cell or tissue.

High radiosensitivity is found in

■ Lymphocytes
■ Blood-forming cells
■ Germ (sex) cells
■ Lens of the eye

Moderate radiosensitivity is seen in

■ Growing bone and cartilage
■ Epithelium of the kidneys, liver, pancreas, thyroid, and adrenal glands

Low radiosensitive tissue is

■ Muscle tissue
■ Mature bone and cartilage
■ Nervous tissue

Weight Factor

Because the human body is made up of various tissues, a weight factor has been studied to give a more accurate probability of possible mutations or induction of cancer caused by radiation. A weight factor accurately calculates doses from exposures to different areas of the body rather than from a whole body dose. Usually radiation exposures are most often very localized, not equally delivered over the entire body.

Some common organs and their weight factors are

Gonads	0.25
Breasts	0.15
Red bone marrow	0.12
Lung	0.12
Thyroid	0.03
Bone surface	0.03
Remainder	0.30
Whole body	1.00

Example:
If the thyroid received a dose of 20 mrad and the breasts received a dose of 60 mrad, the total whole body dose would not be 80 mrad. Partial body doses are calculated as follows:

20 mrad × 0.03 (thyroid) = 0.60 mrad
60 mrad × 0.15 (breast) = 9.0 mrad
0.60 mrad + 9.0 mrad = 9.6 mrad
total dosage

MINIMIZING PATIENT EXPOSURE
Exposure Factors

These determine the overall quality and quantity of the useful beam exposure that produces the radiograph. Generally, the highest practical kVp with the longest acceptable time and the lowest mA will yield the lowest patient exposure dose. This is true because with a higher effective kVp, more energy will pass through the patient rather then become absorbed by the patient. And the human body is better able to recover from a small quantity of radiation over a longer period of time (low mA and long time) rather than a large quantity of radiation (high mA and short time) over a shorter period of time.

Patient exposure doses are usually calculated three different ways: skin entrance dose, gonadal dose, and bone marrow dose. The controlling factors are as follows:

Kilovoltage Peak (kVp). This determines the quality and penetrating ability of the useful beam. A high kVp will produce a useful beam of higher quality and more penetrating ability. Therefore more of the useful beam will pass through the patient and expose the radiographic film, thus decreasing the amount of ionizations occurring within the patient, reducing the energy deposited into the patient, and reducing the absorbed dosage.

Using an excessive kVp will cause an increase in scatter and secondary radiation, thus increasing patient exposure. Secondary and scatter radiation are composed of low-energy photons that are readily absorbed by the patient. The kVp is selected to match the anatomy being examined. The kVp required to radiograph a wrist (45 to 50 kVp) would not penetrate the femur or hip area, but the kVp necessary to penetrate the femur or hip (65 to 70 kVp) would be excessive if used to radiograph the wrist. Either way, if the kVp selected is not appropriate for the anatomical area, the patient's exposure will only increase because a repeat radiograph will be needed.

Milliampere-Seconds (mAs). This factor is divided into two categories, mA and time.

mA is the resultant quantity of photons available at the time of the exposure produced by the tube current.

Time is the actual length of time that the electrons are allowed to travel across the tube to produce x-rays.

Collectively, the mA and time make up the mAs value, and this value is directly related to patient exposure. When times are longer, less mA may be used to maintain density on the radiograph. This will not cause a decrease in overall patient exposure. With reduction of mA and an increase in time, a smaller dosage of radiation is delivered over a longer period of time. The body can withstand a smaller dose over a longer period of time better than a larger dose delivered in a short period of time. But motion must be considered when lengthening exposure times.

Single-Phase, Three-Phase, and High-Frequency Generators. Patient dosage can be reduced by using a high-frequency generator because it produces a monoenergetic beam. In a single-phase machine, the potential kVp rises to the peak and drops down to 0. Therefore, photons are produced in a variety of wavelengths. Low-frequency photons do not contribute to the diagnostic image because they are not highly penetrating. With a three-phase generator, the voltage never drops to 0, therefore low-energy photons are almost eliminated. A three-phase generator will still have some voltage drop-off and allow lower-energy photons to be created, but the voltage drop-off is considerably less than that of a single-phase machine. A high-frequency generator voltage has very little voltage ripple. This prevents most of the lower-energy photons from being produced, reducing the patient's skin exposure. A high-frequency generator will create the most monoenergetic x-ray beam.

The generator types and their efficiency are listed here, *using the same technical factors:*

Single-phase	*Most patient exposure*
Three-phase, six-pulse	
Three-phase, twelve-pulse	
High-frequency generator	*Least patient exposure*

Shielding

Rationale for Use

Because x-radiation is ionizing and has the ability to cause damage within the human body, it is the responsibility of the radiographer to protect the patient. Shielding is used to protect any area of the patient that is not going to aid in the diagnosis of that patient. This is the same rationale as the ALARA concept: allowing an area to be exposed that is not going to contribute to the diagnosis is unnecessary.

Types of Protective Devices

The numerous shielding devices are discussed in Chapter 4. For a shielding device to provide adequate protection, the shielding material must have a high atomic number and be flexible enough to be used in many ways. Presently lead, available in thin, flexible sheets, is the material of choice. Some common shielding devices are

Flat contact shield
Shadow shield
Bucky slot cover
Fluoro drape
Lead-lined walls
Radiographer booth

Placement of Protective Devices

Protective devices must be placed between the radiation source and the patient or person to be protected. With general diagnostic procedures, the shield is usually placed on top of the patient, because the tube is above the patient whereas the image receptor is below the patient. The order is, from the bottom to the top: image receptor, the table, the patient, the x-ray tube.

For an image intensification procedure, the x-ray tube is located below the table and the image receptor is above the table, with the patient between them. In this case the protective shield is placed under the patient so it is between the x-ray tube and the patient. The order is, from the bottom to the top: image intensification tube, the radiographic table, the protective shield, the patient, the image receptor.

During special examinations, such as a computed tomography (CT) scan, in which the x-ray tube travels 360 degrees, around the patient, the shield must be placed completely around the patient to provide radiation protection.

Regardless of the procedure, the shield must be placed between the radiation source and the patient to protect the patient adequately. Care must be used to insure that the shielding material does not interfere with the image quality by attenuating the useful beam that is going to be used to radiograph the anatomy of interest.

Beam Restriction

Purpose

The main purpose of beam restriction is to limit the area being exposed to ionizing radiation. The beam is limited to include only the area of interest, therefore the patient exposure dose is kept to a minimum. Restricting the primary beam also limits the production of scatter and secondary radiation that is able to reach the patient or image receptor, also reducing patient exposure.

Effects on Secondary (Scatter) Radiation

Radiation that is produced at the anode is produced isotopically, in all directions. The majority of the radiation produced is in the direction of the tube port and will contribute to the diagnostic image. The remainder of the radiation produced causes secondary and scatter radiation within the tube housing. Radiation produced in any area of the tube other than the target is referred to as off-focus radiation. Some of the off-focus scatter and secondary radiation produced within the tube will exit from the tube port and travel toward the patient. This type of radiation may lead to exposing the patient, technologist, or radiographic film without contributing to the diagnostic image.

By using devices to limit these types of radiation, the overall image quality increases and the patient exposure decreases. Beam restriction is the best way to limit off-focus radiation.

Types of Beam Restriction

The various types of beam restriction devices are discussed in detail in Chapter 4. In general, cones and cylinders provide the best scatter and secondary radiation reduction, because they are long and absorb the greatest amount of off-focus radiation. However, they are limited in their field sizes and are heavy to work with.

Aperture diaphragms are the least efficient in reducing secondary radiation or scatter, because they are much closer to the production of photons. But they are light and easy to work with and provide some beam restriction. Aperture diaphragms are also limited in size and shape and are not widely used in modern radiology departments.

The most common beam restriction device used today is the *collimator*. This device allows for a wide variety of field sizes and provides the radiographer with a light source and centering cross-hairs. It has four variable shutters that help reduce off-focus and scatter radiation exiting from the tube and exposing the patient or film. Collimators may also be used with cones or cylinders for additional reduction of unnecessary radiation.

Filtration

Filtration is used to remove low-energy photons from the exiting beam. Low-energy photons do not contribute to the diagnostic image; they are absorbed by the patient and/or create secondary or scatter radiation. Filtration may be *inherent* (components of the tube, oil, Pyrex glass, and tube window), *added* (material placed in the pathway of the exiting photons, e.g., the collimator mirror), or *total* (the sum of both added and inherent).

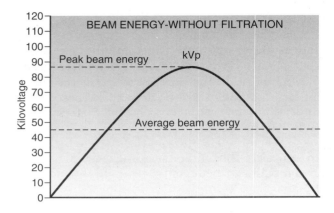

Figure 1-9 ■ Beam energy—without filtration.

A different type of filtration is compensation filters, used with specific body parts to provide a radiograph demonstrating consistent densities when varying body parts are radiographed at the same time, such as the thin area of the upper thoracic spine and the much denser area of the lower thoracic spine.

Effect of Skin and Organ Dose. With the addition of filtration, the lower-energy photons are absorbed by the filter and do not reach the skin or organs of the patient being examined. The more low-energy photons that are filtered out of the useful beam, the lower the dosage to the patient's skin and organs.

Effect on Average Beam Energy. With the addition of a filter, the average beam energy is increased because the low-energy photons are almost eliminated from the beam (Figs. 1–9, 1–10).

NCRP Recommendations. These state that the total beam filtration for generators must be the following:

Below 50 kVp	0.5 Al/eq
50 to 70 kVp	1.5 Al/eq
Above 70 kVp	2.5 Al/eq

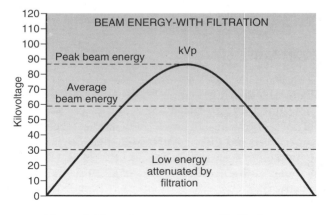

Figure 1-10 ■ Beam energy—with filtration.

This does not include compensating filters that may be used in various examinations.

Patient Positioning and Beam Projection

Beam projection in relationship to patient positioning (anteroposterior [AP] vs. posteroanterior [PA]) is not thought of as a means of patient protection. But the beam projection can determine the exposure to radiosensitive tissues, such as gonads. Before substituting an AP projection for a PA projection, the technologist must consider the anatomical structures being examined and determine whether the reversed projection will depict the anatomy properly. Generally, the farther away the radiosensitive area is from the source, the better it is for the patient.

An example is performing a lumbar spine on a man in the AP projection versus the PA projection. Doing the examination with the patient in the PA projection will reduce the possible exposure dosage to the gonads simply by placing them farther away from the source and allowing the patient's body to attenuate the dangerous low-energy radiation before it reaches the gonads. In other cases, such as a scoliosis series on a young woman, the AP projection would provide better radiation protection to the immature breast tissue. This is true for two reasons: first, the breasts can be collimated out of the useful beam and do not have a chance of being exposed by the diverging beam. Second, the breasts will be farther away from the image receptor; therefore, the body will attenuate most if not all back scatter coming from the film holder.

Beam projection should never be used as a primary method of radiation protection. In every case, common sense must be used to provide a high-quality radiograph with the least exposure to the patient.

Film, Screens, and Film-Screen Combinations

The film used must be spectrally matched to the illumination of the intensifying screen being used. When the sensitivity of the film is increased and the speed of the screen is increased, the quantity of radiation needed is decreased. Faster film-screen combinations require less radiation to form the image, but they also are not able to record as much detail as slower film-screen combinations. The relationship between film-screen combination and exposure is inversely proportional and can be expressed by the following:

$$\frac{mAs^1}{mAs^2} = \frac{RS^2}{RS^1}$$

where mAs means milliampere-second and RS means relative speed.

Example:
An exposure using 80 kVp at 20 mAs with a film-screen combination of 200 yields an acceptable chest radiograph. This technique could be changed to 80 kVp at 10 mAs by using a 400 film-screen system, or 80 kVp at 5 mAs by using an 800 film-screen system.

The higher the film-screen combination, the more efficiently the x-ray photons are converted to visible light photons; therefore, less radiation is used to produce a similar result.

Grids; Air Gap Techniques

Grids are used to attenuate scatter radiation resulting from exposing the radiographic film. Lead strips in the grid filter out scatter as well as some of the useful beam. Grids are available in a variety of efficiencies, which are described by their ratio: 8:1, 10:1, 12:1, and so on. Therefore, technical factors used to produce the radiograph must be increased to compensate for the attenuating quality of the grid. Increasing the technical factors will increase the patient exposure dose. The increased technique, along with the high density of the grid, will cause an increase in scatter production, which will also increase the patient exposure dose.

An air gap technique can be used in place of a grid. The patient is positioned 6 to 8 inches away from the cassette. This helps prevent scatter radiation from reaching the film, by allowing it to diverge or by scattering and missing the film. Basically, the intensity of the beam is reduced from having to travel farther to reach the film. The overall exposure dose is still increased because of the increase in technical factors. The technical factors must still be increased, because of the greater source-to-image distance (SID). To overcome the magnification of the object image distance (the gap), the SID is increased.

Automatic Exposure Control

With AEC, the exposure terminates when optimal density is achieved. If the patient is positioned correctly and the appropriate technical factors, especially kVp, are selected, the AEC will produce a high-quality radiograph. If the patient is not positioned properly, the wrong photocell is selected, or the technique is not within an acceptable range, the patient exposure dose will increase or decrease accordingly. This will result in a suboptimal image and may require repeat exposures to produce an acceptable radiograph, which may increase patient exposure by twofold or more.

Bibliography

Dowd S: Practical Radiation Protection and Applied Radiobiology. Philadelphia, WB Saunders, 1994

Kissane J: Anderson's Pathology International Edition. 9th ed. St. Louis, Mosby–Year Book, 1990

Mettler F, Upton A: Medical Effects of Ionizing Radiation. 2nd ed. Philadelphia, WB Saunders, 1995

Statkiewicz-Sheer MA, Visconti PJ, Ritenour RE: Radiation Protection in Medical Radiography. 2nd ed. St. Louis, Mosby–Year Book, 1993

Chapter 1 **Questions**

1. The length of time required for a radioactive material to reduce its intensity to one half of its original intensity is referred to as:

   A. Half-value layer
   B. The 50% rule
   C. Half-life
   D. This is not measurable.

2. Which of the following factors are used to determine the exposure dose for an individual when the individual's entire body is not exposed?

   A. LET (linear energy transfer)
   B. RBE (relative biological effectiveness)
   C. Wt (weight factor)
   D. QF (quality factor)

3. The amount of a material needed to reduce an x-ray beam to one half its original intensity can be defined as:

   A. Half-value layer
   B. Half-life
   C. The 50% rule
   D. mAs = Distance formula

4. Which regulatory agency makes recommendations for radiation safety?

   A. ICRP (International Council on Radiation Protection)
   B. NCRP (National Council on Radiation Protection)
   C. NAS BEIR (National Academy of Science, Advisory Committee, Biological Effects of Ionizing Radiation
   D. All of the above

5. The acronym ALARA means:

   A. As long as it's reasonable, it's acceptable.
   B. As low as reasonably achievable
   C. As long as the radiation's potential is achieved
   D. None of the above

6. Which of the following enforces radiation protection by making laws?

   A. ICRP (International Council on Radiation Protection)
   B. NCRP (National Council on Radiation Protection)

C. UNSCEAR (United Nations Scientific Community on the Effects of Atomic Radiation)
   D. NRC (Nuclear Regulatory Commission)

7. Why are the effects of radiation difficult to study?

   A. Radiation does not have specific pathology unique to itself.
   B. Large groups of the population need to be studied for extended periods of time.
   C. The effects of radiation are random in nature.
   D. All of the above

8. A graph that describes a response to radiation is referred to as a:

   A. Minimum threshold graph
   B. Probability curve
   C. ALARA curve
   D. Dose response curve

9. Radiation is potentially dangerous because it:

   A. Is invisible
   B. Has the ability to cause chemical and biological changes
   C. Has the ability to cause only biological changes
   D. Has the ability to cause only chemical changes

10. Which of the following graphs would best describe a response to a radiation exposure in direct proportion to that exposure?

    A. Non linear
    B. Linear
    C. Curvilinear
    D. Quadratic

11. If there were no response to a specific quantity of radiation, it would be stated that the exposure fell below the:

    A. Graph numbers
    B. Minimum response time
    C. Threshold
    D. Quadratic formula

12. A nonthreshold dose-effect relationship can be described as:

    A. A response to the dosage regardless of how large or small the dosage is
    B. No response is noted unless the exposure is a specified quantity.
    C. A response that will increase proportionally to the dosage
    D. This type of response is still being studied because it is not well understood.

13. Which of the following best describes a nonstochastic effect?

    A. A dose-response relationship that demonstrates a threshold at which the severity rather than the probability of the response will occur
    B. A dose-response relationship that is nonthreshold, at which the severity of the response will increase rather than the probability of the response will occur
    C. A dose-response relationship that demonstrated a threshold at which the probability rather than the severity of the response will occur
    D. A dose-response relationship that is nonthreshold, at which the probability rather than the severity of the response will occur

14. The LD 50/30 for humans is between 250 and 450 rad. What does LD 50/30 stand for?

    A. Legal dose for the population between 30 and 50 years old
    B. Lethal dose for 50% of the population that is 30 years old or older
    C. Lethal dose for 50% of the population, resulting in death to these people within 30 days
    D. Light dose of radiation for radiation therapy patients that will cure 30% to 50% of all cancers

15. In reference to radiation sickness, which of the following characterizes the period of time that the exposed individual would be asymptomatic?

    A. Hematopoietic formation period
    B. Manifest period
    C. Prodromal period
    D. Latent period

16. The radiation syndrome that is responsible for a gross depletion of epithelial cells resulting in widespread infection of the body's own flora is:

    A. Central nervous system syndrome
    B. Hematopoietic syndrome
    C. Gastrointestinal syndrome
    D. Arnold-Chiari syndrome

17. To experience a central nervous system syndrome due to radiation, the exposed individual would need to receive a dosage of:

    A. 200 to 500 rad
    B. 2000 to 5000 rad
    C. 20 to 5000 rad
    D. 5000 to 8000 rad

18. A somatic effect may be classified as an early effect or a late effect. Which of the following are also true regarding somatic effects?

    A. They become evident only in future generations.
    B. They are dangerous but do not cause cancer.
    C. They become evident in the exposed individual.
    D. More than one but not all the above

19. A late somatic effect is one that manifests:

    A. 3 to 5 days after the exposure
    B. In the evening, after the exposure
    C. 30 to 60 days after the exposure
    D. Several months or years after the exposure

20. An embryonic or fetal effect occurs only with an exposure dosage delivered to:

    A. A pregnant woman
    B. An infant, several hours after delivery
    C. The mother or father of the fetus just prior to conception
    D. Any member of the nuclear family

21. During which period of development is the fetus least radiosensitive?

    A. First trimester
    B. Second trimester
    C. Third trimester
    D. None of the above

22. A radiation exposure to a germ cell may lead to:

    A. An embryonic effect
    B. A fetal effect
    C. A somatic effect
    D. A genetic effect

23. The quantity of radiation required to increase a known disease by twofold in all live births is called:

    A. A genetic effect
    B. A doubling dose
    C. A genetically significant dose
    D. None of the above

24. With regard to the Bergonié-Tribondeau Law of radio-sensitivity, which of the following are true?

    A. The higher the oxygen content, the more radioresistant the tissue
    B. The more mitotic activity, the more radiosensitive the tissue
    C. The least specialized the cell, the more radioresistant the tissue
    D. All of the above

25. Given the following exposure dose, calculate the total exposure for this patient (use the weight factors on page 11):

    1. Four-view mammography—35 mrad
    2. Two views of the chest—15 mrad
    3. One AP view of the cervical spine—20 mrad

    A. 7 mrad total exposure
    B. 18 mrad total exposure
    C. 70 mrad total exposure
    D. 21 mrad total exposure

26. Which of the following exposure factors will yield the lowest patient exposure dose?

    A. 100 kVp and 50 mAs
    B. 75 kVp, 300 mA, and .50 sec
    C. 80 kVp, 1000 mA, and 10 msec
    D. 80 kVp, 10 mA, and 1 sec

27. A high-frequency generator will minimize patient exposure doses by providing a:

    A. More polyenergetic primary beam
    B. More monoenergetic primary beam
    C. High-efficiency filter within the x-ray tube
    D. Widely varying voltage ripple

28. What type of shielding is required in a radiographic room to protect visitors and personnel in rooms and hallways adjacent to the radiographic rooms?

    A. No shielding is needed in these areas.
    B. A Bucky slot cover or fluoro drape is normally used.
    C. Thin sheets of lead imbedded in the walls of the radiographic room
    D. More than one but not all of the above

29. A 20 year old man is going to have an upper GI series. What, if anything, can the technologist do to ensure proper radiation protection for this type of procedure?

    A. Place a gonadal shield over the patient while the fluoroscopic procedure is being performed.
    B. Ask the doctor to use only intermittent fluoro, because of the patient's age.
    C. Carefully place a flat contact shield between the patient and the radiographic table.
    D. Give the patient only half the prescribed barium suspension to drink, hoping that the test will be shortened.

30. One way of limiting the primary beam that is emitted from the x-ray tube is to use beam restriction. Why would beam restriction be an important part of patient protection?

    A. Because it increases the overall beam quality
    B. Beam restriction limits the area of the patient being exposed.
    C. Beam restriction increases the overall area exposed and will optimize all the ionizations within that area.
    D. Beam restriction is not related to patient protection and has no effect on exposure dosage.

31. Increasing the total filtration will have what effect on skin entrance doses?

    A. They will increase.
    B. They will decrease.
    C. They will remain the same.
    D. They will be reduced by half of the distance squared.

32. A stationary radiographic unit operating at an average beam energy of 50 kVp will require _____ filtration to meet the NCRP's recommendations:

    A. 0.5 Al/eq
    B. 1.5 Al/eq
    C. 2.0 Al/eq
    D. 2.5 Al/eq

33. Which of the following technical factors will create the highest skin entrance dose to the patient being examined?

    A. 80 kVp, 300 mA, and .5 sec with no filtration
    B. 80 kVp, 300 mA, and 1/10 sec with no filtration
    C. 80 kVp, 1000 mA, and 1/20 sec with 2.5 Al/eq
    D. 80 kVp, 800 mA, and 1/60 sec with .05 Al/eq

34. In regard to film-screen speed combinations, which of the following statements are true?

    A. The faster the film, the slower the screen needs to be.
    B. Increasing the film-screen speed will increase the mAs needed to produce a quality radiograph.
    C. Decreasing the film-screen speed will decrease the mAs needed to produce a quality radiograph.
    D. Increasing the film-screen speed will decrease the mAs needed to produce a quality radiograph.

35. Utilizing an air gap technique will:

    A. Decrease patient exposure
    B. Increase patient exposure
    C. Not affect patient exposure
    D. More than one but not all of the above

Answers appear at the back of the book.

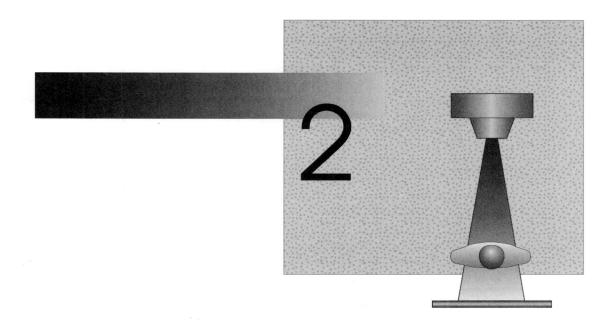

PERSONNEL PROTECTION

Sources of Radiation Exposure
Exposure to Primary X-Ray Beam
Secondary Radiation
Leakage Radiation

Basic Methods of Protection
Time
Distance
Shielding

NCRP Recommendations for Protective Devices

Special Considerations
Portable (Mobile) Units
Fluoroscopy
Guidelines for Fluoroscopy and
Portable Units

SOURCES OF RADIATION EXPOSURE

Exposure to Primary X-Ray Beam

A technologist should never be exposed to the primary x-ray beam. The technologist should not be holding patients. When necessary, this should be handled by family members and nonradiation workers. While assisting the radiologist during a fluoroscopic procedure, technologists should never allow themselves to be exposed to the primary beam, including their hands.

Secondary Radiation

A technologist should always be shielded from scatter and secondary radiation. When performing routine diagnostic procedures, the technologist should be behind the radiographic x-ray booth when the exposure is made.

During a radiographic exposure, the patient is the greatest producer of scatter and secondary radiation and is the origin of most of the exposure that the technologist or doctor will receive. When a primary photon is scattered, it usually has enough energy to cause additional ionizations. Scattering will change a photon's direction, and when it interacts with matter again it will either be absorbed or will cause an additional ionization. This process will occur only twice: after a primary photon has scattered twice, it will not hold enough energy to cause any additional ionizations and is absorbed. The room is designed so that the technologist in the radiographic booth during the exposure will be protected from secondary and scatter radiation.

During a fluoroscopic procedure, technologists cannot always be in the radiographic booth, therefore they need to wear protective apparel to protect themselves during the examination. In this situation, the best method of protection for the technologist is to limit the time in the radiographic room while the x-ray beam is on, remain as far from the source of the radiation as possible, and wear all the protective apparel available, such as a protective apron, eyeglasses, thyroid shield, and, if necessary, gloves. The technologist can also be protected by standing behind the doctor performing the procedure.

Leakage Radiation

Leakage radiation is emitted from the x-ray tube housing. Its primary source is off-focus radiation. This is radiation that is not part of the primary beam and is not necessary to produce the radiographic image. The tube housing is constructed of thick cast steel and will absorb most of the leakage radiation. The tube housing also has a lead lining, usually on the cathode side, because most of the off-focus radiation is there. Leakage radiation that exits from the tube housing must not exceed 100 mr/hr at 1 meter from the housing. Limiting leakage radiation not only reduces the potential exposure to the patient but also reduces the exposure to the technologist.

BASIC METHODS OF PROTECTION

Time

One way technologists are able to protect themselves is by limiting the length of time they are in an area that could potentially expose them to ionizing radiation. This simple action can drastically reduce their cumulative exposure.

Distance

When the technologist moves farther away from the source of the radiation exposure, the exposure dose received is greatly reduced. This concept is mathematically described by the inverse square law. The formula and an example are

$$\frac{I_1}{I_2} = \frac{(D_2)^2}{(D_1)^2}$$

where I means intensity and D means distance.

Example:
A technologist is exposed to 20 mr/hr during a fluoroscopic examination while standing 2 feet from the radiation source. If the technologist moved to 4 feet from the radiation source, the exposure would be reduced by four (5 mr/hr).

Shielding

As noted, technologists should always use the appropriate apparel when they might be exposed to radiation. Shielding incorporates a variety of measures that help protect the technologist, the patient, and the persons in the radiology department.

The design of the radiology suite plays an important role in radiation protection. A primary barrier measuring 1/16″ of lead or lead equivalent is required for any area of the radiographic room that could be exposed to primary radiation. A secondary barrier measuring 1/32″ of lead or a lead equivalent is necessary for all areas that may be exposed to scatter or leakage radiation. Walls that need to be shielded to form primary barriers are lined with 1/16″ lead to 7 feet from the floor, and as secondary barriers from 7 feet to the ceiling. Primary and secondary lead barriers must be overlapped by 1″. The radiographic booth is usually a secondary barrier, with a 1.5 mm lead equivalent window to allow the technologist to view the patient while making the exposure.

Four factors that determine the necessary barrier thickness are discussed next.

Distance

The distance of the x-ray tube from the walls will determine how thick the lead shield within the walls needs to be.

Occupancy Factor

This factor takes into consideration the rooms adjacent to the radiographic room. The type of room will determine the necessary shielding for the adjacent radiographic room's wall. Occupancy factors are full (used every day all day), partial (used intermittently throughout the day), or occasional (used sparingly throughout the day).

Workload

This factor determines the required shielding that depends upon the amount of radiation produced within the room. The numbers of films taken and mA used to produce these films are estimated. These numbers are then used to determine the workload (mA; Min/Week). This would be the mA used to make the exposures; the number of minutes per week that the exposures are made. This number is used as an estimate to determine how heavily the room is used and in what exposure range.

Use Factor

This factor determines the shielding required depending upon the amount of time that the radiographic tube is producing radiation toward the walls, and then that measurement of time is assigned a value depending upon that figure. Usually the walls receive a use factor of one fourth as the primary barrier. The floor, ceiling, radiographic booth, and any other barrier within the radiographic room are assigned a use factor of 1 as a secondary barrier. This factor reflects the fact that secondary radiation and leakage radiation are present every time the radiographic tube is energized.

NCRP RECOMMENDATIONS FOR PROTECTIVE DEVICES

Following is a list of protective devices and the thickness of the lead equivalent required by the NCRP to provide adequate protection.

Contact shields	0.25 mm
Aprons	0.25 mm (minimum) up to 1.00 mm
Eyeglasses	0.35 mm (minimum) up to 0.50 mm
Thyroid shields	0.50 mm
Protective gloves	0.25 mm
Bucky slot cover	0.25 mm
Fluoro drape	0.25 mm
Primary barriers	1/16″ lead sheet
Secondary barriers	1/32″ lead sheet
Tube housing	Enough lead equivalent to prevent leakage radiation 100 mr/hr at 1 meter

SPECIAL CONSIDERATIONS
Portable (Mobile) Units

When using a portable radiographic unit, there are no lead-lined walls or radiographic booth for the technologist. Special considerations are needed. The technologist must be aware of all the people in the vicinity. When making the exposure, a safe distance from the source (tube) is about 6′ to 8′ in any direction, except in the path of the radiation. At this distance most, if not all of the energy contained in the beam, is absorbed. The portable machine is equipped with an exposure cord that is at least 6′ to 8′ feet long to allow the technologist to move to that distance while making the exposure. The safest place for the technologist is at a 90° angle from the tube because the least amount of radiation is scattered at this angle.

It is the technologist's responsibility to move all personnel and patients to a safe area before the exposure is made. The technologist must also announce the exposure to alert all personnel within the general area. Portable machines must provide an audio signal and a visible indicator to acknowledge that the exposure was made. These machines are usually power driven but are limited in the exposure factors that are available.

Fluoroscopy

Because fluoroscopic machines have the ability to remain on, producing radiation for extended lengths of time, special devices are used to protect the patient and technologist.

Protective Drapes

Fluoroscopic machines have special equipment to provide extra protection for the radiographer.

Drapes usually slide between the patient and the operator to minimize the scatter from the patient. The scatter radiation that is produced within the patient is the primary source of exposure to the operator and technologist.

Protective Bucky Slot Cover

This device is in the radiographic table. The space under the table allows the Bucky to be positioned anywhere from the head to the foot of the table. This tract is covered by the Bucky slot cover, preventing scatter from exiting from this area. The Bucky slot cover reduces the amount of scatter radiation that is allowed to pass through this opening to expose the operator or technologist. This means increased radiation protection for the technologist and operator.

Cumulative Timer

Because the x-ray beam may be on for extended lengths of time, a timer is used to tell the operator how long it has been on. The timer is set for 5 minutes and counts down to 0. When the timer reaches 0, an alarm sounds until the timer is reset. The fluoroscopic machine will continue to operate even while the alarm is sounding. The operator may reduce the length of time the beam is on by using intermittent fluoro technique: instead of turning the fluoroscopic beam on and leaving it on for the whole procedure, the beam is turned on and off, therefore limiting the exposure dosage delivered to every person during the procedure's exposure. This technique not only decreases the exposure to the patient but also re-

duces the amount of scatter radiation that the operator and technologist are exposed to.

Guidelines for Fluoroscopy and Portable Units

Because these units are so versatile, guidelines have been established for their use. Both fluoroscopic and portable units must be inspected and follow all quality control requirements that stationary units do. Certain restrictions have been established for source-to-skin distance (SSD) for these units: they may not employ an SSD of less than 12″. They must provide a minimum of 2.5 mm Al/eq filtration. The image intensification unit must be equipped with a dead man type of exposure switch, and the tube output must be limited to 10 rad/min. Both image intensification and portable units must limit leakage radiation to 100 mr/hr at 1 meter. And finally, as with stationary units, portable and image intensification units must provide a beam-on indicator and an audible indicator while x-rays are being produced.

Bibliography

Carlton R, Adler A: Principles of Radiographic Imaging. Albany, Delmar Publishers, 1992

Dowd S: Practical Radiation Protection and Applied Radiobiology. Philadelphia, WB Saunders, 1994

Medical X-Ray, Electron Beam, and Gamma-Ray Protection for Energies up to 50 MeV (Equipment Design, Performance, and Use). NCRP No. 102. Bethesda, MD, National Council on Radiation Protection and Measurements, 1989

Radiation Protection for Medical and Allied Health Personnel. NCRP No. 105. Bethesda, MD, National Council on Radiation Protection and Measurements, 1989

Statkiewicz-Sheer M, Visconti P, Ritenour E: Radiation Protection in Medical Radiography. 2nd ed. St. Louis, Mosby–Year Book, 1993

Chapter 2 Questions

1. Which of the following statements is false?

   A. Technologists are permitted to hold patients as long as they wear protective devices.
   B. Family members are permitted to hold patients as long as they are not pregnant and use protective apparel.
   C. Patients are never held during radiographic procedures by a radiographer or student radiographer.
   D. Patients are not held if specially designed restraining devices are available to prevent the patient from moving.

2. Primary radiation can be defined as radiation:

   A. That the technologist is exposed to
   B. Exiting from the tube port
   C. Interacting with matter and changing direction
   D. That is produced within the tube and becomes part of the leakage radiation

3. Which of the following are true regarding secondary radiation?

   1. It interacts with matter and changes direction.
   2. It is the main exposure for the technologist.
   3. It is 90% bremsstrahlung (braking radiation).
   4. It will cause ionizations within the patient.

   A. 1, 2, and 3
   B. 1 and 3 only
   C. 4 only
   D. 1, 2, and 4

4. The design of the radiographic room will protect the technologist from:

   A. Primary radiation
   B. Secondary radiation after the first interaction
   C. Secondary radiation after the secondary interaction
   D. All of the above

5. What is the primary source of leakage radiation?

   A. Patient
   B. Technologist
   C. X-ray tube housing
   D. Radiographic table

6. What limits the leakage radiation from exiting from the tube housing?

   A. Aluminum and lead
   B. Lead and copper
   C. Distance
   D. Lead and steel

7. What is the source of off-focus radiation?

   A. Anywhere on the surface of the anode's target
   B. Anywhere within the radiographic tube
   C. Anywhere within the radiographic tube, except the anode's target
   D. Anywhere outside of the radiographic tube

8. On which side of the radiographic tube will most of the radiation travel?

   A. Toward the top
   B. Toward the cathode
   C. Toward the anode
   D. Toward the focal track

9. To comply with NCRP guidelines, leakage radiation must not exceed:

   A. 10 mr/hr at 1 meter
   B. 10 rad/hr at 1 meter
   C. 100 mr/hr at 1 foot
   D. 100 mr/hr at 1 meter

10. What are the three ways technologists can protect themselves from an exposure?

    A. Time, distance, and shielding
    B. Time, distance, and technical factors
    C. Shielding, radiographic booth, and technical factors
    D. Moving as far away as possible, high speed film screen combination, and high frequency generator

11. A basic method of technologist shielding is time. Which of the following best describes what is meant by time?

A. Doing only the projection that the technologist feels is important regardless of the order by the physician

B. Minimizing the length of time the technologist is in an area that may be exposed to radiation

C. Working only part-time as a radiographer

D. Doing the least amount of work possible

12. A technologist standing 3 feet from a radiation source receives 5 rad/hr. What would the technologist's exposure dose be if he or she moves 1 foot closer to the source?

A. 11.25 rad/hr

B. 45 rad/hr

C. 11.25 mrad/hr

D. 7.50 rad/hr

13. A wall in the radiographic room is considered to be a primary barrier. What thickness of lead is required to provide adequate shielding?

A. 1/8″ lead equivalent

B. 1/32″ lead equivalent

C. 1/16″ lead equivalent

D. 1/4″ lead equivalent

14. What is a safe distance from a portable machine while making an exposure?

A. 6 feet

B. 6 yards

C. 6 inches

D. 12 inches

15. The safest place for a technologist to stand when making a portable exposure is:

A. At a 90° angle from the tube port

B. At a 180° angle from the tube port

C. 12 inches from the tube port

D. At a 270° angle from the tube port

16. The main purpose of the fluoro drape is to minimize the exposure from:

A. The table

B. The tube

C. The radiologist and radiographer

D. The patient

17. The purpose of a cumulative timer is:

A. To inform the technologist how long the exposure time is

B. To stop the production of x-rays when the timer reaches its limit

C. To allow the doctor to cut the procedure short, even if the diagnosis is not confirmed

D. None of the above

18. A cumulative time for an image intensification tube is:

A. 15 min

B. 10 min

C. 5 min

D. 7 min

19. The minimum source-to-skin distance for an image intensification system such as a C-arm is:

A. 15 cm

B. 12 cm

C. 15 inches

D. 12 inches

20. The total filtration for a high-frequency portable generator is:

A. 2.0 mm Al/eq

B. 2.5 mm Al/eq

C. 3.0 mm Al/eq

D. 3.5 mm Al/eq

Answers appear at the end of the book.

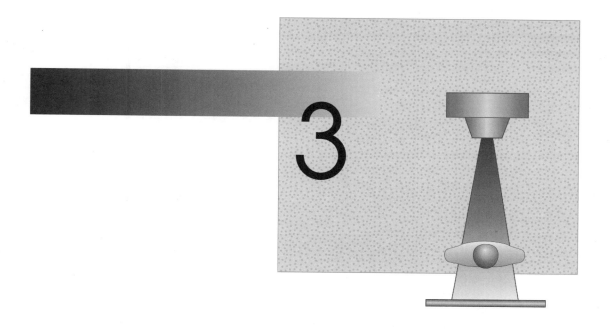

RADIATION EXPOSURE AND MONITORING

Basic Properties of Radiation
　Principles of Radiation
　X-radiation Interactions with Matter
　Radiation Produced at the Target

Units of Measurement
　Rad
　Rem
　Roentgen

Types and Proper use of Dosimeters
　Field Survey Instruments
　Personnel Monitoring

NCRP Recommendations for Personnel Monitoring
　ALARA and Dose Equivalent Limits
　Evaluation of Cumulative Dose
　　Records
　Maintenance of Cumulative Dose
　　Records

BASIC PROPERTIES OF RADIATION

Principles of Radiation

- X-radiation consists of highly penetrating invisible rays.
- X-radiation does not carry an electrical charge.
- X-radiation is part of the electromagnetic spectrum and is available in a variety of energy levels and frequencies.
- X-radiation has the ability to ionize matter and create heat through these ionizations.
- X-radiation travels in a straight line from its point of origin and cannot be focused or converged.
- X-radiation travels at the speed of light, 3×10^{10} cm/sec.
- X-radiation has the ability to cause illumination of certain elements.
- X-radiation has the ability to affect photographic film.
- X-radiation has the ability to cause chemical and biological changes secondary to ionizations.
- X-radiation has the ability to produce secondary and scatter radiation.

X-radiation Interactions with Matter

Coherent Interactions

This type of interaction occurs below 10 kilo electron volts (keV). It is characterized by an incident photon interacting with an orbital electron of an atom. The photon enters the atom and passes next to an electron, causing it to absorb energy. The photon is of low energy, and the energy that is absorbed by the electron is not enough to eject it from its orbit. This is because the energy absorbed is less than the binding energy of the orbital electron. The electron begins to resonate or vibrate because it has more energy than is required to remain in its orbit, and this is called *excitation*. The electron releases this energy in the form of a photon. This photon has exactly the same amount of energy as the incident photon and travels at the same frequency, but it is directed in a different direction. This type of radiation is referred to as scatter radiation (Fig. 3–1).

Photoelectric Interactions

This type of interaction usually occurs at energy levels of about 35 keV. It is characterized by an incident photon interacting with an inner shell electron. The inner shell electron absorbs all the energy of the photon and causes the electron to be ejected from its orbit, because the energy of the photon is greater than the binding energy of the electron. The ejected photon is then referred to as a photoelectron and will be absorbed within a short distance of its ejection. The outer shell electrons within the atom move closer to the nucleus to fill the void of the electron that was ejected. But as these electrons move closer to the nucleus they do not require as much energy to remain in orbit, so they must shed some of their energy. This energy is released as photon energy. This type of radiation is referred to as secondary radiation, because it is created secondary to the initial interaction and not as a direct result. These photons will travel in a different direction from the incident photon. They also travel at lower frequencies because they have less energy than the incident photon (Fig. 3–2).

Compton Interactions

This type of interaction usually occurs at about 100 keV but may occur at up to 1.02 megaelectron volt (MeV). It is characterized by an incident photon interacting with an outer shell electron. The outer shell electron does not absorb all the photon's energy, but it does absorb enough energy to eject the electron from its orbit. The ejected electron is referred to as a recoil electron. The additional energy that is not absorbed by the electron is released as photon energy and directed in another direction; this will not be at an angle greater than 180° from the incident photon. This radiation will travel with less energy than the incident photon, because some of that energy is used to eject the recoil electron. This type of radiation is referred to as scatter radiation and will travel at a lower frequency and have less penetrating ability than does the incident photon (Fig. 3–3).

Pair Production Interactions

This type of interaction will occur at energy levels of 1.02 to 10 MeV. It is characterized by an incident photon interacting with the nucleus or nuclear force field of an atom. With this type of interaction the photon is split into two parts: a *positron* and a *negatron*. The positron carries a positive charge and carries almost all the energy, a minimum of 1.02 MeV. The negatron carries a negative charge and carries only a fragment of the energy. The negatron will travel out of the atom and within a short distance interact with another atom. The positron continues out of the atom and, because of its positive charge, is attracted to another electron, because of its oppos-

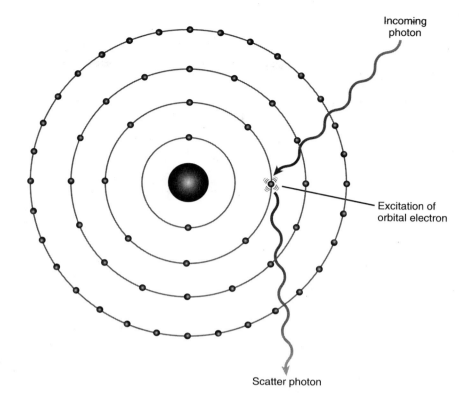

Figure 3-1 ■ Coherent interaction.

ing negative charge, possibly an orbital electron of another atom.

When the positron collides with an electron, it causes an *annihilation reaction*. The annihilation reaction causes the positron and electron to split into two high-energy photons, which have an energy level of 0.51 MeV, or one half the incident photon's energy. These photons continue to interact with other atoms until all their energy is absorbed. The interactions will be primarily

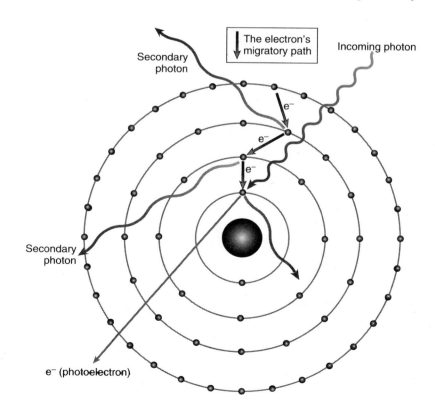

Figure 3-2 ■ Photoelectric interaction.

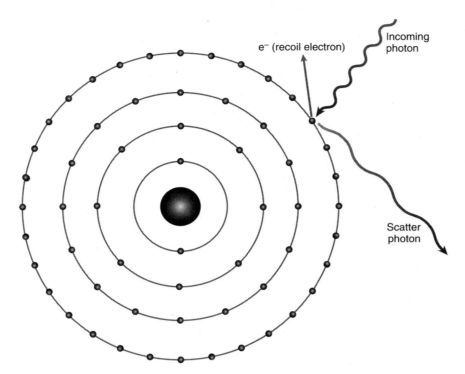

Figure 3-3 ■ Compton interaction.

Compton interactions because of the photons' energy level. This type of interaction with matter is not seen in diagnostic radiography but is a common interaction in radiation therapy because of the energies used in radiation therapy (Fig. 3–4).

Photodisintegration Interaction

This type of interaction begins to occur at energy levels of 10 MeV and greater. It can be characterized by an incident photon that interacts with the nucleus of an atom. The energy of the photon is absorbed by the nucleus and causes the nucleus to eject a neutron or nuclear fragment. These particles are fast moving, highly penetrating, and highly ionizing. This type of interaction is not seen in diagnostic radiography but is seen in radiation therapy because of the higher energy levels used in radiation therapy. The particles that are ejected by the atom's nucleus will continue to cause interactions until all the energy is absorbed (Fig. 3–5).

Radiation Produced at the Target

Characteristic Radiation

This type of radiation is very similar to photoelectric interactions and is named because the radiation produced is characteristic of the target being used. It is characterized by an electron interacting with an inner shell electron of the target atom. The inner shell electron is ejected from its orbit, leaving a void of 1 electron in that orbit. The outer shell electrons within that atom begin to shed energy and move to an orbit closer to the nucleus. The energy that they shed is given off as characteristic radiation. The incoming electron must be of a specific energy level for this to occur at all, because of the target's high atomic number and the binding energy of the orbital electrons.

Bremsstrahlung (Braking Radiation)

This type of radiation is similar to coherent radiation in some respects. It can be characterized by an incoming electron interacting with the nucleus of a target atom. The nucleus has a strong positive charge, whereas the electron has a strong negative charge, so by the laws of electrostatics they are attracted to one another. There is never any contact between the two, but the electron is approaching the nucleus with great velocity. The power of attraction is so great that the electron is slowed almost to a complete stop and loses most, if not all, of its energy. The energy from the incoming electron is released by the atom as x-radiation. The electron can give up so much energy that its velocity is reduced to such an extent that it floats away from the nucleus. This type of radiation can occur at any energy level and makes up the majority of the x-ray beam. It is not characteristic of the target and may be produced equally with a variety of target materials.

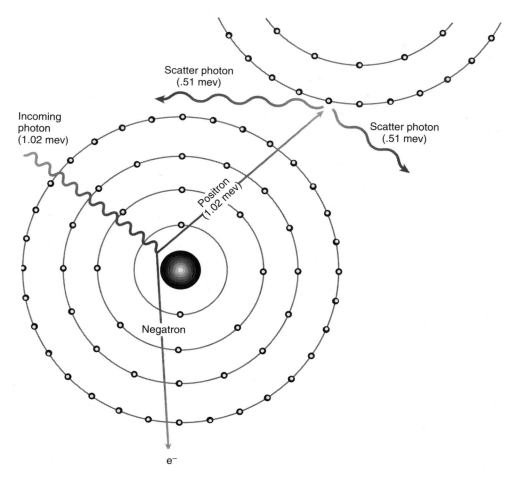

Figure 3-4 ■ Pair production interaction. mev, Million electron volts.

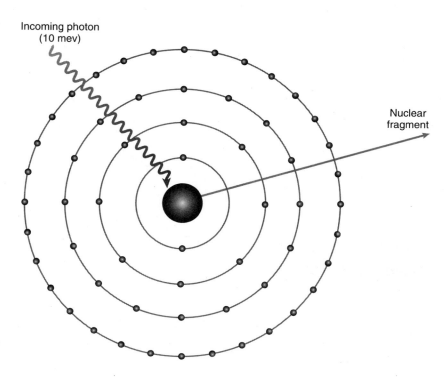

Figure 3-5 ■ Photodisintegration interaction. mev, Million electron volts.

UNITS OF MEASUREMENT

Rad (Radiation Absorbed Dose)

A rad is the amount of energy absorbed in 100 ergs/gram of matter. This unit of measure can be used for any type of radiation and is the one used to quantify patient exposure dose. Dosimeters display their readings in rad: 100 rad = 1 gray (Table 3–1).

Rem (Radiation Equivalent Man)

A rem is used to quantify different types of radiation so that any possible biological effects can be determined. The rem is the unit of measure that expresses occupational exposure dosages. The formula used to determine rem is

Rem = rad × RBE (relative biological effect).

RBE is a method of determining the chance or probability of one type of radiation to cause ionizations when compared with another type of radiation. This will determine the amount of exposure of one type of radiation that is necessary to equal the amount of exposure of a different type of radiation to cause the same amount of biological changes: 100 rem = 1 sievert (see Table 3–1).

Roentgen

A roentgen determines the amount of radiation exposure in air, for energies under 3 MeV. This unit is used to calibrate radiographic equipment and is expressed by a dosimeter: 1 roentgen = 2.58×10^{-4} coulomb/kg air (see Table 3–1).

For x-ray and gamma radiation: 1 rad = 1 rem = 1 roentgen.

TYPES AND PROPER USE OF DOSIMETERS

A dosimeter is a device that detects and quantifies radiation.

Table 3–1 ■ **TRADITIONAL AND SI UNITS OF RADIATION EXPOSURE**

Traditional		SI Units
1 rad	=	0.01 gray
1 rem	=	0.01 sievert
1 roentgen	=	2.58×10^{-4} coulomb/kg air
100 rad	=	1 gray
100 rem	=	1 sievert

Field Survey Instruments

Ionization Chamber

These detectors work by counting ion pairs. Basically they are used for determining an exposure in air per hour. This aids in calculating the length of time a person may be near a patient who has an isotope inside the body. Ionization chambers detect x-ray, gamma, and high-energy beta radiation.

Geiger-Müller Counter

This device works in the same way an ion chamber does, by counting ion pairs. This dosimeter is primarily used for detecting even low levels of x-ray, gamma, beta, and alpha radiation rather than for determining an exposure rate.

Scintillation Counter

This counter uses a sodium iodide crystal that produces a light photon (flashes) when exposed to radiation. This counter is connected to a photomultiplier tube, which converts the light energy into electrical impulses. A specific dose rate is then calculated. A scintillation counter is the most sensitive dosimeter for x-ray and gamma radiation.

Personnel Monitoring

Film Badges

This type of personnel monitoring device is the most commonly used and most cost effective. It is constructed of a plastic housing that has built-in filters, usually of aluminum or copper. They are sensitive to exposures as low as 10 mrem. The film badge is worn at collar level outside any protective garment worn by the technologist.

A special type of film is sealed in a lightproof envelope. The film within the film badge is replaced once every month. From the density of the film a dosage is determined and recorded. These readings are compared with a control badge that measures any environmental radiation in the area.

Thermoluminescent Dosimeter

This type of dosimeter also has a plastic holder, containing lithium fluoride crystals that are sensitive to radiation. The crystals may be used for up to 3 months without being read. When they are exposed to heat, the crystals emit visible light, which corresponds to the quantity of radiation the crystals have been exposed to. The light is then measured and the exposure dosage calculated. The crystals may be reused.

The major disadvantages of the thermoluminescent dosimeter are that a permanent record is not available, as with a film badge; they are expensive; and it is costly to read them. The advantages: they are reusable; immediate readings are available, if necessary; they do not fog easily; and they are highly accurate (5 mrem).

Pocket Dosimeters

This type of dosimeter is a simple ion chamber that determines exposure in air to achieve a dosage. It is filled with a gas, usually argon or neon, that allows electrons to move freely. It has two terminals: a positive wire that is located in the center of the dosimeter and a negative wire in the walls. As the air within the dosimeter becomes ionized, the wire begins to move closer to the walls of the dosimeter while the dosage is recorded and displayed on the face. The pocket dosimeter displays its reading in milliroentgens.

The disadvantage of ion chambers is that they need to be read daily and do not provide a permanent record of the exposure, so the record will be only as good as the method of documentation. These types of dosimeters are also affected by

rough or traumatic handling and dropping. They must be calibrated and charged every day. They are also limited in the quantity of exposure that they are able to read. Once at their limit, there is no way of knowing how much additional exposure is received. Pocket dosimeters read only x-ray and gamma radiation and are not practical for everyday use by the staff radiographer.

NCRP RECOMMENDATIONS FOR PERSONNEL MONITORING

ALARA and Dose Equivalent Limits

ALARA—*As Low as Reasonably Achievable.* This means that all people who may be or are exposed to any type of radiation should be protected by any means possible in order to keep their exposure to an absolute minimum, as long as the means of protection does not interfere with the reason for the exposure. This follows the ideal of a linear nonthreshold dose response curve. All radiation is dangerous regardless of its quantity; even very minute exposures have the ability to cause biological and chemical changes that may lead to biological damage.

Dose Equivalent Limits. Limits have been established and are implemented by the National Council on Radiation Protection Report #116. (Table 3–2).

Table 3–2 ■ NCRP RADIATION EXPOSURE DOSE RECOMMENDATIONS*

Occupational Exposures†
1. Effective dose limits
   - a) Annual — 50 mSv
   - b) Cumulative — 10 mSv × age
2. Equivalent dose annual limits for tissues and organs
   - a) Lens of eye — 150 mSv
   - b) Skin, hands, and feet — 500 mSv

Public Exposures (Annual)
1. Effective dose limit, continuous or frequent exposure† — 1 mSv
2. Effective dose limit, infrequent exposure† — 5 mSv
3. Equivalent dose limits for tissues and organs†
   - a) Lens of eye — 15 mSv
   - b) Skin, hands, and feet — 50 mSv
4. Remedial action for natural sources:
   - a) Effective dose (excluding radon) — >5 mSv
   - b) Exposure to radon decay products — $>7 \times 10^{-3}$ Jh m^{-3}

Education and Training Exposurers (Annual)†
1. Effective dose limit — 1 mSv
2. Equivalent dose limit for tissues and organs
   - a) Lens of eye — 15 mSv
   - b) Skin, hands, and feet — 50 mSv

Embryo-Fetus Exposures† (Monthly)
1. Equivalent dose limit — 0.5 mSv

Negligible Individual Dose (Annual)† — 0.01 mSv

*Excluding medical exposures.
†Sum of external and internal exposures but excluding doses from natural sources.
Reprinted with permission from National Council on Radiation Protection; Limitation of Exposure to Ionizing Radiation. Report #116. Bethesda, Md, 1993.

Evaluation of Cumulative Dose Records

The size of the institution and the type of radiation work performed will dictate whether a radiation safety committee (RSC) or a radiation safety officer (RSO) is needed. All institutions will have one or the other. A radiation safety committee is usually established in very large institutions that perform sophisticated radiation procedures. All committee members should be familiar with radium physics and radiation protection. An RSC may consist of a combination of any of the following people: nuclear medicine physician, radiologist, radiation oncologist, senior hospital administrator, physicist, senior nurse, internist, or investigator who uses radiation in research activities.

In smaller institutions, a radiation safety officer is used. The RSO is usually a health or medical physicist but may be a person with an extensive background in radium physics, radiation protection, and radiobiology, such as a physician. The RSO reports directly to upper management, with access to all levels of the organization.

All exposure records should be evaluated and reviewed by the RSO or RSC. This permits early intervention in identification of any problem areas. If occupational doses are unusually high, the RSO consults with the employee to identify the cause of the excessive exposure. The RSO is also available to counsel and educate all employees in radiation safety and radium physics.

Maintenance of Cumulative Dose Records

The responsibility of record keeping lies with the institution. A record of any and all radiation exposure that an individual receives must be maintained by the employer. When an employee leaves for another institution, the radiation records accompany that person. Then it becomes the responsibility of the new employer to keep not only current records but also the entire radiation history of that employee. Once an exposure is recorded on the employee's permanent record, it cannot be removed. The only exception is for bogus exposures, which may be removed upon the employee's request.

Bibliography

Bushong S: Radiographic Science for Technologists. 5th ed. St. Louis, Mosby–Year Book, 1993

Carlton R, Adler A: Principles of Radiographic Imaging. Albany, NY, Delmar Publishers, 1992

Radiation Protection for Medical and Allied Health Personnel. NCRP No. 105. Bethesda, National Council on Radiation Protection and Measurements, 1989

Selman J: The Fundamentals of X-ray and Radium Physics. 8th ed. Springfield, IL, Charles C Thomas, 1994

Chapter 3 **Questions**

1. All the following are basic properties of x-radiation except:

   A. X-rays are highly penetrating invisible rays.
   B. X-rays are available in a variety of wavelengths.
   C. X-rays travel at the speed of sound.
   D. X-rays have the ability to cause secondary and scatter radiation.

2. This type of interaction is usually caused by a photon with an energy of 10 keV or lower:

   A. Photoelectric interaction
   B. Compton interaction
   C. Pair production interaction
   D. Coherent interaction

3. After a photoelectric interaction has occurred, the resulting photon(s) may be referred to as:

   A. Recoil radiation
   B. Scatter radiation
   C. Secondary radiation
   D. Photoelectric radiation

4. After a coherent interaction with matter, the scatter photon has:

   A. Less energy than the incident photon
   B. More energy than the incident photon
   C. The same energy as the incident photon
   D. Coherent interactions do not produce scatter photons, they produce secondary photons.

5. The ejected photon from a photoelectric interaction with matter results in a secondary radiation and a:

   A. Scatter electron
   B. Photoelectron
   C. Recoil electron
   D. Photoelectric electron

6. A photoelectric interaction is characterized by an incident photon interacting with an:

   A. Inner shell electron
   B. Outer shell electron
   C. Outer shell proton
   D. Inner shell neutron

7. This type of interaction may be characterized by ejection of an outer shell electron:

   A. Coherent
   B. Pair production
   C. Photoelectric
   D. Compton

8. The electron that is ejected during a Compton interaction is referred to as a:

   A. Photoelectron
   B. Recoil electron
   C. Negatron electron
   D. Compton electron

9. Compton interactions will begin to occur at about 100 keV and will continue to occur up to what energy level?

   A. 10 keV
   B. 1.02 keV
   C. 102 MeV
   D. 1.02 MeV

10. During a Compton interaction, what happens to the energy of the incident photon that is not absorbed by the orbital electron?

    A. It becomes a secondary photon.
    B. It becomes a scatter photon.
    C. It is absorbed by a neighboring electron.
    D. It ejects another electron through excitation.

11. When an incoming photon carries an energy level of at least 1.02 MeV, the interaction that will occur will most likely be:

    A. Pair production
    B. Compton
    C. Photodisintegration
    D. Coherent

12. When a photon of 1.02 MeV interacts with the nuclear force field of an atom, it is split into two electrons. What are the names of these two electrons?

    A. Identical scatter electrons
    B. Positive and negative electrons
    C. Positron and negatron electrons
    D. Recoil electrons

13. For a photon to interact with the nucleus of an atom and cause the release of a nuclear fragment, the incident photon must be at which energy level?

    A. 50 MeV
    B. 10 keV
    C. 10 MeV
    D. 3000 keV

14. Characteristic radiation is similar to which type of interaction?

    A. Photoelectric
    B. Coherent
    C. Compton
    D. Pair production

15. Characteristic radiation is produced at higher energies because:

    A. The filament has more atoms to interact with in order to produce the electron cloud.
    B. The material used to construct the anode has a high atomic number.
    C. Characteristic radiation is always of a longer frequency.
    D. All bremsstrahlung is produced first, then the characteristic radiation is produced.

16. Bremsstrahlung is similar to which of the five interactions with matter?

    A. Pair production
    B. Compton
    C. Photoelectric
    D. Coherent

17. Within the diagnostic range, most of the radiation is:

    A. Bremsstrahlung
    B. Characteristic
    C. Compton
    D. Secondary

18. Which unit of measurement is used to measure radiation absorbed dose in matter?

    A. rad
    B. rem
    C. roentgen
    D. RBE

19. The rem (radiation equivalent man) is a measurement used to express exposure doses received by:

    A. Any human
    B. Technologists
    C. Patients
    D. Technologists and patients

20. The unit of measurement for radiation exposure that is used to calibrate radiographic equipment is:

    A. rem
    B. roentgen
    C. rad
    D. roentgen or rad

21. A device to detect and quantify radiation is a:

    A. Spinning top
    B. Oscilloscope
    C. Electronic digital dosimeter
    D. Modified Adrian-Crooks cassette

22. A field survey instrument that determines exposure rates based upon the quantity of ion pairs detected by the unit is a:

    A. Film badge
    B. Geiger-Müller counter
    C. Ionization chamber
    D. Scintillation counter

23. The most widely used personnel monitoring device is a:

    A. Scintillation dosimeter
    B. Thermoluminescent dosimeter
    C. Pocket dosimeter
    D. Film badge

24. Film badges are able to record various types of radiation because:

    A. They have different filters built into the plastic housing that holds the film.
    B. Film badges record only one type of radiation, x-radiation.
    C. Different film thicknesses are used depending upon the type of machines being used (e.g., diagnostic, therapeutic, or mammographic).
    D. They have different sensitivity settings on the plastic housing that can be adjusted to a variety of radiation types.

25. The ALARA concept follows which dose-response relationship?
    A. Nonlinear-threshold
    B. Linear-nonthreshold
    C. Linear-threshold
    D. Nonlinear-nonthreshold

26. The ALARA principle applies to:
    A. Service engineers
    B. Patients only
    C. Technologists only
    D. All people who may be exposed to radiation

27. Which person is responsible for evaluating dosage records for employees?

    A. FDA
    B. RSO
    C. NCRP
    D. UNCEAR

28. The institution responsible for maintaining cumulative dose records for all radiation workers employed by that institution is:

    A. The institution itself
    B. The FDA
    C. The EPA
    D. The dosimetry company (e.g., film badge company)

Answers appear at the end of the book.

1. Which of the following best describes the radiation that exits from the patient?

   A. Primary radiation
   B. Remnant radiation
   C. Leftover radiation
   D. Secondary radiation

2. What factor equalizes different types of radiation when they have different energy transfer rates?

   A. Linear energy transfer
   B. Half-life value
   C. Relative biological effectiveness
   D. Quality factor

3. The term *radiosensitivity* is best described by which of the following?

   A. The radiation that enters the patient's body
   B. Structures that are not very easily affected by radiation
   C. An effect that does not present itself until several weeks after the exposure
   D. Structures that are easily affected by exposure to ionizing radiation

4. A chronic exposure dosage to radiation can be defined as:

   A. A large dosage of radiation delivered over a long period of time
   B. A large dosage of radiation delivered over a period of time no longer than 24 hours
   C. A large dosage of radiation that will cause ill effects 30 days after the exposure
   D. An initial exposure of radiation followed by several repeat exposures during the course of one day

5. Radiation has the ability to cause chemical and biological changes within the human body. These changes may manifest as:

   A. A unique disease that is usually curable
   B. A common illness that is not life threatening
   C. A known disease that may or may not be life threatening
   D. A cold or flu that will most commonly

result in widespread infection and eventual death

6. The effect of a radiation exposure is:

   A. A very random process that will increase with the age of the radiographic tube
   B. A very random process that will increase with the linear energy transfer (LET) of the exposing radiation
   C. A unique process, with easily predictable results
   D. More than one, but not all of the above

7. The ALARA concept is used to protect which of the following people?

   A. The patient
   B. The technologist
   C. The radiologist
   D. All of the above

8. Which cellular component serves to contain and protect the cell?

   A. Cell membrane
   B. Mitochondria
   C. Lysosome
   D. Endoplasmic reticulum

9. On the cellular level, the brain or microprocessor of the cell is the:

   A. Golgi apparatus
   B. Mitochondria
   C. Nucleus
   D. None of the above

10. DNA means:

    A. Deoxyribonucleic acid
    B. Deoxygen nucleus acetone
    C. Division of the nucleic acid
    D. Deoxyribosome nucleus acid

11. The bases that are components of DNA are:

    1. Purines—adenine and guanine
    2. Purines—adenine and thymine
    3. Pyrimidines—guanine and cytosine
    4. Pyrimidines—cytosine and thymine

    A. 1 and 3
    B. 1 and 4

C. 2 and 3

D. 2 and 4

12. The type of cell division that germ cells undergo is referred to as:

    A. Meiosis

    B. Duplication

    C. Mitosis

    D. Telophase

13. In what order does a somatic cell undergo mitosis?

    A. Metaphase, anaphase, telophase, prophase

    B. Prophase, anaphase, metaphase, telophase

    C. Prophase, metaphase, telophase, anaphase

    D. Prophase, metaphase, anaphase, telophase

14. When a radiation photon interacts with a macromolecule of the cell and causes biological damage, it is referred to as:

    A. Point lesion

    B. Indirect effect

    C. Direct effect

    D. Radiolysis

15. Why can irradiated water within the human body be dangerous?

    A. Irradiated water will not cause any biological damage.

    B. It will cause point lesions in most of the cells that contain the irradiated water.

    C. It may lead to the formation of free radicals, which have the ability to cause biological changes within the cell.

    D. Irritating the water within the cell will cause the cell to become hypotonic.

16. Which type of dose response relationship is used when determining safe exposure dose limits?

    A. Nonthreshold model

    B. Threshold model

    C. Curvilinear model

    D. Any or all of the above

17. A dose response relationship in which the response is random and the chance of a response increases with the dosage delivered rather than the severity of the response is classified as:

    1. Threshold

    2. Nonthreshold

    3. Stochastic

    4. Nonstochastic

    A. 3 only

    B. 4 only

    C. 1 and 3

    D. 2 and 3

18. A long-term effect of ionizing radiation will become evident after which of the following lengths of time?

    A. 2 days

    B. 1 week

    C. 2 months

    D. All of the above

19. Ionizing radiation may have a carcinogenic effect. Which of the following dose response relationships best describe the effect?

    A. Quadratic threshold effect

    B. Stochastic effect

    C. Nonstochastic effect

    D. More than one but not all of the above

20. When considering acute radiation syndrome, the period of time that the exposed individual remains symptom-free is referred to as:

    A. Prodromal period

    B. Latent period

    C. Manifest period

    D. Cell deduction period

21. What does LD 50/30 mean?

    A. This is a legal dose that 50% of radiographic units may produce 30% of the time.

    B. This is the lethal dose of radiation that will cause 50% of the exposed population to die from that exposure within 30 days of the exposure.

    C. This is a lethal dose of radiation that will cause 50% of the population to die within 30 feet of where they were exposed

    D. This is a lethal dose of radiation that

will cause death to 30% to 50% of the exposed population

22. The prodromal period after an acute radiation exposure lasts:

    A. 10 to 12 minutes
    B. 5 to 7 days
    C. Not more than 24 hours
    D. Not more than 2 weeks

23. One of the common symptoms of a hematopoietic syndrome is:

    A. A decrease in blood-forming cells
    B. An increase in blood-clotting time
    C. Increased chance of hemorrhage and infection
    D. All of the above

24. Acute radiation exposures up to 1000 rad may result in which of the following syndromes?

    A. Central nervous system syndrome
    B. Gastrointestinal syndrome
    C. Hematopoietic syndrome
    D. All of the above

25. Individuals experiencing a gastrointestinal syndrome may present with dehydration and vomiting. Which of the following would not be characteristic of a gastrointestinal syndrome?

    A. Hemorrhage
    B. Decreased consciousness
    C. Widespread infection
    D. More than one, but not all of the above

26. Exposure doses that are between 2000 and 5000 rad delivered acutely will most likely result in which of the following syndromes?

    A. Hematopoietic syndrome
    B. Gastrointestinal syndrome
    C. Central nervous system syndrome
    D. An exposure of this magnitude will cause instant death.

27. A response to a radiation exposure that presents in the exposed individual within 30 days of the exposure is classified as a:

    A. Somatic—late effect
    B. Somatic—early effect

C. Genetic effect—late onset
D. Embryonic effect

28. An exposed fetus is considered to be the most radioresistant during:

    A. First trimester
    B. Second trimester
    C. Third trimester
    D. A fetus is always radiosensitive.

29. Which of the following blood-forming cells is considered the most radiosensitive?

    A. Yellow bone marrow
    B. Red bone marrow
    C. Thyroid glandular tissue
    D. Immature muscle tissue

30. Under what conditions would a genetic effect become apparent?

    A. An exposure to a germ cell that causes a mutation
    B. An exposure to a somatic cell that causes a mutation
    C. A cell that is used for procreation that has been mutated by radiation
    D. Any egg or sperm cell that is exposed to radiation

31. An exposure dosage that would affect the overall population if the entire population were exposed to the radiation dosage is called

    A. A genetically significant dose
    B. A genetically doubling dose
    C. An embryonic and fetal dose
    D. A total genetic effect

32. The relative radiosensitivity of a tissue is determined by the type of cell and the rate of metabolism. Which of the following would make a cell more radioresistant?

    A. Increased mitotic activity
    B. Undifferentiated stem cell
    C. Low oxygen content
    D. All of the above

33. Which of the following tissue types are the most radiosensitive?

    A. Epithelium of the lens of the eye
    B. Muscle tissue of the lower leg
    C. Cortical bone tissue of the sternum
    D. The nervous tissue of the brain

34. Which of the following factors are used to estimate exposure doses received by localized areas of the exposed individual?

    A. Linear energy transfer
    B. Quality factor
    C. Relative biological effectiveness
    D. Weight factor

35. An individual had three exposures: a chest radiograph (two views) and a lateral soft tissue neck radiograph. The chest films yielded a dosage of 23 mrad with 15 mrad for the neck. Using the weight factors on page 11 in Chapter 1, calculate the total exposure dosage for this patient:

    A. 3.99 mrad
    B. 3.21 rad
    C. 3.21 mrad
    D. 35 mrad

36. Decreasing the kVp used to make a radiographic exposure will have what effect on patient dosage?

    A. Increase patient exposure dose
    B. Decrease patient exposure dose
    C. Have no net effect on patient exposure dose
    D. Patient dosage is directly related to mAs and unrelated to kVp

37. Using excessive kVp will result in a patient exposure dosage that will:

    A. Decrease the overall patient exposure
    B. Increase the scatter production and decrease the patient exposure dose
    C. Increase penetrability of the primary beam, the radiographic density, and the patient exposure
    D. Raise the overall radiographic quality, decrease the patient dosage

38. Why do patient exposure dosages decrease with high-frequency generators?

    A. They decrease voltage ripple.
    B. They increase the heterogeneous primary beam.
    C. They increase voltage ripple.
    D. None of the above

39. Which of the following generators is considered the least efficient?

    A. Single-phase
    B. Three-phase, six-pulse generator
    C. Three-phase, twelve-pulse generator
    D. High-frequency generator

40. For a protective shield to provide maximum protection from the effects of ionizing radiation, it would need to be placed:

    A. Between the patient and the radiographic film
    B. Between the radiographic tube and the film
    C. Between the radiographic tube and the radiographer
    D. Between the patient and the primary radiation

41. Why is beam restriction an important aspect of patient protection?

    A. Beam restriction limits the area exposed to ionizing radiation.
    B. Beam restriction increases the penetrating ability of the primary beam.
    C. Beam restriction eliminates scatter and off-focus radiation exiting from the tube housing.
    D. Beam restriction minimizes the scattering effects of excessive kVp while optimizing the mAs used to make the exposure.

42. During an esophagogram, while the doctor is performing the image intensification portion of the examination, where should the technologist place the protective shield?

    A. On top of the patient's reproductive organs
    B. Between the patient and the overhead tube
    C. Under the radiographic table in the same plane as the patient's reproductive organs
    D. Between the patient and the radiographic table in the plane of the patient's reproductive organs

43. Which type of beam-restrictive device removes the most scatter and off-focus radiation produced within the radiographic tube?

A. A collimator
B. An aperture diaphragm
C. A 6″ cone
D. An 18″ cylinder cone

44. Total filtration includes which of the following components?

1. Collimator mirror
2. Tube (Pyrex glass)
3. Oil
4. Tube window (plastic)

A. 1, 2, and 4
B. 2 and 4 only
C. 1, 3, and 4
D. 1, 2, 3, and 4

45. Which of the following best describes why a compensating filter is used?

A. To equalize different anatomical structures and provide an even density throughout the radiograph
B. To make the anatomical structures change size
C. To allow the radiographic machine to compensate for a technical error by filtering out unwanted, highly penetrating photons
D. It adjusts for anatomical densities, making structures of equal density widely varying.

46. What is the relationship between skin dose and filtration?

A. Increase skin dosage and decrease filtration.
B. Increase filtration and increase skin exposure.
C. Decrease filtration and increase skin exposure.
D. No relationship exists between filtration and skin exposure.

47. Total tube filtration above 70 kVp must be at least:

A. 1.0 Al/eq
B. 1.5 Al/eq
C. 2.0 Al/eq
D. 2.5 Al/eq

48. What does the addition of filtration do to the average energy of the primary beam?

A. Filtration decreases the overall beam energy.
B. Filtration increases the overall beam energy, over 90 kVp.
C. Filtration will not change the overall beam energy.
D. Filtration increases the overall beam energy.

49. The relative film-screen speed is increased from 200 RS to 400 RS. If the mAs to make the first exposure is 45, what will the new mAs value be?

A. 90 mAs
B. 45 mAs
C. 22 mAs
D. 180 mAs

50. An exposure made with a grid produces a radiograph with optimal density. If the exposure is repeated without the grid and the technique adjusted to have the same density as the first radiograph, what will happen to the dosage received by the patient?

A. The dosage will remain the same.
B. The dosage delivered to the patient will decrease.
C. The exposure dosage delivered to the patient will increase.
D. The skin entrance dose will decrease, but the overall dosage delivered to the patient will increase.

51. When used properly, what effect will automatic exposure control have on patient dosage?

A. AEC will always increase the dosage delivered to the patient.
B. AEC will sometimes increase the dosage delivered to the patient.
C. AEC is specially designed to increase the dosage to the patient.
D. AEC is specially designed to decrease the dosage to the patient.

52. Primary radiation can be defined as:

A. Radiation that is produced within the radiographic tube
B. Radiation that exits from the patient
C. Radiation that interacts with matter but does not change direction
D. Radiation that exits from the tube port

53. Under what circumstances is it acceptable for a technologist to be exposed to the primary beam?

    A. When the technologist needs to hold a patient
    B. During an image intensification examination
    C. Never
    D. During a portable examination

54. Which of the following is true regarding secondary or scatter radiation?

    A. It is radiation that is produced within the tube but does exit from the tube port.
    B. It is primary radiation after it interacts with matter.
    C. It is radiation that is attenuated by the patient.
    D. More than one, but not all of the above

55. Which source exposes the majority of technologists to occupational radiation?

    A. The x-ray tube
    B. The radiographic booth
    C. The patient
    D. The radiographic table along with the Bucky or film holder

56. How many interactions with matter are required for an x-ray photon, within the diagnostic range, to be reduced to an energy level low enough to be completely absorbed and cease to exist?

    A. One
    B. Two
    C. Three
    D. Four

57. Which of the following are shielding devices that are designed to protect only the technologist:

    A. Flat contact shield
    B. Radiographic booth
    C. Lead-lined walls
    D. More than one, but not all of the above

58. Why must the tube housing provide shielding as a primary barrier?

    A. To absorb primary radiation
    B. To absorb secondary and scatter radiation

    C. To absorb off-focus radiation
    D. More than one, but not all, of the above

59. Which end of the radiographic tube provides the maximum amount of shielding?

    A. The top of the tube housing
    B. The cathode side of the tube housing
    C. The right side of the tube housing
    D. The anode side of the tube housing

60. In order for the tube housing to provide adequate shielding from leakage radiation, the exposure in air must not exceed

    A. 100 r/hr at 1 meter
    B. 10 mr/hr at 1 meter
    C. 100 mr/hr at 1 meter
    D. 100 mr/hr at 1 meter

61. Which of the following are considered basic methods of protection for the technologist?

    A. Time
    B. Distance
    C. Shielding
    D. All of the above

62. While assisting in a radiologic procedure, a technologist receives an exposure of 15 mr/hr at 2.5′ feet from the source. How would the technologist's exposure change if he or she doubled the distance from the source?

    A. Increase by two times
    B. Decrease by two times
    C. Increase by four times
    D. Decrease by four times

63. Using the answer to question 62, what would the actual exposure dosage received by the technologist be?

    A. 7.5 r/hr
    B. 37.5 mr/hr
    C. 7.5 mr/hr
    D. 3.75 mr/min

64. What law of physics describes the relationship in question 62?

    A. Inverse square law
    B. mAs distance law
    C. Law of conservation
    D. Distance-intensity law

65. What determines whether a barrier is a primary barrier?

    A. Any surface exposed to secondary radiation 50% of the time
    B. Any surface that may be exposed to primary radiation
    C. Any surface that is exposed to primary radiation less than 50% of the time
    D. More than one, but not all

66. A wall that is shielded as a primary barrier must have a shielding thickness of at least:

    A. 1/32″ Pb/eq
    B. 1/16″ Pb/eq
    C. 1/16″ Al/eq
    D. 1/4″ Pb/eq

67. A wall that is not exposed to the primary beam can be shielded as a secondary barrier. How far from the floor must the shielding extend?

    A. To the ceiling
    B. 7′ from the floor
    C. 9 to 10′ from the floor
    D. 7′ from the ceiling

68. A wall that can be exposed to primary radiation must be shielded with:

    A. A 1/16″ lead sheet 7′ from the ceiling and a 1/32″ lead sheet the rest of the way
    B. A 1/16″ lead sheet 7″ from the floor and a 1/32″ lead sheet the rest of the way
    C. A 1/16″ lead sheet 7′ from the floor and a 1/32″ lead sheet the rest of the way
    D. A 1/16″ lead sheet from the floor to the ceiling, because it is a primary barrier

69. Lead sheets that are used as primary and secondary barriers must overlap a minimum of:

    A. 1/4″
    B. 1/2″
    C. 1″
    D. 2.5″

70. The radiographic booth is shielded as a _____ barrier and would require _____ Pb/eq:

    A. Primary—1/16″
    B. Primary—1/32″
    C. Secondary—1/16″
    D. Secondary—1/32″

71. In determining shielding requirements, the workload is one factor considered. What is meant by workload?

    A. How much work will be required to shield the room
    B. How many cases will be done in the room per hour
    C. The number of exposures taken in the room and the mAs used to produce the exposure, yielding a mA-Min/week
    D. The length of time radiation will be produced toward a specific barrier, determining the workload of a specific barrier

72. According to the NCRP, what is the minimum thickness of a flat contact shield that would be used for patient protection?

    A. 1/32″ Pb
    B. 0.50 mm Pb
    C. 0.25 mm Pb
    D. 0.35 mm Pb

73. Which of the following will provide adequate shielding protection with a minimum thickness of 0.35 mm of lead?

    A. Flat contact shields
    B. Protective gloves
    C. Eyeglasses
    D. Bucky slot cover

74. At what distance should the technologist stand when making a portable exposure?

    A. 6 to 8′ from the patient
    B. 6 to 8′ from the portable unit
    C. 6 to 8′ from the source
    D. As far as reasonably achievable

75. At what angle from the tube port will the technologist be exposed to the least amount of scatter radiation?

    A. 270°
    B. 45°
    C. 180°
    D. 90°

76. The main function of a protective drape used during an image intensification procedure is to:

    A. Protect the patient
    B. Protect the patient and the technologist
    C. Protect the machine operator and the technologist
    D. Provide patient privacy

77. The cumulative timer serves what purpose?

    A. To remind the user how long the beam has been on for patient exposure
    B. To annoy the machine operator every 5 minutes
    C. To stop the machine after 5 minutes of use
    D. To protect the operator from overexposure

78. Which of the following are requirements for an image intensification unit?

    1. Dead man exposure switch
    2. Maximum exposure of 100 mr/min
    3. Minimum source-to-skin distance of 12″
    4. Maximum tube leakage of 100 mr/hr at 1 meter

    A. 1, 2, 3, and 4
    B. 1, 3, and 4
    C. 1 and 4
    D. 1 only

79. The minimum source-to-skin distance for a portable or mobile unit is:

    A. 2′
    B. 15″
    C. 1′
    D. 1.5′

80. Which of the following are considered basic properties of x-ray?

    1. Highly penetrating invisible rays
    2. Affects photographic film
    3. Travels at the speed of sound
    4. Has the ability to cause biological but not chemical changes

    A. 1, 2, 3, and 4
    B. 2, 3, and 4
    C. 1, 3, and 4
    D. 1, 2, and 4

81. What type of interaction with matter is characterized by a photon interacting with an orbital electron and changing direction without ejecting the electron?

    A. Photoelectric
    B. Coherent
    C. Pair production
    D. Compton

82. During a coherent interaction, why isn't the orbital electron ejected from the atom?

    A. Because the energy contained within the photon is below the binding energy of the electron
    B. Because it does not interact with an orbital electron
    C. Because it interacts with the nucleus of the atom and there are no electrons within the nucleus
    D. The electron is ejected and is called a recoil electron.

83. Which of the following is true concerning a coherent interaction with matter?

    A. The scatter photon contains more energy than the incoming photon.
    B. The incoming photon contains more energy than the scatter photon.
    C. The process of ionization subtracts most of the energy from the incoming photon.
    D. The incoming photon and the scatter photon have equal amounts of energy, and the interaction with the atom yields no net change in energy.

84. Photoelectric interactions with matter usually occur at what kiloelectron volts?

    A. 10 keV
    B. 35 keV
    C. 100 keV
    D. 1.02 keV

85. A photoelectric interaction with matter is characterized by an incident photon interaction with:

    A. An inner shell electron
    B. An outer shell electron
    C. Any electron orbiting the atom
    D. Both inner and outer shell electrons

86. After a photoelectric interaction with matter, the result is:

    A. A negative atom and a photoelectron
    B. A positive atom and a recoil electron
    C. A positive atom and a photoelectron
    D. A positive atom and a negatron

87. During a photoelectric interaction with matter, the electrons from outer shells migrate toward the nucleus and release energy. This energy is referred to as:

    A. Electron energy
    B. Photon energy; scatter radiation
    C. Atomic electron energy
    D. Photon energy; secondary radiation

88. The radiation that is produced from a photoelectric interaction with matter is:

    A. A higher-frequency radiation
    B. A more penetrating radiation
    C. A lower-frequency radiation
    D. The same frequency, but less penetrating radiation

89. The ejected electron in a photoelectric interaction is referred to as:

    A. Recoil electron
    B. Photoelectron
    C. Positron
    D. Negatron

90. Which of the following is the most common with a photon energy of 120 kV?

    A. Coherent
    B. Photoelectric
    C. Compton
    D. Pair production

91. During a Compton interaction within matter, the incident photon interacts with:

    A. An inner shell electron
    B. An outer shell electron
    C. A nuclear electron
    D. Any available electron

92. A Compton interaction results in:

    A. The production of secondary radiation
    B. The production of scatter radiation
    C. An ionized atom
    D. More than one but not all of the above

93. Scatter radiation that is produced as a result of a Compton interaction with matter is:

    A. Highly energetic and highly penetrating
    B. Of a lower frequency than the incident photon
    C. Not highly penetrating but does have the ability to cause additional ionizations
    D. More than one but not all of the above

94. The minimum amount of energy that is required for a pair production interaction to occur is:

    A. 1.02 keV
    B. 100 Mev
    C. 1.02 Mev
    D. 102,000 eV

95. A pair production interaction is characterized by a highly energetic photon interacting with:

    A. The nucleus of the atom
    B. The electrons closest to the nucleus
    C. The protons within the nucleus
    D. The neutrons within the nucleus

96. Which of the following is true regarding a pair production interaction with matter?

    A. The positron contains most of the energy whereas the negatron contains only a fraction of energy.
    B. The negatron contains most of the energy whereas the positron contains only a fraction of energy.
    C. The positron and negatron contain exactly the same amount of energy.
    D. None of the above

97. The positive charge of the positron will cause it to travel:

    A. Toward the negatron
    B. Away from any orbital electrons of other atoms
    C. Toward orbital electrons of another atom
    D. Positrons are stationary spins and do not move.

98. If a positron interacts with an orbital electron, what type of interaction occurs?

    A. Compton interaction
    B. Photodisintegration
    C. Annihilation reaction
    D. Photoelectric

99. An annihilation reaction between a positron and an orbital electron causes:

    A. Two high-energy photons, each 0.51 Mev in strength
    B. One high-energy photon of 0.51 Mev
    C. More than three photons, each containing at least 0.51 Mev
    D. Once this reaction occurs, both cease to exist.

100. Which of the following interactions would not occur in the diagnostic range?

    A. Coherent
    B. Photoelectric
    C. Compton
    D. Pair production

101. Which interaction results in the production of a highly penetrating, fast-moving, and highly ionizing radiation?

    A. Annihilation reaction
    B. Photoelectric
    C. Photodisintegration
    D. Pair production

102. At what energy level will a photodisintegration interaction with matter occur?

    A. 10 Mev
    B. 100 Mev
    C. 10 keV
    D. 1.02 Mev

103. Characteristic radiation is similar to which of the following interactions with matter?

    A. Pair production
    B. Coherent
    C. Photoelectric
    D. Compton

104. One factor that determines the frequency and penetrability of characteristic radiation is:

    A. The material of the target
    B. The angle of the anode
    C. The speed at which the anode rotates
    D. None of the above have anything to do with the frequency or penetrability of the photons produced.

105. With reference to Bremsstrahlung, the energy of the electron is:

    A. Absorbed by the atom and redirected as photon energy with 50% net loss of energy
    B. Absorbed by the atom and redirected as photon energy with little or no net loss of energy
    C. Absorbed by the atom and redirected as photon energy with a moderate increase in frequency
    D. Absorbed by the atom and ceases to exist

106. The unit of measure that is used to describe the amount of energy absorbed in matter is:

    A. Ram
    B. Rad
    C. Rem
    D. Roentgen

107. Which of the following units of radiation measurement is used to depict radiation exposures that occur on the job?

    A. Ram
    B. Rad
    C. Rem
    D. Roentgen

108. What does the abbreviation rem stand for?

    A. Radiation equivalent man
    B. Radiation exposure toward man
    C. Relative exposure man
    D. Radiation emitted toward man

109. When considering x-ray and gamma radiation, which of the following is true?

    A. 1 rad + 1 rem = 1 roentgen
    B. 20 rad = 1 rem = 20 roentgen
    C. 1 rad = 1 rem = 1 roentgen
    D. 2 rad = 1 rem + 5 roentgen

110. What unit of measure is used to determine an exposure rate in air?

    A. Ram

B. Rem

C. Rad

D. Roentgen

111. Which of the following survey meters would determine the exposure rate by the number of ion pairs detected?

   A. Ionization chamber
   B. Geiger-Müller counter
   C. Scintillation counter
   D. More than one but not all of the above

112. Which type of survey meter is the most sensitive meter for the detection of x-ray and gamma radiation?

   A. Ionization counter
   B. Geiger-Müller counter
   C. Scintillation counter
   D. All of the above have the same level of efficiency.

113. Which type of personnel monitoring device requires the use of a control device to determine the level of background radiation?

   A. Film badges
   B. Thermoluminescent dosimeter
   C. Pocket dosimeter
   D. All of the above

114. A device that is used to determine personnel exposure, using lithium fluoride crystals and heat, is a:

   A. Film badge
   B. Thermoluminescent dosimeter
   C. Pocket dosimeter
   D. Scintillation detector

115. The personnel monitoring device that is the most cost efficient is the:

   A. Geiger-Müller counter
   B. Thermoluminescent dosimeter
   C. Pocket dosimeter
   D. Film badge

116. A personnel monitoring device that needs to be read every day is the:

   A. Geiger-Müller counter
   B. Pocket dosimeter
   C. Thermoluminescent dosimeter
   D. Film badge

117. Which personnel monitoring device provides a permanent record of exposure doses?

   A. Scintillation counter
   B. Pocket dosimeter
   C. Film badge
   D. Ionization chambers

118. The personnel monitoring device consisting of a gas-filled chamber that converts the number of ionizations into an exposure dosage is the:

   A. Ionization chamber
   B. Scintillation counter
   C. Film badge
   D. Pocket dosimeter

119. Which of the following survey instruments is the most sensitive in detecting gamma radiation?

   A. Pocket dosimeter
   B. Geiger-Müller counter
   C. Film badge
   D. Scintillation counter

120. What is the annual dose equivalent limit for a radiologic technologist?

   A. 5 mrem
   B. 0.01 rad
   C. 5 rem
   D. None of the above

121. The dose-equivalent limit per month for a developing fetus must not exceed:

   A. 0.5 rem
   B. 0.05 mrem
   C. 0.05 rem
   D. 0.01 rem

122. NCRP has determined that the negligible risk level is 0.001 rem per year. What does this mean?

   A. An exposure this low would cause only minimal cellular damage.
   B. An exposure dose of this level would not cause cancer.
   C. An exposure dose of this level is not considered to be dangerous to humans.
   D. Exposures of this magnitude can induce a mild radiation syndrome.

123. What is the maximum cumulative dose exposure limit for a 36-year-old radiologic technologist working as a technologist for 12 years, including fluoroscopic procedures?

    A. 12 mrem
    B. 12 rem
    C. 36 rem
    D. 48 rem

124. The person or persons responsible for maintenance of cumulative dose records is:

    A. The company evaluating the film badges
    B. The institution of employment
    C. The individual technologists
    D. There is no need to keep records unless there is a large exposure.

125. Annual dose equivalent limits for the general public must not exceed:

    A. 0.1 rad
    B. 0.05 mrad
    C. 1 rem/year
    D. 0.1 mrem

126. What person would handle any employee receiving exposure doses in excess of the maximum permissible dose (DEL) as established by the NCRP?

    A. The chief technologist
    B. The individual receiving the exposure
    C. The radiation safety officer/committee
    D. The state in which the exposure was received

127. Which of the following radiographic units is required to have the following:

    1. Visual beam on indicators
    2. An audio signal at the time of the exposure
    3. A maximum leakage of 100 mr/hr at 1 meter

    A. Portable units
    B. Fluoroscopic units (stationary and portable)
    C. Stationary radiographic unit
    D. All of the above

128. What is the dose equivalent limit for a secretary working in a busy radiology department?

    A. 0.1 rem annually
    B. 0.5 rem annually
    C. 0.5 mrem annually
    D. 0.005 rem annually

129. What is the annual MPD for a diagnostic radiographer?

    A. 10 rem
    B. MPD is not used anymore.
    C. 5 rem
    D. 2 rem

130. What is unique about the exposure switch on fluoroscopic units?

    A. It glows in the dark
    B. It is a dead man type.
    C. It is a toggle switch.
    D. None of the above

Answers appear at the end of the book.

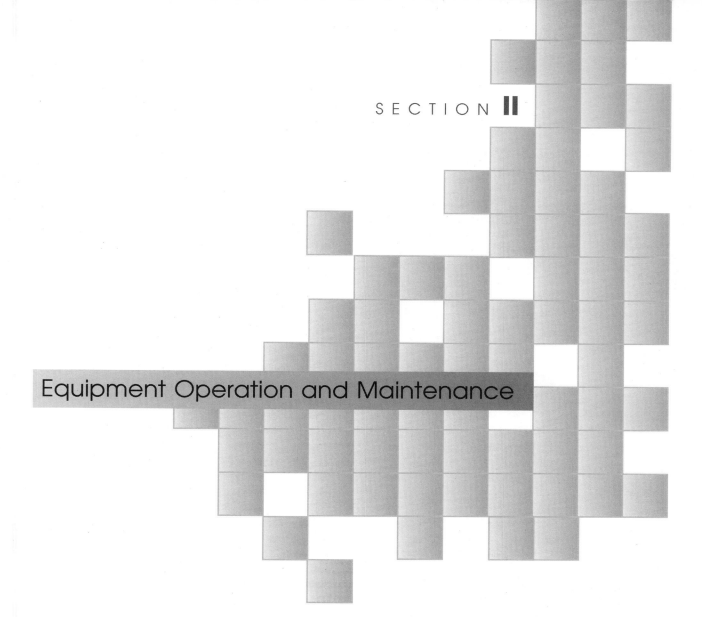

Equipment Operation and Maintenance

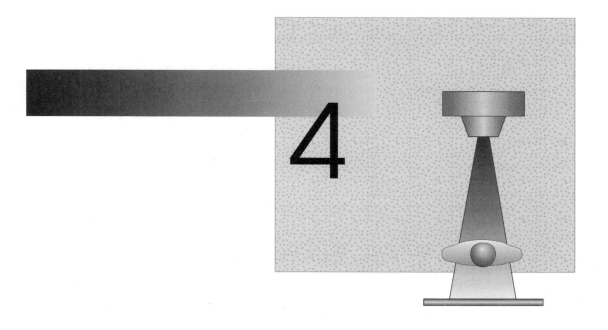

RADIOGRAPHIC EQUIPMENT

COMPONENTS OF A BASIC RADIOGRAPHIC UNIT

Operation Console

The operation console, located inside the radiographer's booth, consists of the control panel. It is connected to the low-voltage side of the x-ray circuit and allows for the selection of all technical factors (kVp, milliampere [mA], time, milliampere-second [mAs] read-out, focal spot size, Bucky/non-Bucky).

The X-Ray Tube

This component is located on the high-voltage side of the x-ray circuit (Fig. 4–1).

The Three Major Components

CATHODE—NEGATIVE POLE

The negative pole cathode consists of the tungsten filament and the (nickel) focusing cup. The filament "boils off" electrons through a process called *thermionic emission*. This negatively charged electron cloud, referred to as a *space charge*, is formed within the focusing cup. Thermionic emission occurs during the preparatory stage of the radiographic exposure.

Tungsten is the material of choice because it has a high melting point (3410 C°), which enables the filament to reach the temperature necessary to boil off electrons without melting. Most modern x-ray tubes have two filaments, one small and one large. The technologist can select a large or small focal spot depending upon the examination to be done. The cathode is connected to both the high voltage and filament circuit of the x-ray circuit.

ANODE—POSITIVE POLE

The positive pole anode consists of a stationary or rotating target for x-ray production. The anode is connected to the high-voltage portion of the x-ray circuit, giving it a large positive charge. This charge increases the electrons' attraction toward the anode. The filament is aligned to the angled edge of the target. This provides an area for the electrons from the electron cloud to strike in order to produce x-rays; this is the actual *focal spot*, or *focal tract*. The anode's angle is a very important factor in resolution of the resulting radiograph. The anode's angle is discussed further in Chapter 6. There are two types of anodes:

Stationary. This is a fixed structure made of tungsten imbedded in a copper shaft. Stationary anodes are limited in their uses because of their poor heat conductivity. Generally, stationary anodes are used only in dental units and in some older mammography units (the target would then be made of molybdenum).

Rotating. This type of anode rotates to increase its efficiency. It is constructed of a tungsten-rhenium alloy with a molybdenum shaft,

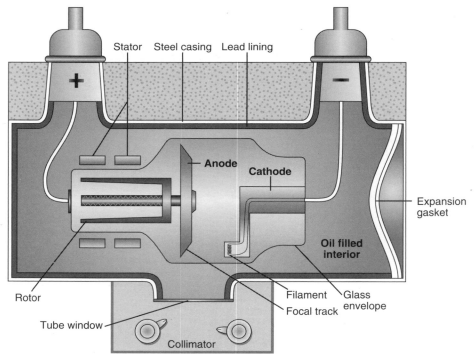

Figure 4-1 ■ Basic x-ray tube.

which dissipates the large amount of heat incurred during x-ray production. Molybdenum provides excellent heat conductivity, rhenium allows for rapid expansion of the metals and prevents cracking, and tungsten provides x-ray photons within the diagnostic range.

Because the anode is rotating, it can receive electrons at extremely high speeds without overheating and pitting. Standard anodes rotate at speeds of 3000 to 4000 rpm, and high-speed anodes rotate at speeds of between 10,000 and 12,000 rpm. If the anode fails to rotate or rotates at a speed slower than it has been designed for, a condition known as *anode pitting* will develop, in which actual divots are melted into the focal tract by the electrons coming from the cathode. This extreme amount of heat builds up because the anode is not rotating at its designed speed. In a properly rotating anode, the heat is evenly distributed over the entire surface of the anode, thus minimizing this problem.

Another common problem is *anode cracking*. This occurs when a cool anode is bombarded with electrons. The heat the anode receives is more than it is able to handle, and the metal is not able to expand quickly enough, resulting in cracking. Proper warm-up procedures are different for every manufacturer, but in general low kVp, low mA, and a long period of time will allow the anode to heat evenly without cracking. If either pitting or cracking occurs, the radiographic tube must be replaced.

GLASS ENVELOPE

A glass envelope provides a vacuum in which electrons travel from cathode to anode. This environment allows the electrons to flow from the cathode to the anode without impedance; therefore, with the applied kVp, the electrons will achieve the speed necessary to be converted into photon energy. The glass envelope is constructed of Pyrex glass for its strength and excellent heat conductivity. The glass envelope is also surrounded by oil to increase the thermal conductivity of the x-ray tube. The Pyrex glass and the oil both contribute to the tube's inherent or built-in filtration because the radiation produced at the anode must pass through the envelope and oil. Thus very low energy photons are prevented from exiting from the tube housing as they become attenuated in the oil.

A condition known as tube sunburn occurs when the tungsten of the filament evaporates and is deposited on the inside of the glass envelope. When the tungsten builds up within the tube, it causes the tube to arc and burns the tube out. It also causes the glass to turn a sunburnt color.

Tube Rating Charts

Tube Limit. This determines the maximum amount of kV, mA, and time allowed for a single exposure, without overloading the radiographic tube. Less than 1% of the electrical energy is converted into x-ray energy; more than 98% is converted into heat energy (Fig. 4–2).

Anode Cooling Curve. This represents the thermal capacity of the anode and the time necessary for it to cool. The anode is constructed to provide a high melting point because of the materials used—tungsten (atomic number 74, and rhenium, atomic number 75). The anode cooling curve also determines the amount of serial exposures that are safe for a particular unit; its thermal capacity is expressed in heat units (HU) (Fig. 4–3).

Tube Housing Cooling Curves. This curve represents the maximum amount of HU the tube housing is able to receive and the length of time required for it to cool to a safe level, to prevent overheating. This is also expressed in HU (Fig. 4–4).

Formulas for Determining Heat Units
Single-phase:

$$kV \times mA \times time \times 1 = HU$$

Three-phase:

Six-pulse: $kV \times mA \times time \times 1.35 = HU$
Twelve-pulse: $kV \times mA \times time \times 1.41 = HU$

Automatic Exposure Control

The automatic exposure control (AEC) is a mechanism programmed to terminate the exposure time. It measures a preset quantity of radiation and breaks the timer circuit when this amount has been reached. This mechanism controls the exposure time only.

Phototimer

The primary beam passes through the patient, table, and cassette to a fluorescent screen, which converts photon energy into light energy. The light photons then excite a photo-multiplier tube, which establishes a charge in a capacitor. When the capacitor reaches a certain charge, it discharges an electric current that breaks the timer circuit, therefore terminating the exposure.

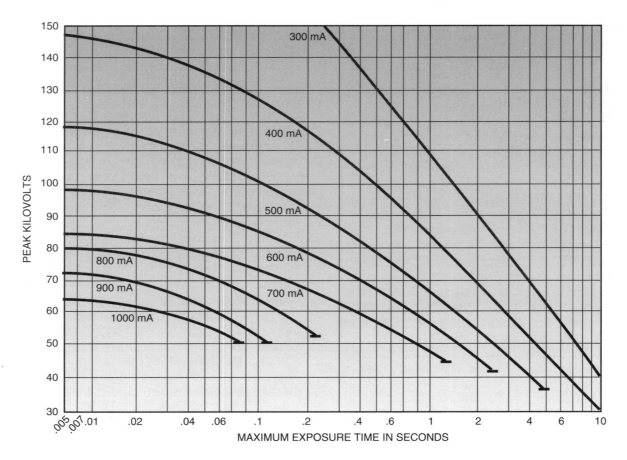

Note: Exposures that are below and to the left of the mA line are safe exposures.

Figure 4-2 ■ Radiographic tube rating chart.

Ionization Chamber

The primary beam passes through the patient and table, then it enters an ion chamber (before the cassette). Inside the chamber, ions are collected or counted. When the pre-set limit is reached, the timer circuit is broken and the exposure terminated.

In using AEC, radiographic quality is directly proportional to the accuracy of the radiographic positioning. If the area of interest is not centered or the wrong ionization chamber is selected, then the resulting radiograph will be either underexposed or overexposed.

Minimum Response Time

This refers to the time required for the AEC to react to the radiation and terminate the exposure. In a *photomultiplier*, the duration is 0.05 sec or less; in *ionization chambers*, as low as 0.001 sec. Problems can occur at high kVp techniques with imaging systems that employ fast film-screen combinations. A condition called *quantum mottle* is caused by an insufficient amount of radiation to excite the intensifying screen, resulting in a radiograph that is not evenly exposed.

Backup Time

This mechanism terminates the exposure if the ion chambers fail to work or if they are being used improperly. It may be used manually or connected to an interlock system. It prevents tube overload and unnecessary radiation exposure to the patient. The timer circuit is broken, thus terminating the exposure. Backup times, by law, cannot exceed 150% of the anticipated mAs value, generally 600 mAs at 50 kVp or above, and 200 mAs at 50 kVp or less.

Another problem arises when the exposure factors used create an excessive amount of scatter radiation (high kVp techniques). Ion chambers cannot differentiate between remnant radiation (exiting from the patient) and scatter radiation, therefore the exposure may be terminated early because of the increase in scatter radiation.

Exposure Controls (kVp, mAs (mA × Time))

Kilovoltage Peak (kVp)

This controls the penetrating ability of the primary beam or the force used to move the space charge or electrons across the x-ray tube from the cathode to the anode. An increase in kVp equals an increase in frequency and penetrating ability of the resultant photons. As the kVp increases, the amount of ionizations that it potentially can cause in matter will also increase. The kVp control adjusts the autotransformer located in the primary, low-voltage circuit.

Milliamperage (mA)

mA controls the amount of electrons available at the time of the exposure. An increase in mA equals an increase in electrons (in the space charge) and the number of photons produced at the time of the exposure. The mA control adjusts

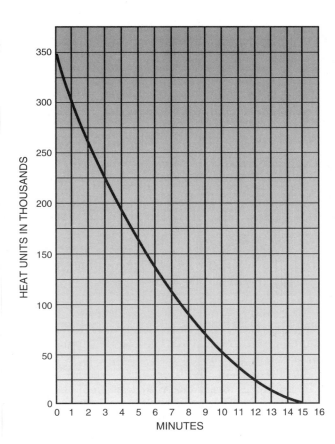

Figure 4-3 ■ Anode cooling curve.

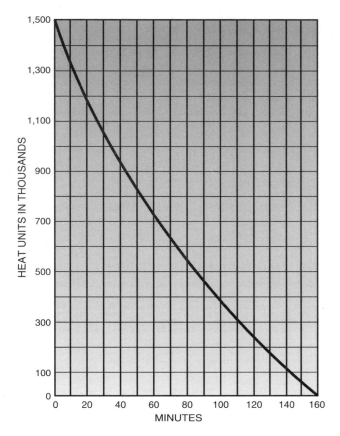

Figure 4-4 ■ Tube housing cooling curve.

the variable resistor in the filament circuit, thus increasing or decreasing the thermionic emission occurring at the filament.

Time

Time refers to the amount of time the kilovoltage is applied, allowing electrons to move from the cathode to the anode, or the length of time x-ray photons are being produced.

Milliampere-Seconds (mAs). mA and time are inversely proportional to one another and may be described by the formula

$$mA \times time = mAs$$

Therefore,

$$\frac{\text{Time (first exposure)}}{\text{Time (second exposure)}} = \frac{\text{mA (second exposure)}}{\text{mA (first exposure)}}$$

Beam Restriction Devices

Aperture Diaphragm

This is a flat piece of metal with different sizes of hole cut in it. It is the simplest type of beam-restrictive device in design and use. An aperture diaphragm is placed between the x-ray tube port and the patient, therefore limiting the area that would be exposed to x-radiation. Advantages include the ease of use and the cost. Disadvantages include the increased off-focus radiation reaching the film (Fig. 4–5).

The equation for determining field size:

$$\frac{\text{SID} \times \text{diameter of diaphragm}}{\text{Distance from focal spot to diaphragm}} = \frac{\text{Projected}}{\text{image size}}$$

Cones/Cylinders

The shape is the major difference between cones and cylinders, although cylinders may also have extensions. These devices are usually used with collimators, but they may be used alone. They are suspended from the x-ray tube port, therefore limiting the area of exposure the patient receives. Advantages of cones/cylinders are their ease of use and cost. Disadvantages include their weight, which may compromise patient safety, along with an increased penumbra and limited field sizes. Extension cylinders provide better absorption of scatter and off-focus radiation because they are located farther away from the focal spot (Fig. 4–6).

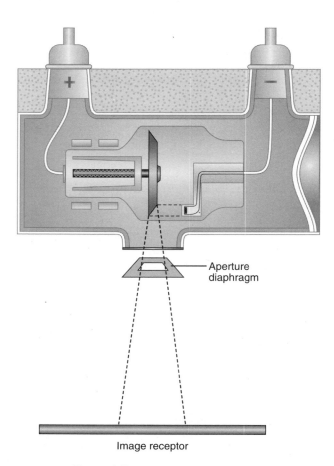

Figure 4–5 ■ Aperture diaphragm.

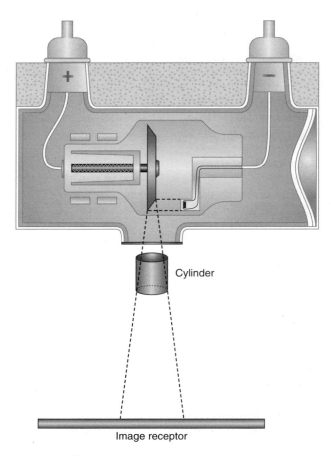

Figure 4–6 ■ Cones and cylinders.

The equation for determining field size:

$$\frac{\text{SID} \times \text{lower diameter of cone/cylinder}}{\substack{\text{Distance from focal spot to the bottom} \\ \text{of the cone/cylinder}}} = \frac{\text{Projected}}{\text{image size}}$$

Collimators

A collimator is a box-shaped device permanently attached over the tube port. It has two pairs of adjustable shutters, allowing for any square or rectangular field size. It is the most modern and most widely used device. The upper shutters reduce the quantity of off-focus radiation that reaches the film. The lower shutters reduce the penumbra of the resulting image.

One major advantage of collimators is that they provide a light source (cross-hairs, AEC ion chamber outlines). This light source is provided by a small light bulb that projects onto a mirror. The mirror is in the direct field, positioned at a 45° angle. In order for the light field to correspond to the radiation field size, the distance between the mirror and light source (light bulb) must be the same as the distance between the radiation source and the mirror. The mirror also adds to the added filtration of the primary beam, which is equivalent to 1 mm of aluminum.

Another advantage of a collimator is PBL (positive beam limitation). This mechanism adjusts the radiation field size to correspond to the film size when the Bucky is used, to prevent an exposure area larger than the film size being used. The amount of scatter reaching the film is reduced as well as the patient exposure dose.

Major disadvantages of collimators are the complexity of their construction and use. Collimators are also expensive to purchase and require additional maintenance (Fig. 4–7).

Other Devices

Other devices include any material that is used to block the primary beam or scatter radiation from reaching the radiographic film. Contact shields, which are lead-impregnated rubber sheets, are one example. These are either in sheets, or they may be cut into any shape desired. Shadow shields are wedge-shaped pieces of lead that are suspended from the tube housing or collimator; they shield by casting a shadow on the area, limiting the radiation that is received by that area.

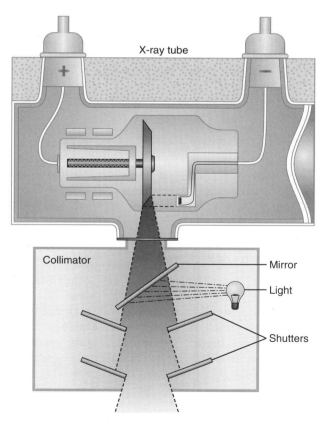

Figure 4-7 ■ Collimator.

X-RAY GENERATORS, TRANSFORMERS, AND RECTIFICATION SYSTEMS

Basic Principles of Electricity

Electrostatics

Electrostatics is the physics of the electrostatic phenomena. It involves the study of the distribution of fixed electric charges or electrons that are at rest.

The Five Laws of Electrostatics

1. *Repulsion-attraction.* Like charges attract, unlike charges repel.
2. *The inverse square law (see Chapter 2).* The force between two like charges is directly proportional to the product of their magnitudes and inversely proportional to the square of the distance between them.

$$\frac{I_1}{I_2} = \frac{(D_2)^2}{(D_1)^2}$$

Where I means intensity and D means distance.

3. *Distribution.* Charges reside on the external surfaces of conductors and equally throughout nonconductors.
4. *Concentration.* The greatest concentration of charges is on the surfaces where the curvature is the greatest.
5. *Movement.* Only negative (electrons) charges move along solid conductors.

Three Methods of Electrification

1. *Friction.* One object is rubbed against another, and because of differences in the number of electrons available and their binding energy (valence), electrons are able to travel from one material to the other.
2. *Contact.* When two objects touch, they permit electrons to move from a high concentration to a lower concentration until an equilibrium is met.
   a. *Static discharge.* When two strongly opposite charges come within close proximity to one another, creating a potential difference, electrons will jump the gap and the excess energy will be emitted as light photons, a spark.
3. *Induction.* The process of electric fields acting on one another without any physical contact, thus resulting in electron movement without electrons moving from one material to another.

Electrodynamics

Electric current is defined as electrons within a conductor that are predominantly moving in the same direction.

Metallic Conductors. Metal is the most common pathway for electrons to travel. Metal allows valence, or outer shell, electrons to drift or move across the conductor's surface.

Vacuum. A vacuum is a space from which all air has been removed, therefore there are few available atoms to oppose the flow of electrons. This allows electrons to reach the speed necessary, within the x-ray tube, to produce x-ray photons when the electrons decelerate or are stopped by the anode (target).

Gases. Gases, such as neon, promote the drift of electrons from a negative electrode to a positive electrode.

Ionic Solutions. These cause electrons to migrate to positive or negative poles during electrolysis, when they are subjected to an electric current.

Electric Circuit

An electric circuit is a pathway that permits electrons to move in a complete circle from their source through resisting electrical devices and back to the source. An excess of electrons at one end of the pathway will permit or facilitate their movement.

Describing Current Flow. Electrons move from a region of higher concentration to a region of lower concentration and will stop flowing when an equilibrium is met.

Ampere (Amp). The quantity of electrons flowing. An ampere is 1 coulomb of electrical charge per second (6.24×10^{18}/sec); 1 amp = 1 coulomb/sec.

Voltage (Potential Difference, Electromotive Force, EMF). The actual maximum difference of potential between the positive and negative poles of the electron source. The force that the electrons are pushed by as they travel from cathode to anode. Flowing electrons are not needed to have a potential difference. 1 joule of work done on 1 coulomb of charge; 1 volt = 1 joule/coulomb.

Resistance. The amount of opposition to the current in the circuit.

Four things influence resistance:

1. *Ability to conduct.* Material being used: insulator, semiconductor, conductor, superconductor.
2. *Length of the conductor.* Directly proportional to the resistance: the longer the conductor, the greater the resistance.
3. *Diameter (cross-section).* Inversely proportional: as the diameter increases, the resistance decreases.
4. *Temperature.* Directly proportional: as the temperature of the conductor increases, the resistance in that conductor also increases.

Ohm's Law. This law defines the mathematical relationships between amps, volts, and resistance:

1. R/V = I   Volts   = V
2. V × I = R   Amperes   = I (intensity)
3. R/I = V   Resistance = R

Types of resistance:

1. *Series:* Electrons pass through resistive devices all connected in a row, one after another:

$R_1 + R_2 + R_3$ = TOTAL RESISTANCE

2. *Parallel:* Electrons pass through individual branches, providing various resistive devices:

$1/R_1 + 1/R_2 + 1/R_3 =$
$$\text{TOTAL CONDUCTANCE } (R_T)$$

Note: Invert total conductance to get total resistance.

$R_T/1$ = TOTAL RESISTANCE

Power Formula:
   P = V × I
   P = power (watts)
   V = volts
   I = intensity (amps)

Magnetism

When a charged particle is in motion, a magnetic force field perpendicular to the motion will be created (orbital magnetic moment). Magnetism is a force that is able to attract or repel magnetic bodies.

Three Types of Magnets

1. Natural magnet. The lodestone within the Earth.
2. Artificial permanent magnet. Manmade steel magnets that hold their charge forever.
3. Artificial temporary magnet. Magnet made with electricity (electromagnet).

Laws of Magnets

1. Repulsion-attraction. Like poles repel, unlike poles attract.

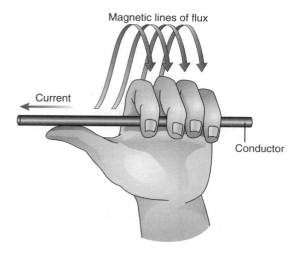

Figure 4-8 ■ Left hand thumb rule.

2. Inverse square law. The force of the magnetic fields is directly proportional to their magnitudes and inversely proportional to the square of the distance between them.
3. Magnetic poles. Every magnet has two magnetic poles, one north and one south.

Electromagnetism

The name for the magnetic phenomenon associated with electric current is electromagnetism. Whenever an electric current flows in a wire, a magnetic field is created around that wire.

Left Hand Thumb Rule. The magnetic field travels around the wire, as the fingers, while the thumb shows the direction of the flow of electrons (Fig. 4–8).

Electromagnetic Induction. The induction of a potential difference (EMF) voltage in a solid conductor. There are three methods:

1. Move a wire across a stationary magnetic field.
2. Move a magnetic field across a stationary wire.
3. Vary the magnetic field strength while a stationary wire lies within the field.

Four Factors That Regulate the Induced Current:

1. Speed—at which the wire cuts the magnetic field
2. Strength—of the magnetic lines of flux
3. Number—of turns or coils within the wire
4. Angle—at which the wire cuts the magnetic field. Maximum potential difference, or voltage, is achieved when there is a 90° angle between the wire and the magnetic lines of flux.

Generators

Mechanisms that convert mechanical energy into electrical energy are called generators.

Components

1. Wire (loop/armature)
2. Magnet (magnetic lines of flux)
3. Power source—some type of mechanical energy to rotate the wire.

Principle: Left Hand Generator Rule

(Fig. 4–9)

1. Thumb—points in the direction the conductor is moving.
2. Index finger—points in the direction of the magnetic line of flux.
3. Middle finger—points in the direction of the current or electron flow.

How a Simple Generator Works

(Fig. 4–10)

Position 1. The wire is parallel to the magnetic lines of flux; therefore no current is induced in the conductor.

Position 2. The wire is passing through the magnetic lines of flux. As the angle between the conductor and the magnetic lines of flux increases, the current induced in the conductor increases, peaking when the conductor reaches 90° or is perpendicular to the magnetic lines of flux.

Position 3. The wire is continuing through the magnetic lines of flux, but now the angle between the magnetic lines of flux and the conductor is decreasing; therefore the current induced in the conductor is gradually decreasing until the wire is at a 0° angle or parallel to the magnetic lines of flux.

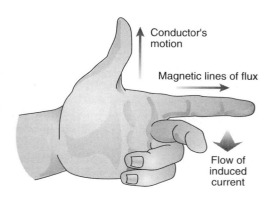

Figure 4-9 ■ Left hand generator rule.

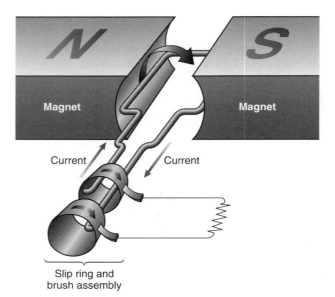

Figure 4-10 ■ Simple generator.

Position 4. The wire again begins to cut the magnetic lines of flux at an increasing angle, resulting in an increase in current induced in the conductor. The current will again peak when the conductor cuts the lines of flux at 90°, but because the conductor is passing through the lines of flux in the opposite direction, the current will travel through the conductor in the opposite direction, as described by the left hand generator rule.

Position 5. As the conductor continues to pass through the lines of flux, the angle at which the conductor cuts the lines of flux decreases; therefore the amount of current continues to decrease until it reaches 0 and the conductor is parallel to the flux lines. This process continues over and over, each time creating a wave form called a *sine wave*, and the rate at which this process occurs is the frequency.

Sine Wave

This is a graph that represents the amount of EMF (voltage) induced by a magnetic field as a conductor (armature) is passed through it. When the wire is parallel to the magnetic field, no EMF is induced in the wire, but as the angle between the wire and the magnetic field increases, EMF is induced in the wire. The maximum EMF is induced when the wire is perpendicular to the magnetic field (90°).

As the current is induced, it will flow in one direction, as described by the left hand generator (dynamo) rule. Once the conductor has reached 90° it begins descending through the field again.

As this happens, the angle is now decreased, causing the EMF also to decrease (refer to Fig. 4–11). The conductor has now traveled 180° through the magnetic field; as it continues to move through the magnetic field, EMF is again induced. The EMF peaks and then returns to 0. This also occurs as the angle increases and decreases between the conductor and magnetic field. The current is induced in the opposite direction (left hand generator rule). This results in the second arc of the sine wave, below the 0 line.

What the graph is actually showing is a positive and a negative flow of current. This type of reversing electricity is referred to as *alternating current* (AC). Each time the EMF is induced, peaks, and drops back to 0, the current is induced in the opposite direction, peaks, and drops to 0 again. One cycle has occurred (rotating the wire 360°).

Alternating current is expressed in *hertz*; a hertz is the frequency of the sine wave, or the amount of cycles per second. In the United States, there are 60 cycles per second, resulting in a 60-hertz alternating current. It is important to remember that for every 1 hertz the EMF is induced and peaks twice, equally in opposite directions, each peak taking 1/120 of a second (see Fig. 4–11).

Motors

A motor is an electrical device that converts electrical energy into mechanical energy.

Components

1. Wire (armature or loop of wire)
2. Magnet (may be an electromagnet)
3. Electrical energy

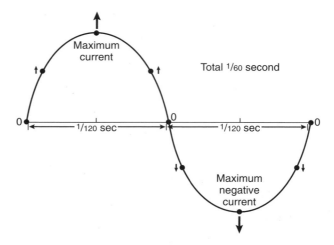

Figure 4-11 ■ Sine wave.

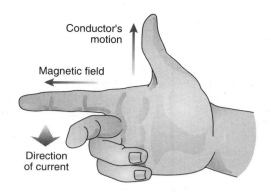

Figure 4-12 ■ Right hand motor rule.

Principle: Right Hand Motor Rule

(Fig. 4–12):

1. Thumb—points in the direction the wire will move
2. Index finger—points in the direction of the magnetic field
3. Middle finger—points in the direction of the electrical current of the wire

Types of Motors

1. Synchronous (time). The armature of the motor will rotate at the same speed as the loop of wire in the generator (x-ray impulse timer).
2. Induction motor. A stator, the stationary part of a motor, consists of an even number of stationary electromagnets distributed around the sides of a motor. The center is a rotating part called the rotor; it consists of bars of copper arranged around a cylindrical iron core. It resembles a squirrel cage (this rotates the anode's target).

Meters

Meters quantify electrical activity within a circuit. There are two types:

1. *Galvanometer*. Measures direct current; if connected in series within the circuit it will measure amperage; if connected parallel within the circuit it will measure voltage.
2. *Dynamometer*. Measures alternating current; if connected in series it will measure amperage; if connected parallel in the circuit it will measure voltage.

Transformers

These are devices that regulate the amount of voltage within a circuit.

Basics

1. Must have alternating current
2. There are no moving parts and no electrical connection.
3. Principle: electromagnetic mutual induction

Operation

The magnetic field created by the flowing current on the primary side of the transformer will fluctuate with the alternating current. This induces the same amount of current flowing at the same voltage on the secondary side of the transformer.

Types

Air Core. Two coils of wire with no iron core. The primary side of the transformer is supplied with AC (Fig. 4–13).

Open Core. Two coils of wire with an iron core within each coil. There is no attachment between the cores; the primary coil is attached to an AC supply (Fig. 4–14).

Closed Core (Doughnut). Two coils of wire wrapped around a square iron core. This design is more efficient by preventing a loss of lines of flux. This type is found within the x-ray circuit (Fig. 4–15).

Closed Core Step-Up. More windings on the secondary side than on the primary side; results in an increase in voltage from the primary side to the secondary side.

Closed Core Step-Down. More windings on the primary side than the secondary side; results in a decrease in voltage from the primary side to the secondary side.

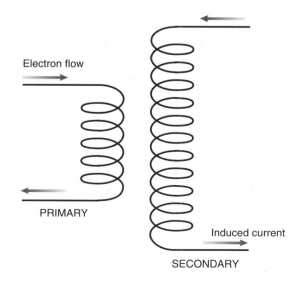

Figure 4-13 ■ Air core transformer (step-up transformer).

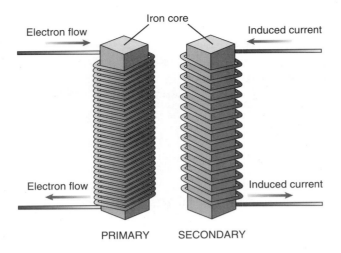

Figure 4-14 ■ Open-core transformer (step-down transformer).

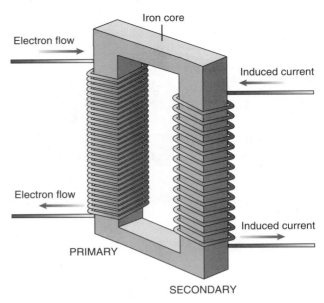

Figure 4-15 ■ Closed-core transformer (step-down transformer).

Shell Type. A laminated core is used, consisting of alternating steel and silicon sheets with two rectangular holes. The primary and the secondary coils are wound around the center section for maximum efficiency. This type is the most efficient; however, it is not used due to the energy levels of the x-ray circuit (Fig. 4–16).

Transformer Law

The voltage induced in the secondary coil is proportional to the voltage in the primary coil as the number of turns in the secondary coil is to the number of turns in the primary coil.

$$\frac{V_1}{V_2} = \frac{W_1}{W_2}$$

where V means voltage and W means windings.

Transformer Losses

Copper Loss. (True Resistance). The loss of electrical power due to the resistance of the coils.

Eddy Current Loss. (Swirling Currents). The fluctuating magnetic fields set up in the

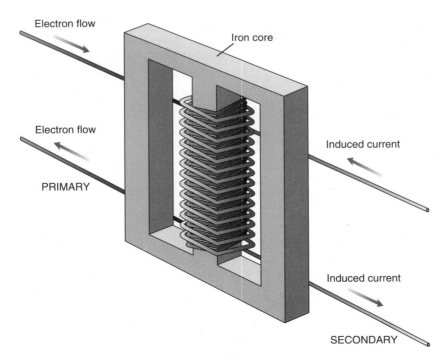

Figure 4-16 ■ Shell-type transformer (step-up transformer).

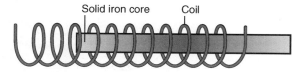

Figure 4-19 ■ Choke coil.

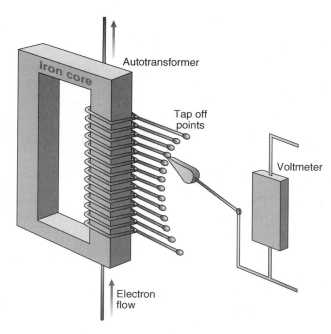

Figure 4-17 ■ Autotransformer.

transformer core by the AC in the coils induce electrical eddy currents (swirling of electrons within the core itself, electromagnetic induction). Eddy currents produce heat, therefore electrical energy is lost because resistance increases. This effect is minimized by the use of laminated silicon steel.

Hysteresis Loss. The rearrangement of magnetic domains, due to the AC, causes heat production and increases resistance, therefore decreasing electrical energy.

Current and Voltage

These are inversely proportional to one another in order to keep the total energy within a conductor constant (the law of conservation).

1. Step-up transformer: Increase voltage, decrease amperage.
2. Step-down transformer: Decrease voltage, increase amperage.

Voltage-Controlling Devices

Autotransformer. A coil of wire with a large iron core. The coil has tap or break-off points at

various locations along the wire. These tap-off points make it possible to vary the amount of voltage reaching the secondary side of the transformer. The greater the windings located before the tap-off point, the greater the voltage induced within the circuit. This makes it possible to select a predetermined amount of kVp. The principle that it works on is electromagnetic self-induction. The coil of wire acts as both the primary and secondary side of the transformer, with the tap-off points allowing a variable voltage to be selected.

The autotransformer is located on the primary low voltage side of the x-ray circuit and allows a predetermined amount of kVp to be selected (Fig. 4–17).

Rheostat. This is a coil of wire with a sliding tap, found in the filament circuit. As the tap slides across the coil, the resistance varies. As the resistance increases, the amperage decreases; therefore the amount of voltage increases (Fig. 4–18).

Choke Coil. A coil of wire with a movable iron core. As the core is inserted into the coil, the resistance within the coil increases, due to back-EMF. The principle of electromagnetic self-induction allows the choke coil to work (Fig. 4–19).

Saturable Reactor. Same design as a choke coil, but the iron core is supplied with a direct current. The principle that allows a saturable reactor to work is electromagnetic self-induction (Fig. 4–20).

The Basic X-Ray Circuit

(Fig. 4–21)

- What it does
- Principle by how it works
- Where it is located in the circuit

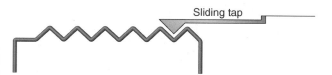

Figure 4-18 ■ Rheostat.

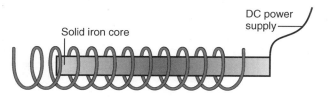

Figure 4-20 ■ Saturable reactor.

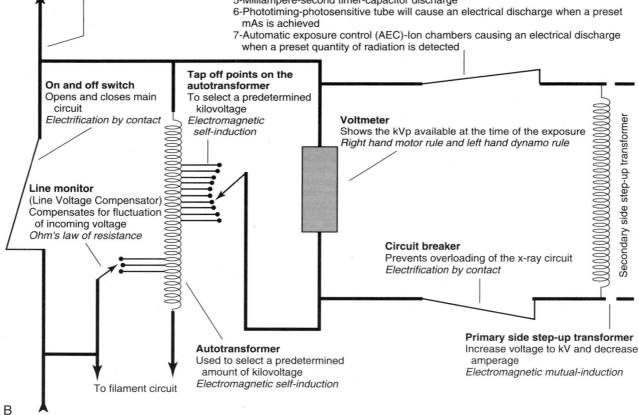

Primary low-voltage circuit   Primary high-voltage circuit

Filament circuit

A

Timer Circuit
Regulates the length of time x-ray production is allowed to occur
TYPES:
1-Synchronous timer-right hand motor rule and left hand thumb rule
2-Motor driven or mechanical timer-right hand motor rule and left hand thumb rule
3-Electronic impulse timer-silicon controlled rectifier (capacitor) and a microprocessor
4-Impulse timer-electrical discharge (thyratron) synchronized with electrical impulses
5-Milliampere-second timer-capacitor discharge
6-Phototiming-photosensitive tube will cause an electrical discharge when a preset mAs is achieved
7-Automatic exposure control (AEC)-Ion chambers causing an electrical discharge when a preset quantity of radiation is detected

Electric source
Alternating current (60 Hz-210-220 volts)
Electromagnetic induction and contact

On and off switch
Opens and closes main circuit
Electrification by contact

Tap off points on the autotransformer
To select a predetermined kilovoltage
Electromagnetic self-induction

Voltmeter
Shows the kVp available at the time of the exposure
Right hand motor rule and left hand dynamo rule

Line monitor
(Line Voltage Compensator)
Compensates for fluctuation of incoming voltage
Ohm's law of resistance

Secondary side step-up transformer

Circuit breaker
Prevents overloading of the x-ray circuit
Electrification by contact

To filament circuit

Autotransformer
Used to select a predetermined amount of kilovoltage
Electromagnetic self-induction

Primary side step-up transformer
Increase voltage to kV and decrease amperage
Electromagnetic mutual-induction

B

Figure 4-21 ▪ *A,* Basic x-ray circuit. *B,* Primary circuit—low voltage.

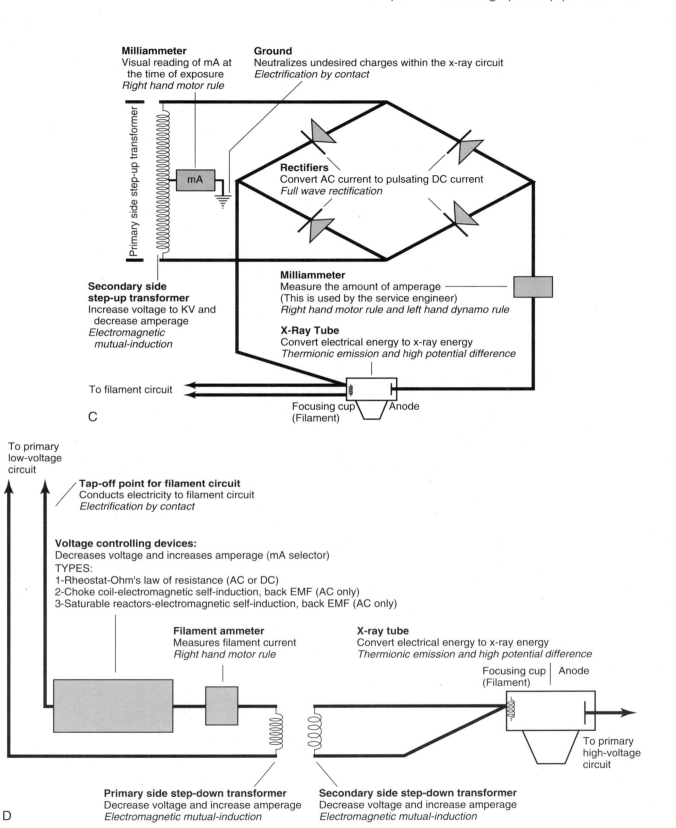

Milliammeter
Visual reading of mA at
the time of exposure
Right hand motor rule

Ground
Neutralizes undesired charges within the x-ray circuit
Electrification by contact

Primary side step-up transformer

mA

Rectifiers
Convert AC current to pulsating DC current
Full wave rectification

**Secondary side
step-up transformer**
Increase voltage to KV and
decrease amperage
*Electromagnetic
mutual-induction*

Milliammeter
Measure the amount of amperage
(This is used by the service engineer)
Right hand motor rule and left hand dynamo rule

X-Ray Tube
Convert electrical energy to x-ray energy
Thermionic emission and high potential difference

To filament circuit

Focusing cup   Anode
(Filament)

C

To primary
low-voltage
circuit

Tap-off point for filament circuit
Conducts electricity to filament circuit
Electrification by contact

Voltage controlling devices:
Decreases voltage and increases amperage (mA selector)
TYPES:
1-Rheostat-Ohm's law of resistance (AC or DC)
2-Choke coil-electromagnetic self-induction, back EMF (AC only)
3-Saturable reactors-electromagnetic self-induction, back EMF (AC only)

Filament ammeter
Measures filament current
Right hand motor rule

X-ray tube
Convert electrical energy to x-ray energy
Thermionic emission and high potential difference

Focusing cup | Anode
(Filament)

To primary
high-voltage
circuit

Primary side step-down transformer
Decrease voltage and increase amperage
Electromagnetic mutual-induction

Secondary side step-down transformer
Decrease voltage and increase amperage
Electromagnetic mutual-induction

D

Figure 4-21 ■ *Continued. C,* Primary circuit—high voltage. *D,* Filament circuit.

Rectification

Rectification is the process by which AC is converted into pulsating DC with the use of valve tubes or solid state diodes (Fig. 4–22).

Types

Self-Rectification. In this type, the x-ray tube itself is the only diode in the circuit. One half of the sine wave is suppressed, resulting in pulsating DC instead of AC. Of all the rectification systems, this one is the least efficient, and it is not used in modern x-ray machines.

Half-Wave Rectification. Two diodes are located in the circuit. These act to suppress one half of the sine wave or AC. This also results in pulsating DC.

Full-Wave Rectification. This type includes four diodes located within the x-ray circuit, which allows current to flow to the x-ray tube without interruption. This system converts AC into DC. This is the most efficient system, and it is standard throughout radiology.

There are three types of full-wave rectification:

1. Single-phase generator. This has four diodes and uses 1-phase, 2-pulse AC. One phase equals 1/60th sec, and there are two pulses in that 1/60 sec. The efficiency conversion factor is 1.00.
2. Three-phase, 6-pulse generator. This type of rectification includes six diodes and uses 3-phase, 6-pulse AC. The AC is supplied in three phases, thus preventing the voltage from dropping to 0. Within the three phases there are six pulses, each one occurring in 1/360 sec. The step-up is in a star/Y or delta configuration. The efficiency factor is 1.35.

3. Three-phase, 12-pulse generator. This includes 12 diodes and uses 3-phase, 12-pulse AC. The current is supplied in three phases and twelve pulses, with each one lasting only 1/720 sec. This results in a voltage ripple and is usually measured in milliseconds. The step-up also is a star/Y or delta configuration. This type is the most efficient and has an efficiency conversion factor of 1.41.

FLUOROSCOPIC UNIT

Image Intensifier

Two Types of Vision

Photopic. This type of vision requires light and is the function of the cone cells within the eye. The cone cells respond to many light wavelengths (a minimum of 100 light photons) and provide the best visual acuity and contrast perception.

Scotopic. This type provides vision in dim light, called night vision, and is a function of the rod cells of the eye. The rod cells respond to small quantities of light (as few as 15 light photons) and also provide peripheral vision. They respond to only a few light wavelengths and therefore do not provide a high level of visual acuity.

Fluoroscopic Unit Versus Image Intensification

Fluoroscopic Unit. This type of unit is no longer used. It required the radiologist to allow a minimum of 10 to 15 minutes of darkness adaptation, so he or she would be able to view images. Therefore, the radiologist was relying solely on rod vision. The images were projected onto a screen and the radiologist needed to wear red-tinted glasses to view them. These units also increased the quantity of radiation needed to produce images and therefore increased the exposure to the radiologist, radiographer, and patient.

Image Intensification. The terms *fluoro* and *image intensification* are commonly interchangeable. This type of unit takes the remnant radiation that exits from the patient and intensifies it so that it may be viewed with the use of the cone cells of the eye, therefore eliminating the need for darkness adaptation or special glasses. This enables radiologists to interpret the examination with an increased amount of visual acuity, providing a more accurate diagnosis. Also, the examination can be done with less radiation exposure to the patient, radiographer, and radiologist.

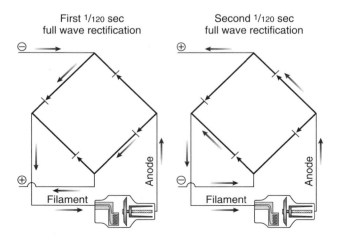

Figure 4-22 ■ Rectification (single phase).

Basic Components of an Image Intensification Unit

- X-ray production occurs under the examination table.
- X-ray tubes operate on 0.5 to 5.0 mA, which allows for longer exposures without the threat of overheating the tube.
- An audible alarm will sound after 5 minutes of usage but will not terminate x-ray production.
- The x-ray source to the patient may not be closer than 15 inches for a stationary unit and 12 inches for a portable unit.

COMPONENTS AND OPERATION OF IMAGE INTENSIFICATION TUBES (Fig. 4–23)

The X-ray Photon. This comprises the radiation that exits from the patient—remnant radiation.

Input Screen. Concave in construction, this screen converts x-ray energy into light energy and fluorescence; many light photons are created for each x-ray photon.

Photocathode. Concave in construction, the photocathode absorbs light energy and releases electron energy. The electrons travel toward the anode and output screen.

Electrostatic Lenses. These have a negative charge and focus the electrons to a convergence point. At this point the image is inverted (left to right and up-side-down). The lenses not only focus the electrons but also accelerate them toward the anode and output screen.

Anode. The positively charged (25-kV) anode allows the electrons to reach the maximum speed (repulsion-attraction law). It is constructed with a hole in the middle to allow the electrons to pass through and strike the output screen.

Output Screen. This screen converts the electrons into light energy, which becomes the visible image. This image is inverted and backward, but it is bright enough to be viewed by cone cells within the eye.

Glass Envelope. A jug-shaped tube made of Pyrex; the tube is a vacuum.

MULTIFOCUS TUBES

These types of tubes provide magnification of images, usually 6″ or 9″. The actual focal point is moved from a point farther or closer to the output screen—the closer it is to the output screen, the more magnification it provides. This feature is controlled by increasing or decreasing the strength of the negative charge on electrostatic lenses, therefore causing the electron stream to converge closer or farther from the output screen. Most modern tubes provide a dual focus, which is controlled by the operator (Fig. 4–24).

Four Types of Viewing Systems

Optical Mirror

This consists of a series of mirrors that project an image that is viewed by the radiologist (user). This type of viewing mechanism is very limited, because the user is not able to move around and still view the image. Also, only one person at a time can view it. It does allow imaging to occur in real time, but with a significant increase in radiation exposure to the patient. Basically, this

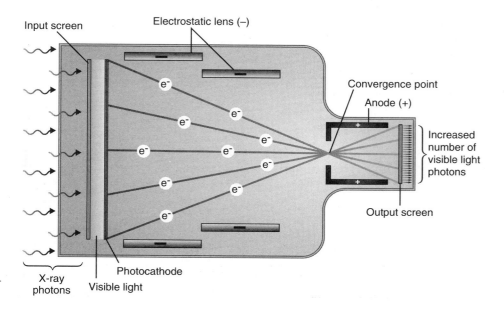

Figure 4-23 ■ Image intensification tube.

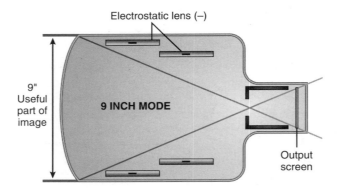

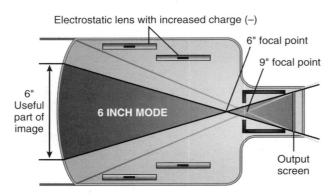

Figure 4-24 ■ Multifocus image intensification tubes.

type of viewing system is outdated and no longer in use in today's modern departments.

Video

This modern type of viewing system allows many people to view the images at once, does not significantly increase the radiation exposure to the patient, and allows simultaneous viewing of dynamic images as well as static and dynamic imaging.

Some of the disadvantages include the complexity of the equipment and the expense to purchase and maintain it. Also, when exposing static images the dynamic picture is interrupted.

MAJOR COMPONENTS (Fig. 4–25)

Video Tubes. These are tubes that transform visible light into a video signal. The two major types are

- *Vidicon tube,* composed of antimony trisulfide
- *Plumbicon tube,* composed of lead oxide

These photosensitive materials are arranged in globules on a matrix that forms the signal plate. When struck by light, they release electrons pro-

portional to the intensity of the light photon. The images' resolution depends upon the size of the globules: the smaller the globules, the better the resolution. Plumbicon tubes are faster than vidicon tubes.

Cathode. This is located within the video tube and heats to cause thermionic emission. Electrons are released and travel toward the anode. Electrons are focused by a control grid and formed into an electron beam.

Deflecting Coils. These coils have a negative charge; they direct the electron beam and cause it to scan the signal plate in a specific manner. This scanning pattern is referred to as a raster pattern (525 lines per 1/30 sec). To avoid a flickering that is detectable by the human eye, the electron gun scans half the signal plate, then goes back and scans the other half. First, it scans all the even lines (262.5 lines per 1/60 sec), then returns to scan all the odd lines (262.5 lines per 1/60 sec).

Focusing Coils. These coils have a negative charge and keep the electron beam in a tight stream, as well as accelerating electrons toward the signal plate.

Anode. This component is a wire mesh that has a positive charge that brings the electrons to a near-standstill. This allows them to be straightened and hit the signal plate closer to 90°, which increases the resolution of the resultant image.

Signal Plate. This thin graphite layer with a positive charge is thin enough to allow light to pass through but thick enough to conduct an electrical current. The signal plate is made from a photosensitive, photoconductive material (globules) suspended on a matrix that absorbs light and releases electrons proportional to the light photons' intensity, therefore leaving the plate with a positive charge. When the electron beam scans across the matrix, it causes electrical dis-

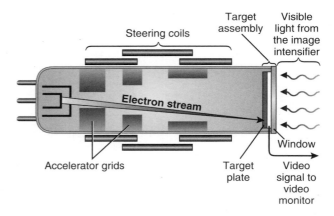

Figure 4-25 ■ Video tube.

charges in pulses. These pulses are conducted and become the video signal.

Video Camera Charged Coupled Devices

These use a semiconducting material that allows storage and discharge of a latent image through the positive/negative (P/N) junctions. The charges are stored and discharged in a raster pattern. These units are very durable and allow viewing on a video monitor with very little image lag.

Video Monitor

This basic television tube is also called a cathode ray tube (CRT). Its function is to turn the pulsating video signal into a visible image. The electron gun emits a tight stream of electrons by the negative charge of the focusing coils. They are "boiled off" from the filament by thermionic emission. The electrons are formed into a thin stream by the negative charge of the control grid. They are accelerated toward the video screen by the positive charge of the anode. The deflecting coils control the electron stream, allowing it to scan each line of the video monitor evenly.

The video screen is composed of a fluorescent phosphor laminated into the inside of a glass envelope, which illuminates as it is struck by the electrons. The brightness of the illumination corresponds to the velocity at which the electrons are traveling (Fig. 4–26).

Recording Systems

Dynamic Recording

This type of recording allows the fluoroscopic procedure to be recorded in real time. Once recorded,

it can be played back and viewed in real time or live action. There are two types:

Cine Film. This film is 16 or 35 mm movie film. A beam-splitting device is necessary for this viewing system, therefore increasing the patient exposure dose. Cine film requires about 90% of the visible light from the output phosphor to be adequately exposed. The images are recorded at high speed (30 or 60 frames/sec) and played back at about 24 frames/sec. Each frame is shown twice, totaling 48 frames/sec. At 48 frames/sec, the human eye cannot detect an individual frame and it looks like one continuous picture, without any stop in the action. For this effect, the camera must be synchronized with the pulses of the image intensifier (60 hertz), and this is why 30 or 60 frames/sec is used.

The major advantage of cine film is the increased resolution of the resulting images. A big disadvantage is that the x-ray tube must be able to withstand a tremendous amount of heat. Usually, a high-efficiency, 3-phase, 12-pulse, grid bias, liquid-cooled tube is used and synchronized with the shutter of the camera.

Videotape Recording. Two types of magnetic videotape are available for dynamic image recording: 1/2 inch VHS (VHS-s) or 3/4 inch U-Matic videotape. The video signal is magnetically encoded onto the videotape and can be retrieved and played back with the use of a video recorder. This type of recording medium provides high resolution, the ability to stop and start the tape any where in the recording, a reliable record of the procedure, and compact storage.

Static Recording Devices

These types of imaging systems are the most widespread; they are usually referred to as spot filming devices. They are the closest imaging system to plain overhead filming. Spot filming provides an accurate record of the procedure and is easily viewed and stored with other films within a patient's x-ray folder. There are three basic types:

Cassettes. These are usually 9×9" or 8×10", but any radiographic cassette with an intensifying screen may be used. The cassette is held by the machine and stored within a lead-lined compartment. When an exposure is desired, the machine slides the cassette into position in the primary beam. At the same time the radiographic tube's mA is increased to about 100 to 200 mA to provide adequate exposure of the desired area. Spot film cassettes may be exposed many different ways (full film, halves, thirds, or quarter exposures).

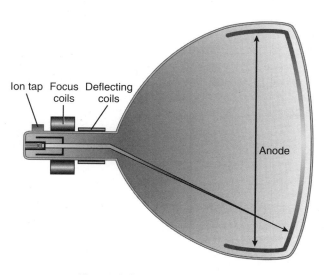

Figure 4–26 ■ Video monitor.

Some disadvantages of spot film cassettes: at the time of exposure the cassette is within the primary beam so the image cannot be viewed at the time of exposure, and using cassettes greatly increases the patient exposure dose. This dose exceeds that of any other imaging medium, solely because it is a direct exposure, similar to an overhead radiograph.

105 mm Chip Film. This type of image recording device uses individual pieces of film to record the images. Unlike cassettes, the chip film is not a direct exposure—it uses a beam-splitting device that allows the image to be viewed and recorded simultaneously. A chip film imaging system may expose up to 12 frames/sec.

70 mm Roll Film. This type of imaging system is very similar to the chip film system. The major difference is that instead of individual pieces of film, it is one roll of film. It too can expose up to 12 frames/sec. It may be viewed as a roll or cut to any length desired.

Videodisc Recording. This type of recording medium provides an excellent method of recording, viewing, and storing fluoroscopic procedures. By use of a laser, the procedure is encoded onto the surface of a disc. This process is extremely fast and reliable. The major disadvantage of the laser disc imaging system is the cost of both the initial purchase and the maintenance of the equipment.

Automatic Brightness Control

Total Brightness Gain

Magnification and flux are the factors that determine total brightness gain. It is a measurement of the overall boost in image intensity after the image intensification. The formula for determining total brightness gain is

Flux gain $\times$ minification gain =
Total brightness gain

As the image intensifier ages, total brightness gain will decay; this decrease may be as much as 10% per year.

Minification Gain. This occurs because the electrons from the input screen (larger diameter) are directed toward the output screen (smaller diameter) and forced to converge to fit onto it. The number of electrons is the same, but the area they cover is much smaller. The output phosphor is therefore excited to a greater extent, causing an increased amount of illumination. The mathematical formula for determining magnification is

(Input diameter)^2/(output diameter)^2 =
Minification gain

Flux Gain. This is an actual measurement of the conversion efficiency of the output phosphor. What is measured is the quantity of light photons emitted from the output phosphor per electron striking the output phosphor. The better the conversion efficiency is, the brighter the intensified image will be, decreasing the amount of radiation needed. However, as the conversion efficiency increases, the resolution of the resultant image decreases.

Brightness Control

Other terms for brightness control are automatic brightness control (ABC), automatic dose control (ADC), and automatic brightness stabilization (ABS). Brightness is controlled by varying the kVp, mA, and electrical pulses (time) during image intensification. As the density of the anatomical part changes, the technique will adjust automatically to accommodate the density change. This results in high-quality diagnostic images for all densities within the patient.

Important Image Quality Considerations

CONTRAST

Contrast is influenced by the amplitude, or force, of the video signal. This is controlled by the kVp and influenced by the scatter radiation produced by the high kVp technique that is normally used. Contrast is also influenced by the inherent penumbra of the visible light within the image intensification tube. This penumbral light may be compared with the base plus fog of radiographic film. As this inherent penumbra increases within the image intensification tube, the contrast of the image decreases.

RESOLUTION

The greatest limitation of using image intensification is the viewing system. The most common viewing systems provide only a 525-raster pattern on the video monitor; some specialized units have raster patterns as high as 1000 lines per frame. As video technology advances and larger matrices become available, the image quality will increase proportionally. Image resolution is also affected by the electrostatic lenses, focal point, magnification gain, and multifield or multifocus image intensifiers.

DISTORTION

This factor is greatly affected by the tube-part alignment, but there are also inherent tube considerations within the image intensifier that cause a certain amount of distortion, usually in shape. A usual cause is inverting the image, regard to transforming and converging the electrons, and light photons.

QUANTUM MOTTLE

This problem occurs when there is an insufficient amount of radiation to produce an image with an even distribution of radiation. The resultant image is patchy and undiagnostic. The most common solution is increasing the amount of mA. Some other factors that influence quantum mottle are remnant radiation exiting from the patient, the conversion efficiency of the input screen, magnification gain, flux gain, and total brightness gain.

TYPES OF UNITS

Stationary

This type of radiographic unit is fixed in one room. The room is designed with an adequate power supply, radiation shielding, and lighting. Specialized uses may require special equipment and markers in the room.

Portable (Mobile)

This type of equipment is not fixed in any one location and is designed to maneuver in tight areas. Usually these machines have motors to move them along because they would be extremely difficult to push manually. Standard radiographic portable machines are available in several different types, such as DC and capacitor discharge machines. It is important to know what kind of machine you are working with to avoid repeat exposures.

Specialized or Dedicated

A specialized or dedicated unit is one designed and calibrated to produce high-quality images of a specific nature. These units may also be coupled with dedicated processors to ensure the quality of the resultant radiographs. Some examples of these types of units are

- Head/skull units
- Chest stands/units
- Mammography units
- Tomography units
- Portable units
- Portable image intensification units (C-arm)
- Image intensification units
- Podiatry (foot) units
- Dental units
- Panorex units

Bibliography

Bushong S: Radiologic Science for Technologists. 5th ed. St. Louis, Mosby–Year Book, 1993

Carlton R, Adler A: Principles of Radiographic Imaging. Albany, NY, Delmar Publishers, 1992

Selman J: The Fundamentals of X-Ray and Radium Physics. 8th ed. Springfield, IL, Charles C Thomas Publisher, 1994

Chapter 4 **Questions**

1. The filament is made of a material with a high melting point called tungsten. This is the material of choice because tungsten's melting point is:

   A. 4310°C
   B. 3712°C
   C. 7443°C
   D. 3410°C

2. Some radiographic tubes have anodes that rotate at high speeds. These speeds may reach:

   A. 3000 to 7000 rpm
   B. 20,000 to 30,500 rpm
   C. 11,500 to 25,500 rpm
   D. 10,000 to 12,000 rpm

3. The formula for determining the heat units for a 3-phase, 12-pulse, high-efficiency generator is as follows:

   A. $kV \times Time \times mA = HU$
   B. $kV \times Time \times mA \times 1.35 = HU$
   C. $kV \times Time \times mA \times 1.41 = HU$
   D. $kV \times Time \times mA \times 1.00 = HU$

4. The amount of time necessary for automatic exposure control (AEC) to respond to radiation and terminate the exposure is referred to as:

   A. Backup time
   B. Exposure time
   C. Minimum response time
   D. None of the above

5. A beam restriction device is primarily used to:

   A. Limit the field size
   B. Protect the technologist
   C. Prevent an exposure
   D. Limit a tube overload

6. Within the collimator, the upper shutters serve to:

   A. Reduce off-focus radiation from reaching the film
   B. Reduce penumbra reaching the film
   C. Reduce the force of the radiation reaching the film
   D. All of the above

7. Electric charges reside on which surfaces of solid conductors?

   A. Internal surfaces
   B. External surfaces
   C. External surfaces in a helical configuration
   D. In an alternating fashion from the internal surface to the external surface

8. The formula given here is used to determine the total resistance in what type of circuit?

   $$R_1 + R_2 + R_3 = T_R$$

   A. Series circuit
   B. Parallel circuit
   C. Quad circuit
   D. An old circuit

9. Amperage is a unit of measure that is used to describe the:

   A. Direction of electrons
   B. Quantity of electrons
   C. Quality of electrons
   D. All of the above

10. As described by the left hand thumb rule, the fingers represent:

    A. Strength of the electrons
    B. Direction of the magnetic field
    C. Direction of the flowing electrons
    D. Strength of the magnetic field

11. Generators are used to convert what type of energy into what type of energy?

    A. Mechanical energy to electrical energy
    B. Electrical energy to mechanical energy
    C. Electrical energy to x-ray energy
    D. Mechanical energy to x-ray energy

12. As described by the left hand generator rule, the middle finger represents the:

    A. Direction of the magnetic flux
    B. Direction of the flowing electrons
    C. Direction of conventional current flow
    D. Direction the conductor is moving in the magnetic field

13. A sine wave is designed to graphically display:

    A. Direct current

B. Alternating current

C. The inverse of cos

D. More than one, but not all of the above

14. The primary use of a motor is to convert:

    A. Electrical energy to mechanical energy

    B. Mechanical energy to electrical energy

    C. Mechanical energy to x-ray energy

    D. Electrical energy to x-ray energy

15. As described by the right hand motor rule, the middle finger represents the:

    A. Direction the conductor is moving

    B. Strength of the magnetic field

    C. Direction of electron flow

    D. Direction of the current as it passes from the cathode to the anode across the x-ray tube

16. An induction motor is used in which part of the x-ray circuit?

    A. Autotransformer

    B. Rectifier/solid state diodes

    C. Rotor

    D. Filament

17. A meter that is connected in series within an alternating current circuit and measures the amperage within that circuit is called:

    A. Alternating current ammeter

    B. Dynamometer

    C. Galvanometer

    D. Voltmeter

18. A device that is used to regulate the amount of voltage within a circuit is called:

    A. Thermionic emission at the filament

    B. On/off switch

    C. Rectification

    D. Transformer

19. The type of transformer that is most commonly used in an x-ray circuit is:

    A. Air core

    B. Closed core

    C. Shell type

    D. Solid core

20. The rearrangement of magnetic domains due to the rapid fluctuation of the pulses of the alternating current is referred to as which of the following transformer losses?

A. Voltage loss

B. Copper loss

C. Eddy current loss

D. Hysteresis loss

21. The voltmeter is located in the radiographic circuit:

    A. Before the autotransformer, primary low voltage circuit

    B. After the rectifiers, filament circuit

    C. After the autotransformer, primary low voltage circuit

    D. At the x-ray tube, high voltage circuit

22. The main function of a step-up transformer is to:

    A. Increase amperage; decrease voltage

    B. Increase voltage; decrease amperage

    C. Decrease amperage; decrease voltage

    D. Increase voltage; increase amperage

23. An autotransformer works on which law of electromagnetism?

    A. Electromagnetic mutual induction

    B. Electromagnetic self-induction

    C. Electrification by contact

    D. Capacitor discharge

24. The device that controls the voltage that goes to the filament, such as a choke coil, is located in the:

    A. Filament circuit, high voltage

    B. Filament circuit

    C. Primary low voltage circuit

    D. This is a separate circuit.

25. The step-up transformer's location within the x-ray circuit is:

    A. Before the rectifiers and after the autotransformer

    B. Before the rectifiers and before the autotransformer

    C. Before the exposure timer and after the rectifiers

    D. After the exposure timer and after the rectifiers

26. How many rectifiers are required for a full-wave, 3-phase, 12-pulse generator?

    A. Four

    B. Six

C. Eight

D. Twelve

27. Once rectified, the current may be described as:

A. Direct current

B. Alternating current

C. Electromagnetic direct current

D. Pulsating direct current

28. The exposure timer is located in which portion of the x-ray circuit?

A. High-voltage primary circuit

B. Low-voltage primary circuit

C. Primary timer circuit

D. Filament circuit

29. In an old fluoroscopic procedure, the radiologist would need 10 to 15 minutes of dark adaptation. This is because he or she was basically using which type of vision?

A. Photopic vision

B. Dim light vision

C. Scotopic vision

D. Night vision

30. The image intensification unit operates on what range of mA values?

A. 0.05–15 mA

B. 0.5–5 mA

C. 10–50 mA

D. 8.3–80 mA

31. Remnant radiation describes:

A. Radiation after exiting from the patient

B. Radiation after exiting from the tube port

C. Radiation that is produced as off-focus radiation and exits from the tube port

D. Radiation after it has exited from the image intensifier

32. A viewing system that allows for only one person viewing at a time and is composed of a series of reflective mirrors is called a:

A. Video relay mirror system

B. Optical mirror system

C. Direct exposure system

D. There is no such viewing system.

33. The major difference between a static viewing system and a dynamic viewing system is:

A. There is no difference.

B. The dynamic system allows for real time viewing.

C. The two systems use different types of x-ray tubes.

D. The static system allows for real time viewing.

34. Total brightness gain is a multiple of:

A. Flux gain × minification gain = Total brightness gain

B. Flux gain × magnification gain = Total brightness gain

C. Input diameter squared × minification gain = Total brightness gain

D. None of the above

35. Which component varies the actual technique used by the image intensification tube to compensate for varying densities?

A. Anode

B. Total brightness gain

C. Automatic exposure control (AEC)

D. Automatic brightness control (ABC)

Answers appear at the back of the book.

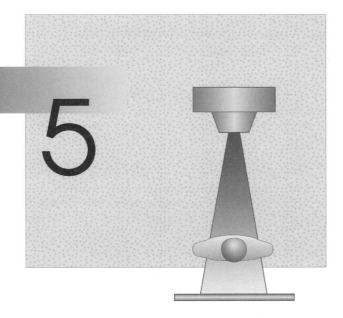

EVALUATION OF RADIOGRAPHIC EQUIPMENT AND ACCESSORIES

EQUIPMENT CALIBRATION

Performance improvement programs have become an extremely important aspect of the radiology department. It is important to understand the difference between performance improvement and quality control. Performance improvement is the overall plan that includes quality control. Performance improvement also includes all matters dealing with patients, such as scheduling, readings/reports, and the accuracy of the diagnosis. Performance improvement also governs the radiographer's outcomes through reject/repeat analysis and optimal/suboptimal programs.

Quality control deals only with the equipment. This means that the machines are tested for every possible variable to make a system that will provide consistently high-quality results (Table 5–1). It has nothing to do with technologists, radiologists, or patients.

Kilovoltage Peak (kVp)

During the exposure time kVp is the force that moves electrons from the cathode to the anode. As the radiographic tube and generator components age, the settings become less accurate. Kilovoltage settings can be checked by either a kVp cassette (Adrian-Crookes or Wisconsin cassette) or an electronic digital dosimeter. The advantage of a dosimeter is obtaining immediate readings with a higher accuracy. The kVp setting may not drift more than +/−5 kVp; if it does, the generator needs to be recalibrated. kVp accuracy will affect not only the density but also the scale of contrast because it directly affects the overall beam quality; this will be evident on the resulting radiograph. kVp testing should be done at least annually.

Filtration

Radiographic tubes that operate within the diagnostic range are required to have 2.5 mm of aluminum (Al) equivalent (0.5 mm/Al equivalent for mammography). This is a combination of inherent filtration and added filtration for a total filtration of 2.5 mm/Al. The purpose of the filtration is to filter out low-energy, low-frequency photons (so they never reach the film). The test used to determine whether the total filtration is adequate is the half value layer (HVL) test: an exposure is made, then thin sheets of aluminum are placed between the tube port and a dosimeter until the beam's intensity is reduced to half. When the beam is reduced to half of its original intensity, that particular thickness of aluminum sheets has determined the HVL.

Milliamperage (mA)

The mA is a measurement of the tube current or the quantity of electrons in the space charge that are available at the time of the exposure. As a result of tube aging, mA settings may begin to vary; therefore, the mA accuracy needs to be checked. This accuracy may be tested three ways: (1) an mR/mAs test, (2) an mA linearity; and (3) an mAs reproducibility. For these tests to be checked accurately, the time and the kVp must be within acceptable limits.

mR/mAs

This test evaluates the actual x-ray production or exposure in air in comparison with the mAs setting. It is performed with the generator set at a specific kVp and mAs. The geometry of tube alignment and dosimeter placement must also remain consistent for accurate readings.

At least three exposures are made, and dosimeter readings are recorded. These readings are then divided by the mAs used at the time of the exposure. The result is the mR/mAs ratio.

This test is performed annually in each of the radiographic rooms within the department. From one room to another the readings should be within +/−10% mR/mAs. The accuracy of the rooms' outputs will greatly affect the number of repeat exposures that radiographers will have to perform. This also allows accurate technique charts to be formulated, aiding in the reduction of repeat examinations.

mA Linearity

In this test, the mR/mAs is measured for a given mAs, then the mA and time stations are varied to check the linearity of the mA station. A linearity test is employed to determine the accuracy of the mA stations from a low mA to a high mA.

Before the linearity test, the timer accuracy must be within normal limits. This is tested by utilizing different mA and time stations to yield the same mAs value. Any combination of mA and time equalling a given mAs should yield consistent mAs density and radiation production. This is described by the reciprocity law, which states that the total energy is responsible for producing the latent image regardless of the combination of the technical factors (mA/time) used to achieve that quantity of radiation.

The accuracy of the tube's mA linearity is checked by recording dosimeter readings at dif-

Table 5-1 ■ **EQUIPMENT CALIBRATION**			
Component	**Testing Method**	**Acceptable Range**	**Frequency of Testing**
Kilovoltage peak (kVp)	Special cassette or a special digital dosimeter	Not more than +/−5 kVp	Annually
Filtration (HVL)	Aluminum sheets and a digital dosimeter	Mammography unit: 0.5 mm/Al equivalent Diagnostic units: 2.5 mm/Al equivalent	Annually
Exposure/tube current mR/ mAs	Digital dosimeter (exposure in air)	Not more than +/−10% from unit to unit	Annually
mA linearity	Different mA stations yielding the same mAs and a digital dosimeter	Not more than +/−10% for adjacent mA stations and not more than +/−50% from the lowest to the highest	Annually
Exposure reproducibility	Utilizing the same kVp, mA, and time, but changing them between exposures	Not more than +/−5%	Annually
Effective focal spot size	Slit camera or pinhole camera (same units may use resolution star pattern)	Focal spots 0.8–1.5 mm: up to 40% larger Focal spots 1.5/mm: up to 30% larger	Tested on new machines as part of acceptance, not necessary at any other time
Timers	Spinning top (single-phase only) Motorized synchronous top (3-phase and single-phase) Electronic timing device— counts the number of pulses	+/−5% for times >10 ms +/−20% for times <10 ms	Annually
Light field congruence	May be as simple as 9 coins to special templates	Not more than +/−2% SID	Semiannually
Central ray alignment	Central ray aligned to a lead marker	Not more than +/−1% of the light field central ray	Semiannually
Positive beam limitation (PBL)	This can be examined visually or measured	Not more than +/−3% of the SID to image receptor dimensions (both longitudinally and transverse)	Semiannually
Manual collimation	This can be examined visually or measured	Not more than 2% of the SID to image receptor dimensions (both longitudinally and transverse)	Semiannually
Visual examinations	Cables, collimators, crane, tracks, SID interlocks, deadlock switches	All these components should operate properly	Annually

ferent mAs values. These readings should not vary more than +/−10%. For example, a technique that uses 50 mA at 2 sec (100 mAs) should yield the same quantity of radiation and provide the same radiographic density as a technique using 200 mA at 0.5 sec (100 mAs).

mA Reproducibility

This is a test of the tube's ability to reproduce the same technique, using several different exposures with the same technical factors (mA, time, and kVp). An exposure is made at a set technique and a dosimeter reading is taken, then the technical factors are changed to a randomly selected technique. The exposure factors are then adjusted back to the original technical factors, and another exposure is made, and a dosimeter reading is made and compared with the first. These readings should not vary more than +/−5%.

Effective Focal Spot Size

The effective focal spot size greatly affects the resultant detail on the finished radiograph. A measure of the effective focal spot can be done with a slit camera or pinhole camera. Resolution can be evaluated with a star pattern or by imaging a line pattern. Focal spot sizes are usually measured with a slit camera but may also be evaluated with a star test pattern for focal spots 0.3 mm or smaller, or a pinhole camera for focal spots larger than 0.3 mm. Because of tube construction and variations, the latitude allowed for variation between the actual and effective focal spot is fairly great. The acceptable limits are:

0.8 mm	May be 50% larger
0.8 to 1.5 mm	May be 40% larger
Over 1.5 mm	May be 30% larger

than stated by the manufacturer.

Time

Time is defined as the length of time that electrons are allowed to travel from the cathode to the anode, permitting x-ray production. This factor tends to vary as the tube and the timer age. Timer accuracy can be tested with a spinning top test for single-phase generators or a synchronous timer or oscilloscope for 3-phase generators.

Spinning Top Test

A top is placed on a radiographic cassette and set in motion. An exposure is then made; the resulting radiograph demonstrates a certain number of dots, depending upon the exposure time. Since the radiograph machine operates on 60-hertz current and it is a single-phase, full-wave, rectified system, there are 120 different phases per second (60 normal cycles plus 60 rectified cycles equals 120). Therefore, if the number of dots on the radiograph is multiplied by the constant 1/120, the product will be the exposure time used.

> ### Example:
> A radiograph showing 12 dots was made at what exposure time? Use the formula
>
> (# of dots) × 1/120 (constant) = exposure time
>
> therefore, 12 dots multiplied by 1/120 equals 1/10 sec (12 × 1/120 = 1/10). This should be the exposure time set on the control panel.

Synchronous Timer

This is used only with 3-phase machines, but the basic principle is the same. An exposure is made, and the resultant radiograph demonstrates an arc, instead of dots. The arc is then measured and the exposure time determined by the length of the arc.

Automatic Exposure Control

The AEC test includes backup times, minimum response times, and sensor positioning and function. The accuracy of the AEC circuit directly affects the ability to produce quality radiographs. AEC relies greatly upon the radiographer's ability to position the desired anatomy accurately, but the unit's ability to produce a high-quality radiograph of properly positioned anatomy should be tested annually.

Other Timing Devices

With the emergence of total performance improvement programs, advanced timing devices such as electronic digital dosimeters and oscilloscopes are being purchased by more and more radiology departments. These testing devices can also be used to test the rectification circuit to ensure that all rectifiers are operating properly. If exposure times at all time stations are allowing only one half the selected exposure time, rectification may be identified as a possible problem. The readings must be within +/−5% for times greater than 10 ms and +/−20% for times less than 10 ms of the selected times. Timer circuits should be tested annually.

BEAM RESTRICTION DEVICES
Light Field to Radiation Field Alignment

A test for light field congruence is as simple as placing nine lead markers in the corners of the light field. An exposure is then made. The resulting radiograph will reveal the congruence of the radiation field to light field. Any radiographic unit with positive beam limitation (PBL) should be evaluated to ensure that the radiation field is not larger than the actual film size. Without use of the manual override, the PBL should limit the radiation field to film size or smaller to comply with federal law. The Bucky tray is also evaluated at this time to ensure that the center of the light/radiation field is aligned with the center of the Bucky tray/film. The radiation field to light field alignment should not vary +/−2% of the selected source-to-image distance (SID). These tests should be performed semiannually.

Central Ray Alignment

The test for this is performed by suspending two markers above the film that represent the center or cross-hairs of the light field. An exposure is made; the resulting radiograph will demonstrate where the markers are in relation to the center of the film. This should not vary more than 1% of the light field central ray.

RECOGNITION OF MALFUNCTIONS

Technologists must be able to recognize various types of equipment malfunctions to prevent repeats exposures, thus reducing the radiation exposure to patient and technologist. Although technologists are not responsible for repairing the radiographic equipment, they must be able to narrow down the possible problems. The technologist is responsible for reporting problems and aiding the engineer in a possible solution. This is a scientific process that eliminates one possible problem at a time, by manipulating one variable factor at a time until the problem surfaces. Obviously, this review is done with phantoms, not actual patients.

SCREENS AND CASSETTES

A cassette and screen consist of many layers and components that allow for the most efficient x-ray photon conversion into visible light photons while providing a safe, lightproof environment for the radiographic film (Fig. 5–1).

Screens

Base

A base material is usually made of a plastic material about 1 mm thick, attached to the inside of the cassette. This material must be flexible and tough, resist discoloration, and be chemically inert. If this material reacts with or discolors the film/phosphors, it may act as a filter or absorb the valuable light photons, resulting in a decreased light exposure to the radiographic film.

Reflective Layer

This is a thin layer of a foil-like material (25 μm thick) that is used to direct the light photons

toward the radiographic film. The phosphors emit light isotopically or in all directions equally. The reflective layer directs the light back toward the film and increases the light exposure to the film by as much as twofold. This maximizes the x-ray photon conversion to light photons reaching the film, therefore the quantity of radiation needed to produce the latent image is less than with a cassette without a reflective layer.

Phosphor Layer

This is a unique crystal that is able to convert x-ray energy into visible light energy. This layer is between 150 and 300 μm thick, depending upon the phosphor type and screen efficiency. When selecting a phosphor, some major considerations include

Atomic Number. A thin phosphor with a high atomic number is preferred because the photons are very energetic, which is necessary for them to work efficiently. The majority of the photon interactions with the phosphors must be photoelectric and Compton interactions to allow for maximum illumination of the phosphor.

Conversion Efficiency. This is a measurement of light emission per x-ray photon and is labeled as the *screen speed*. This ratio of radiation to visible light must be very high in order for this material to be efficient. The higher the conversion efficiency, the lower the amount of radiation required to maintain density.

Spectral Emission. Different phosphors have the ability to release light photons of specific wavelength (color), most often green or blue. This spectral emission must match the spectral sensitivity of the radiographic film being used to maximize the exposure to the radiographic film from the visible light.

Luminescence. This is the ability of a material to emit light in a particular wavelength when exposed to x-ray energy. This occurs in two ways:

1. *Fluorescence:* The type of luminescent emission that occurs immediately upon exposure to radiation. Once the exposure to

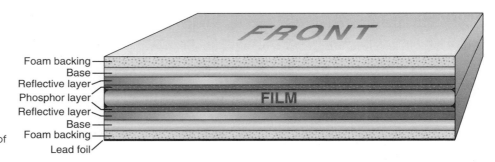

Figure 5-1 ■ Cross-section of a radiographic cassette.

Foam backing
Base
Reflective layer
Phosphor layer
Reflective layer
Base
Foam backing
Lead foil

radiation has ceased, the emission of light photons by the phosphor also ceases, occurring almost immediately.

2. *Phosphorescence:* This type of luminescent emission also occurs immediately but light continues to emit after the photon exposure has ceased. (This prolonged light emission may last long enough to expose another radiographic film when the cassette is reloaded in the darkroom.) The condition is referred to as screen lag or afterglow. It may produce unwanted density on the resultant film, which may be caused by the phosphor type or could occur as screens age (screen life = 7 to 10 years).

Cassettes

These must be constructed to accommodate a variety of film sizes. They must have a uniformly radiolucent front and a surface for attachment of the intensifying screen. The back cover of the cassette must also provide an area for the attachment of an intensifying screen. At least one of the intensifying screens must have a foam backing to provide tight contact against the film. The back cover also has a lead foil backing to prevent back scatter from reaching the film. The cassette must provide a lightproof space for the film. It must also be rigid and provide enough support for the body part being imaged.

Most cassettes have a little window that has a sliding, lightproof door. This space is used for a permanent record of pertinent patient information by using a flash machine (name, date, medical record number, institution name). Some cassettes also have grids incorporated into the front cover. They usually provide a visible center line in the middle of the cassette, along with information such as grid ratio and focal range.

When using grid cassettes, be careful to follow the manufacturers' recommendations for SID or focal range and to keep the x-ray tube perpendicular to the cassette to prevent grid cut-off.

Handling

Cassettes should never be thrown, dropped, or misused—they are tough but not indestructible. When loading cassettes, do not open fully. They need to be opened only 2 to 3 inches to allow films to be unloaded and loaded. This will help prevent foreign objects from coming in contact with the screen, such as dust or anything else that might damage it. This approach will also help to prevent foreign objects from forming artifacts on the resulting radiographs.

One way these artifacts are minimized is by using a daylight processing system. In this system, the film is loaded and unloaded inside the machine, which greatly minimizes any possible artifacts affecting image quality and helps prolong cassette life.

Artifacts

A compromised cassette or screen may result in a variety of artifacts on the resultant radiograph.

Light Leaks. If a cassette's structure is compromised and light is allowed in, it will expose the unexposed radiographic film, obliterate (fog) any latent image, and render the radiograph useless.

Asymmetric Screens. When highly efficient screens are used, they must be matched so the fronts and backs of the screens emit the same quantity of light, otherwise one portion of the film may be exposed more than another portion. This condition is not the same as quantum mottle.

Poor Film-Screen Contact. Poor or traumatic handling may lead to warping of the cassette and screens. This will prevent the film from accurately depicting the area of interest and compromise the radiographic detail.

Maintenance

Cassettes as well as intensifying screens should be cleaned on a routine basis. Cassettes that become soiled or come in contact with bodily fluids should be cleaned immediately with the appropriate solutions. Generally, cassette exteriors should be wiped clean with alcohol or a recommended germicide spray after each use. These cleansers should in no way damage or change the integrity of the cassette or leave any type of residue. Intensifying screens need to be cleaned with an approved solution that will not damage the screens' integrity or leave residue, and must be wiped clean with an approved cloth that will not leave any dust particles or scratches on the screen. Cassettes should always be stored empty, closed but not locked, on their edges. (Although this is the manufacturer's recommendation, in the average radiology department it is impossible to store cassettes empty.)

Film-screen contact needs to be checked annually. This is done with the wire mesh test. Place a wire mesh on the top of a cassette and take an exposure. If the resulting radiograph shows any distortion of the wire mesh, then the film and the intensifying screen are not in complete contact with each other. Intensifying screens should also be checked for screen lag. This can be done by placing the open cassette on the radiographic table, and without any radiographic film. Open up the light field to include the entire intensifying screen. Make an exposure—choose an exposure with a long time for better visibility, for when the radiation strikes the intensifying screen it will emit visible light. Once the exposure has ended, the screen should cease emitting light; if it does not then there is a problem with the screen and it needs to be replaced.

SHIELDING ACCESSORIES

All protective garments should be surveyed by the physicist or the radiation safety officer at least once a year. This is a visual inspection to assure that all the garments' seams and straps are intact. This also includes a fluoroscopic inspection to assure that there are no cracks or discontinuations in the lead lining of the garments. Lead is a very soft metal, and because it is used in such thin sheets for garments it is prone to crack when subjected to constant bending. If any problem with a garment is found, it should not be used until the necessary repairs have been made.

Along with the physical and fluoroscopic inspection of the garments, the equipment used to store the garments should also be inspected. This may include a rack that is hung on a wall or a table utilized for the storage of contact shields. If shields are not stored properly or the devices that are used to store lead-lined garments are not intact, the integrity of the protective garments may be compromised.

These inspections should be performed annually in every room in the department and on every protective device in use in the department.

Bibliography

Bushong S: Radiographic Science for Technologists. 5th ed., St. Louis, Mosby–Year Book, 1993

Carlton R, Adler A: Principles of Radiographic Imaging. Albany, NY, Delmar Publishers, 1992

Quality Assurance for Diagnostic Imaging Equipment. NCRP Report No. 99. Bethesda, MD, National Council on Radiation Protection and Measurements, 1989

Selman J: The Fundamentals of X-Ray and Radium Physics. 8th ed. Springfield, IL, Charles C Thomas, Publisher, 1994

Chapter 5 **Questions**

1. A quality control plan deals primarily with:

   A. Repeat/reject analysis
   B. Patient scheduling and patient readings/reports
   C. Equipment calibration and maintenance
   D. A combination of all of the above

2. Kilovoltage accuracy must be within $+/-5$ kVp from the selected kilovoltage. This may be evaluated by what method?

   A. kVp linearity test
   B. Total kVp HVL test
   C. kVp or Wisconsin cassette
   D. Sensitometer

3. Assuming that kVp is accurate and the timer is working properly, which type of evaluation would be used to check the accuracy of different mA stations?

   A. mA reproducibility test
   B. mA linearity test
   C. Densitometer
   D. mA spinning top test

4. The mA linearity becomes less accurate with tube aging and must be recalibrated if the mA linearity drifts more than:

   A. 2%
   B. 10%
   C. 15%
   D. 20%

5. Exposure reproducibility is evaluated by making several exposures all with the same technical factors. What device is used to take readings and evaluate the accuracy of the tube's ability to reproduce an exposure?

   A. Densitometer
   B. Sensitometer
   C. Dosimeter
   D. Spinning top test

6. Focal spot size may be evaluated by using which of the following device(s)?

   A. Slit camera
   B. Star test pattern
   C. Line pair test
   D. It may be evaluated with any of the above devices.

7. For focal spots between 0.8 and 1.5 mm, the actual size may vary up to:

   A. 20%
   B. 30%
   C. 40%
   D. 50%

8. A timer for a single-phase unit may be evaluated with which device?

   A. A spinning top test
   B. Timer Reproducibility
   C. Dosimeter
   D. Synchronous timer test

9. An exposure is taken with a spinning top in place on a single-phase, fully rectified generator at an exposure time of 1/20 sec. If the timer circuit is working correctly, the radiograph should yield:

   A. 3 dots
   B. 4 dots
   C. 5 dots
   D. 6 dots

10. In evaluating the timer circuit for a single-phase, fully rectified generator at an exposure time of 1/5 sec, the resulting radiograph demonstrates 12 dots. What, if any, is the most likely problem with the x-ray circuit?

    A. The exposure button was released too soon.
    B. There is a problem with the circuit's rectification.
    C. The timer is burnt out.
    D. The anode was not brought up to full speed before the exposure was made.

11. The device used to evaluate the timer circuit on both a 3-phase, 6-pulse and a 3-phase, 12-pulse generator is:

    A. A synchronous timer
    B. A spinning top
    C. A 3-phase spinning top
    D. With a 3-phase generator, there is no reason to check the timer's accuracy.

12. Timer accuracy for a 3-phase, 12-pulse, high-efficiency generator, for exposures

greater than 10 ms, should not vary more than:

A. 5%
B. 10%
C. 15%
D. 20%

13. A test in which nine lead markers are placed in the corners of the light field is used to evaluate:

    A. Central ray alignment
    B. Light field to radiation field alignment
    C. Film-screen contact
    D. There is no such test.

14. Phosphors emit visible light isotopically, therefore a thin layer of a material is placed behind the phosphor layer to utilize the light photons with higher efficiency. This layer is called:

    A. A base layer
    B. A reflective layer
    C. An aluminum foil layer
    D. This material is built into the phosphor layer.

15. When an x-ray photon interacts with the phosphor layer, the majority of the interactions with the phosphors are:

    A. Annihilation reactions
    B. Bremsstrahlung and characteristic
    C. Photoelectric and coherent
    D. Photoelectric and Compton

16. The arbitrary number that represents screen speed is directly related to the phosphors':

    A. Atomic number
    B. Overall size
    C. Spectral emission
    D. Conversion efficiency

17. Different types of phosphors emit visible light in different frequencies, called spectral emission. What is the importance of this?

    A. The spectral emission must be the direct opposite of the radiographic film to maximize the exposure.
    B. The spectral emission of the intensifying screen must match the sensitivity of the radiographic film to maximize the exposure.

    C. The spectral emission of the intensifying screen must be at a lower frequency than the sensitivity of the radiographic film to maximize the exposure.
    D. The spectral emission of the intensifying screen must be at a higher frequency than the sensitivity of the radiographic film to maximize the exposure.

18. The type of illumination that is most desirable for a radiographic intensifying screen is:

    A. Luminescence
    B. Phosphorescence
    C. Fluorescence
    D. White light

19. A thin piece of lead foil is attached to the inside back cover of a radiographic cassette. This serves to:

    A. Prevent exposure of the radiographic film from remnant radiation
    B. Prevent the exposure of the radiographic film from back scatter radiation
    C. Strengthen the cassette for tabletop examinations
    D. Aid in preserving the integrity of the cassette

20. When highly efficient intensifying screens are used and the front screen and the back screen do not emit the same quantity of light, an uneven exposure of light to the radiographic film will result. This type of artifact can be classified as:

    A. Poor film-screen contact
    B. Asymmetric screens
    C. Insufficient light quality
    D. Quantum mottle

21. When cleaning the intensifying screens, it is standard procedure to use screen cleaner and:

    A. A 4×4″ or 8×8″ gauze pad
    B. A special towel that will not scratch or leave dust on the screen
    C. A towel that was used in special procedures the day before
    D. Any paper towel

22. Film-screen contact is evaluated with a wire mesh test that determines whether the film

and intensifying screen are in direct contact with one another. As part of a quality control program, this test should be performed:

A. Monthly
B. Quarterly
C. Semiannually
D. Annually

23. Intensifying screens may be evaluated for screen lag by:

A. Using a specially designed dosimeter
B. Opening up the cassette and exposing it to radiation
C. Using a device that times the spectral emission
D. Opening up the cassette to examine the phosphor layer

24. When lead garments are tested under fluoroscopy to evaluate the integrity of the garments, it is important that

A. Only all lead aprons are tested
B. All lead aprons and thyroid shields are tested
C. Any garments, including protective shields for patients, are tested
D. Only aprons and contact shields that have been misused are tested, because they are most likely to be cracked

25. Which of the following people are responsible for actually performing quality control tests on lead-lined garments?

A. Radiologist
B. Radiographer
C. Radiation safety officer
D. Physician

Answers appear at the end of the book.

Section II Questions

1. In a basic radiographic unit, the operation console is used to select:

   1. Kilovoltage
   2. Milliamperage-seconds
   3. Focal spot size
   4. Ion chambers for AEC exposures

   A. 1 and 2
   B. 1 only
   C. 1, 2, and 3
   D. 1, 2, 3, and 4

2. The cathode boils electrons off the filament's surface through a process called thermionic emission. This process occurs during what stage of x-ray production?

   A. At the time of the exposure
   B. Immediately after the exposure
   C. During the prep stage after the application of the kVp
   D. During the prep stage prior to the application of the kVp

3. Where in a basic x-ray circuit is the operation console located?

   A. Primary side—low voltage
   B. Primary side—high voltage
   C. Secondary side—low voltage
   D. Secondary side—high voltage

4. The filament must be made of a material with a high atomic number and a high melting point to prevent filament burnout. Which material is best suited for the filament?

   A. Cesium iodine
   B. Tungsten-rhenium alloy
   C. Molybdenum
   D. Tungsten

5. In a basic radiographic circuit, where is the filament located?

   A. Primary side—high voltage and the filament circuit
   B. Primary side—low voltage
   C. Secondary side—high voltage and the filament circuit
   D. Secondary side—low voltage and the filament circuit

6. Tungsten makes a very good material for the filament because it has a high atomic number and a melting point of:

   A. 5431°
   B. 4310°
   C. 3410°
   D. 1043°

7. The modern x-ray tube is surrounded by oil. What purpose does the oil serve?

   1. Increases thermal conductivity
   2. Adds to the inherent filtration
   3. To prevent a short between the cathode and anode
   4. Increases the added filtration

   A. 1 and 4
   B. 1 and 2
   C. 2 and 3
   D. 1 and 3

8. When a rotating anode fails to rotate or rotates at a speed slower than the designed speed, what condition occurs?

   A. Pitting of the anode
   B. Less radiation than expected will be produced.
   C. More radiation than expected will be produced.
   D. The radiation produced will be less penetrating.

9. A stationary anode is basically used for which type of radiographic procedure?

   A. Chest x-rays made at a chest unit
   B. Extremities (e.g., feet, ankles, hands)
   C. Mammography
   D. Dental

10. What is the purpose of having a tungsten-rhenium alloy versus a pure tungsten anode?

    A. Rhenium allows better heat conductivity.
    B. Rhenium allows the metal to expand at a rapid rate to prevent anode cracking.
    C. Tungsten-rhenium alloy is a cost efficient alloy.
    D. More than one, but not all of the above

11. In the modern radiographic circuit, where is the anode located?

    A. High voltage—negative terminal
    B. Low voltage—negative terminal
    C. High voltage—positive terminal
    D. Low voltage—positive terminal

12. The most common problem with stationary anodes is that they do not provide:

    A. An accurate target
    B. A large enough target
    C. An adequate amount of heat conductivity
    D. A strong enough negative charge to boil off electrons

13. When electrons are ejected from the surface of the filament, what holds them in a tight cloud and prevents them from dissipating?

    A. The vacuum of the x-ray tube
    B. A grid bias tube prevents this from happening.
    C. The negative charge of the focusing cup
    D. The positive charge of the focusing cup

14. If the improper warm-up procedure is used on a cold anode, it may lead to:

    A. Anode overheating
    B. Anode cracking
    C. Anode pitting
    D. Anode melting, changing its overall shape

15. Why is it important for the x-ray tube to be a vacuum?

    A. This allows electrons to flow without any impedance.
    B. To prevent tube arcing
    C. To hold the space charge close to the filament
    D. To allow photons to exit from the tube port

16. Which of the following items make up the inherent filtration?

    1. Oil
    2. Pyrex glass
    3. Tube window (plastic)
    4. Aluminum

    A. 1 and 4
    B. 1, 2, and 4
    C. 1, 2, and 3
    D. 1, 3, and 4

17. Less than 1% of electrical energy is converted into photon energy. What happens to the rest of the electrical energy?

    A. It remains electrical energy to complete the circuit.
    B. It is converted to x-ray energy.
    C. It is converted to ionic energy.
    D. It is converted to heat energy.

18. A tube rating chart is used to:

    A. Prevent patient overexposure
    B. Provide a safe range of exposure factors that may be utilized
    C. Provide a guideline for technologists, but only as a guide, and exposures made in excess of this guide are still relatively safe
    D. Allow the service engineer to calibrate the machine adequately

19. Referring to Figure 4–2, which of the following would not be safe?

    A. 120 kVp—400 mA—0.2 sec
    B. 140 kVp—300 mA—0.3 sec
    C. 80 kVp—700 mA—0.03 sec
    D. 40 kVp—500 mA—4 sec

20. Referring to Figure 4–2, which of the following techniques would be within acceptable limits?

    A. 70 kVp—700 mA—0.2 sec
    B. 100 kVp—500 mA—0.2 sec
    C. 130 kVp—400 mA—0.008 sec
    D. 60 kVp—500 mA—3 sec

21. An anode cooling curve is a chart that is used to determine:

    A. A safe technique that would not overload the anode
    B. The thermal characteristics of the anode
    C. The amount of heat produced by a series of exposures
    D. The amount of heat produced by quantum mottle

22. Referring to Figure 4–3, if a series of exposures was made resulting in 200,000 HU, how long would it take before the anode would be completely cool?

    A. 3.5 minutes
    B. 4 minutes
    C. 12.5 minutes
    D. 18.5 minutes

23. During an angiography procedure, one exposure produces 150,000 HU. How many serial exposures could be safely made by referring to Figure 4–3?

    A. 3 exposures
    B. 2 exposures
    C. 4 exposures
    D. 2.5 exposures

24. A lumbar spine examination was performed that resulted in the anode receiving 200,000 HU. Using Figure 4–3, how long would it take for the anode to cool before another examination of 200,000 HU?

    A. 3.5 minutes
    B. 1.5 minutes
    C. 4 minutes
    D. 5 minutes

25. Referring to Figure 4–3, if a PA and lateral chest x-ray (100,000 HU), an AP pelvis (50,000 HU), and an AP and lateral hip (100,000 HU) were performed on the same radiographic unit, assuming there was no anode cooling between exposures, how long would it take before the anode was cool enough to repeat the entire examination?

    A. 2 minutes
    B. 7 minutes
    C. 5 minutes
    D. 3.5 minutes

26. Calculate the heat units for the following technique:

    100 kVp
    10:1 reciprocating grid
    1000 mA
    Small focal spot
    0.03 sec
    3-Phase, 12-pulse unit

    A. 30,000 HU

    B. 4230 HU
    C. 3000 HU
    D. 42,300 HU

27. The tube housing cooling curve is designed to prevent:

    A. Exposures that would cause a nuclear meltdown
    B. The tube housing from receiving its thermal capacity in heat units from heat produced by exposures
    C. Radiographers from burning their hands on a hot tube housing
    D. Overheating the filament due to multiple exposures in series

28. Calculate the following for a single-phase, fully rectified unit:

    54 kVp
    Large focal spot
    8:1 portable grid
    35 mAs
    0.10 sec
    72″ source-to-image distance (SID)

    A. 20,000 HU
    B. 18,900 HU
    C. 1,890 HU
    D. 1890 HU

29. When an automatic exposure control unit reaches a predetermined quantity of radiation, the:

    A. Filament is allowed to cool and stop thermionic emission
    B. Timer circuit terminates the exposure, causing x-ray production to cease
    C. Rectification circuit switches to self-rectification and stops x-ray production
    D. kVp is redirected to another circuit

30. The ion chambers of an automatic exposure control unit are located:

    A. Under the table, above the cassette
    B. Under the table, under the cassette
    C. In the table, above the cassette
    D. Under the table, in the cassette

31. A minimum response time refers to the length of time:

    A. The phosphors emit visible light, exposing the radiographic film

B. The anode needs to reach maximum speed
C. The AEC circuit needs to terminate the exposure
D. Necessary to heat the filament to a temperature hot enough to cause thermionic emission

32. By law, generators that utilize automatic exposure control must have an interlock system to ensure that back-up times do not exceed:

A. Double the selected mAs
B. Double the overall technique, including kVp
C. 150% of the selected mAs
D. 150% of the anticipated mAs

33. The technical factor that describes the penetrating ability or quality of the x-ray beam exiting from the tube port is:

A. mAs
B. kVp
C. mA
D. 60- or 120-hertz fully rectified current

34. High kVp techniques may cause AEC systems to terminate exposures prematurely because:

A. kVp is calibrated in AEC units
B. All the radiation passes through the ion chambers, undetected
C. The ion chambers detect a greater amount of radiation due to the increased amount of secondary and scatter radiation
D. High kVp techniques tend to increase the mAs values to almost double their original values

35. A photon that is produced at 130 kVp and 50 mAs may be classified by the following:

1. Highly penetrating
2. High frequency
3. Ability to cause many ionizations
4. Produces a minimal amount of secondary and scatter radiation

A. 1 and 2
B. 1, 2, and 3
C. 1, 2, 3, and 4
D. 3 only

36. What method is used to regulate the amount of thermionic emission that will occur at the filament?

A. Pulse oximeter
B. Line flux compensator
C. Variable resistor
D. Autotransformer

37. mA may be defined as:

A. The amount of electrons available at the time of the exposure
B. The amperage necessary to heat the filament to the appropriate temperature
C. The positive portion of the space charge
D. The time required for the electrons to move from the cathode to the anode

38. Which technical factor regulates how long the applied kilovoltage is allowed to move from the cathode to the anode?

A. mAs
B. Time
C. kVp
D. mA

39. The product of milliamperage and time make up the mAs factor of a radiographic technique. These factors may be altered by which of the following mathematical relationships resulting in the same net mAs?

A. A direct proportion
B. An inverse proportion
C. A relative log proportion
D. Inversely proportional relative logarithm

40. Which of the below techniques would yield the same radiographic density as the following:

100 kVp
10:1 portable grid
Small focal spot
1 second
300 milliamperes

A. 100 kVp—1000 mA—3 sec—no grid—small focal spot
B. 100 kVp—600 mA—0.25 sec—8:1 grid—large focal spot

C. 100 kVp—1200 mA—0.25 sec—10:1 grid—small focal spot
D. 100 kVp—1200 mA—0.4 sec—10:1 grid—small focal spot

41. If motion is to be minimized and the technologist elects to double the mA, what other technical factor needs to be adjusted in order to obtain the same radiographic density?

    A. Decrease the kVp factor by 50%.
    B. Increase the time factor by 50%.
    C. Use a small focal spot and keep all other factors the same.
    D. Decrease the time factor by 50%.

42. Which type of beam restriction device is the simplest to use but also the least effective?

    A. Cone
    B. Collimator
    C. Cylinder
    D. Aperture diaphragm

43. Calculate the following projected image size for an aperture diaphragm:

    72″ SID
    3″ diameter of aperture diaphragm
    5″ from focal spot to diaphragm
    Small focal spot

    A. 43.2 cm
    B. 46.0 mm²
    C. 42.2″
    D. 43.2″

44. Modern radiographic units have collimators to limit the field size. Within the collimator the upper shutters serve to:

    A. Reduce light exposure to the radiographic film
    B. Reduce secondary or scatter radiation
    C. Reduce off-focus radiation
    D. Reduce the amount of penumbra

45. Many collimators are equipped with a device that limits the field size to the film size being used if the Bucky is used. This device is referred to as:

    A. Primary beam limitation (PBL)
    B. Positive beam limitation (PBL)
    C. Automatic beam limitation (ABL)
    D. Corrective beam limitation (CBL)

46. For the light field to correspond to the radiation field size, the light source is placed:

    A. The same distance from the mirror as the radiation source
    B. At the left side under the anode at a right angle
    C. 1.25 cm closer than the distance from the radiation source
    D. Twice the distance from the radiation source

47. The mirror within the collimator is placed within the primary beam and adds to the total filtration of the beam. For the mirror to depict the radiation field accurately, it is positioned:

    A. At a right angle
    B. At an obtuse angle
    C. At a 45° angle
    D. At a 22.5° angle

48. A protective shielding device that is attached to the collimator and has the ability to shield the patient by casting a shadow is a:

    A. Suspension shield
    B. Collimator shield
    C. Contact shield
    D. Shadow shield

49. Electrons along a solid conductor move in which direction?

    A. This depends on whether it is AC or DC.
    B. From positive to negative
    C. From negative to positive
    D. From a higher concentration to a lower concentration regardless of positive or negative charge

50. One of the basic laws of electrostatics states that the highest concentration of electron charges is found on:

    A. The thickest part of the wire
    B. The surface of the conductor with the greatest curvature
    C. The area of the wire with no insulation
    D. Equally through the entire length of the conductor regardless of size or shape

51. One method of electrification is by friction. Which of the following best describes electrification by friction?

    A. Touching a highly charged terminal to a battery
    B. Rubbing a balloon on a piece of carpet
    C. Turning a light switch on and off rapidly
    D. The influence a varying magnetic field has on a solid conductor

52. When two objects with strongly opposing charges come within close proximity of one another, electrons may bridge the gap. This type of electrification is referred to as electrification by:

    A. Induction
    B. Close proximity contact
    C. Static discharge
    D. Electrodynamic

53. The unit that is used to describe current flow is a:

    A. Volt
    B. Ampere
    C. Ohm
    D. Joule

54. Which of the following best describes resistance?

    A. The number of resistors within the circuit
    B. 1 joule/coulomb of energy
    C. 1 coulomb of energy/second^2
    D. The amount of impedance to the flow of electrons

55. The mathematical relationship between volt, ampere, and resistance is described by Ohm's law. Which of the following is the mathematical formula for Ohm's law?

    A. V/R = I
    B. I/R = V
    C. R/V = I
    D. (R × V) = 1/2 I

56. Calculate the following for amperage:

    120 volts
    30 ohms
    60 hertz

    A. 50 amps
    B. 0.241 amp

C. 360 amps
D. 40 amps

57. Calculate the following for voltage.

    80 ohms
    45 amps
    60 hertz

    A. 3600 volts
    B. 360 volts
    C. 1.7 volts
    D. 0.5625 volts

58. Calculate the following for resistance.

    80 amps
    120 volts
    60 hertz

    A. 0.666 ohm
    B. 1.5 ohms
    C. 96 ohms
    D. 9600 ohms

59. Resistors connected one after the other in a row within the same circuit are said to be connected in:

    A. Parallel resistors
    B. Series resistors
    C. Multiple resistors
    D. Line resistors

60. Calculate the total resistance for the following circuit if the resistors are connected in parallel.

    #1 = 5 ohms
    #2 = 15 ohms
    #3 = 45 ohms

    A. 65 ohms
    B. 11.2 ohms
    C. 1.12 ohms
    D. 0.2889 ohms

61. Using the same resistors as in question number 60, calculate the total resistance for a series circuit.

    A. 65 amps
    B. 25 amps
    C. 25 ohms
    D. 65 ohms

62. Using the power formula, calculate the watts for the following:

    100 volts

20 amps
30′ of solid copper wire
Series resistors
   #1 = 5 ohms; #2 = 3 ohms;
     #3 = 6 ohms

A. 28,000 watts
B. 2000 watts
C. 84,000 watts
D. 143 watts

63. The type of magnet that has the ability to be turned on and off is a:

A. Natural magnet
B. Artificial permanent magnet
C. Artificial temporary magnet
D. Electron temporary magnet

64. The magnet law stating that the force of the magnetic field increases proportionally to the distance between them is called the:

A. Electromagnetism law
B. Repulsion-attraction law
C. Inverse square law
D. Diamagnetic law

65. What does the thumb represent in the left-hand thumb rule?

A. Conventional current
B. Electron flow
C. The direction of the magnetic field
D. The direction the conductor moves

66. Which of the following regulates the amount of induced current in a conductor?

1. Speed at which the wire cuts the magnetic field
2. Strength of the magnetic field
3. Number of batteries in the circuit
4. Angle at which the wire cuts the magnetic field

A. 1 and 2
B. 1, 2, 3, and 4
C. 2, 3, and 4
D. 1, 2, and 4

67. The index finger of the left-hand generator rule represents:

A. Direction of electron flow
B. Direction of the conductor's movement
C. Direction of induced current
D. Direction of magnetic flux lines

68. A generator converts which type of energy into electrical energy?

A. X-ray
B. Mechanical
C. Electrical
D. Light

69. As the angle between the magnetic lines of flux and the conductor increases, what happens to the induced current?

A. It changes direction
B. It increases
C. It decreases
D. It remains the same

70. How long does it take for the completion of one sine wave representing 60 hertz of current?

A. 60 seconds
B. 6 seconds
C. 1/6 second
D. 1/60 second

71. The middle finger of the right hand **motor** rule represents:

A. The direction of the wire
B. The direction of the magnetic flux
C. The direction of the current in the **wire**
D. The direction the armature will **move**

72. Which type of motor uses electromagnets in its operation?

A. Synchronous motor
B. Impulse motor
C. Inductance motor
D. Rotor (induction) motor

73. Which type of meter is used to measure amperage in a circuit operating on alternating current?

A. Oscilloscope
B. Sphygmomanometer
C. Galvanometer
D. Dynamometer

74. What is a basic function of a transformer?

A. To regulate amperage within a circuit
B. To transform DC to AC
C. To regulate voltage within a circuit
D. To vary resistance within AC circuits

75. The type of step-up transformer that is most commonly used in a radiographic unit is:

    A. Shell type
    B. Closed core
    C. Open core
    D. Air core

76. Which type of transformer is the most efficient?

    A. Shell type
    B. Closed core
    C. Open core
    D. Air core

77. Which formula best describes the transformer law? V, voltage; W, transformer windings.

    A. $\dfrac{V_1}{V_2} = \dfrac{W_1}{W_2}$

    B. $\dfrac{V_2}{V_1} = \dfrac{W_1}{W_2}$

    C. $\dfrac{V_1}{V_2} = \dfrac{W_2}{W_1}$

    D. $\left(\dfrac{V_1}{V_2}\right)^2 = \left(\dfrac{W_1}{W_2}\right)^3$

78. A hysteresis transformer loss can be characterized by the following:

    A. Swirling of currents caused by fleck magnetic fields
    B. The resistive force of the copper wire within a magnet
    C. The true resistance of the direct current
    D. The rapidly changing magnetic domain due to alternating current

79. According to the law of conservation of energy, voltage and amperage have which type of relationship?

    A. A square relationship
    B. Directly proportional to one another
    C. Inversely proportional to each other
    D. The square root of the voltage multiplied by the amperage

80. Which type of transformer works on the principle of electromagnetic self-induction?

    A. Rheostat
    B. Choke coil

C. Autotransformer
D. Saturable reactor

For the following five questions, select the proper location within the x-ray circuit from this list:

    A. Primary, high voltage
    B. Primary, low voltage
    C. Secondary, high voltage
    D. Filament circuit

81. The line voltage compensator is located:

82. The solid state diodes are located:

83. The step-down transformer is located:

84. The exposure timer is located:

85. The autotransformer is located:

86. Which of the following components work on electromagnetic mutual induction?

    A. Step-up transformer
    B. Solid state diodes
    C. Autotransformer
    D. Electromagnetic timer

87. The step-up transformer is located in the x-ray circuit between which two components?

    A. Ground wire and rectifiers
    B. Rectifiers and x-ray tube
    C. Choke coil and rectifiers
    D. Autotransformer and milliammeter

88. The type of transformer that is utilized in the filament circuit is:

    A. Step-up transformer
    B. Step-down transformer
    C. Autotransformer
    D. Saturable reactor

89. The function of the autotransformer is to:

    A. Regulate the voltage of the incoming line voltage
    B. Select the appropriate kilovoltage
    C. Select a predetermined amount of kilovoltage
    D. Automatically change AC to pulsating DC

90. Which of the following radiographic exposure timers are accurate to times as low as 1 ms?

A. Synchronous timer
B. Electronic impulse timer
C. Mechanical timer
D. Synchronous electronic timer

91. Which of the following components serves as a safety device that greatly reduces the possibility of electrification:

    A. Step-down transformer
    B. Electronic impulse timer
    C. Ground wire
    D. Rheostat

92. What is the main purpose of the x-ray tube and where in the circuit is it located?

    A. To convert x-ray energy to electrical energy—primary, high voltage
    B. To convert and conceal radioactivity of electrons—primary, high voltage
    C. To convert electrical energy to x-ray energy—primary, low voltage
    D. To convert electrical energy to x-ray energy—primary, high voltage

93. The purpose of the valve tube rectifiers is to convert:

    A. Alternating DC into pulsating DC
    B. AC into DC
    C. AC into pulsating AC
    D. AC into pulsating DC

94. Calculate the number of rectifiers necessary for a 3-phase, 12-pulse unit to be fully rectified:

    A. Four
    B. Six
    C. Eight
    D. Twelve

95. In comparison with a single-phase, fully rectified system, a 3-phase, 12-pulse machine is how much more efficient?

    A. 1.53 times more efficient
    B. 1.35 times more efficient
    C. 1.14 times more efficient
    D. 1.41 times more efficient

96. The type of vision that is controlled by cone cells and is responsible for visual acuity and contrast perception is:

    A. Photophobic

B. Photopic
C. Scotopic
D. Photoscopic

97. What is the range of milliamperage used by a modern image intensification unit?

    A. 5–50 mA
    B. 0.5–50 mA
    C. 0.5–5 mA
    D. 0.05–0.5 mA

98. In a portable image intensifier unit such as a C-arm, the source-to-skin distance cannot be less than:

    A. 12″
    B. 15″
    C. 15 cm
    D. 12 meters

99. In the image intensification tube, the anode serves to:

    A. Provide a target of the electrons
    B. Focus the electrons into a stream
    C. Accelerate the electrons across the tube
    D. Invert the electrons to allow them to travel faster

100. What component in the image intensification system allows images to be magnified?

    A. Multifilament
    B. Anode's heel
    C. Electrostatic lenses
    D. Electron gun

101. How does the image intensification system make an image larger or magnified?

    A. By increasing the positive charge to the anode's heel
    B. By decreasing the positive charge to the filament
    C. By moving the convergence of the electrons farther from the anode's surface
    D. By decreasing the charge of the electrostatic lenses

102. Which type of the image intensification viewing system is considered to be the most modern, allowing many people to view at the same time?

    A. Optical mirror system

B. Movie screen
C. Cine screen coupled with an optical illusion
D. Video system coupled with a CRT

103. One of the components within a video system is a video tube. What function does the cathode have within the video tube?

    A. Directs a stream of electrons toward the video tube's anode
    B. Provides a supply of electrons through a process called thermionic emission
    C. Provides a method of converting visible light into a video signal
    D. More than one but not all of the above

104. The steering coils or focusing coils that are used in conjunction with the video tube are located:

    A. Inside the video tube
    B. Outside the video tube
    C. Next to the anode
    D. Next to the signal plate

105. The resolution of the video signal is directly proportional to:

    A. The size of the photoconductive globules
    B. The size and strength of the electron stream
    C. The density of the photoconductive material
    D. The gas that fills the video tube (antimony trisulfide or lead oxide)

106. Which of the following recording systems requires an increase in patient exposure?

    1. Cine recording system
    2. Video recording system
    3. Cassette recording system
    4. Videodisc recording system

    A. 1 and 2
    B. 1 and 3
    C. 2 and 4
    D. 1, 2, and 3

107. The total brightness gain for an image intensification system is directly dependent upon:

    A. Minification and flux gain
    B. Magnification and flux gain
    C. Brightness gain and flux gain
    D. Minification gain and brightness gain

108. What causes magnification gain?

    A. A dual focused tube
    B. A grid bias tube
    C. The diameter of the input screen divided by the diameter of the output screen
    D. The overall speed of the electrons striking the input screen

109. Which component of an image intensification system is responsible for automatically adjusting the technique to maintain an optimal density?

    A. Automatic brightness control
    B. Phototimer density control
    C. Automatic brightness stabilization
    D. More than one, but not all of the above

110. In respect to resolution, the weakest link in an image intensification system is/are:

    A. The video components
    B. The operator
    C. The quality of the input screen
    D. The area of convergence of the electrons

111. If an insufficient quantity of radiation is detected by the image intensification tube, the resultant image will suffer from a condition called:

    A. A high amount of diagnostic quality
    B. Chemical fog, caused by underexposure
    C. Complete overexposure
    D. Quantum mottle, a patchy exposure of the film

112. A portable unit that needs to be plugged into a wall outlet and charged before each exposure is referred to as:

    A. An image intensification unit
    B. A DC unit
    C. A capacitor discharge unit
    D. A high-frequency unit

113. The force that pushes electrons from the cathode to the anode during the times of exposure may be referred to as:

    A. Kilovoltage peak

B. Milliamperage

C. Milliampere-seconds

D. Kilovoltage minor

114. The kVp accuracy may be evaluated with a digital dosimeter. What is an acceptable range for these readings?

A. +/−5% of the selected kVp

B. +/−10% of the selected kVp

C. +/−5 kVp of the selected kVp

D. +/−3 kVp of the selected kVp

115. According to the NCRP, what is the required amount of total filtration for an x-ray generator operating at 93 kVp?

A. 4.5 mm/Al equivalent total filtration

B. 3.0 mm/Al equivalent total filtration

C. 2.0 mm/Al equivalent total filtration

D. 2.5 mm/Al equivalent total filtration

116. The x-ray tube current is defined as:

A. The quantity of electrons available at the time of the exposure

B. The amount of time electrons move across the tube

C. The amount of the charge at the filament, held in the focusing cup

D. The force that is applied at the time of the exposure

117. Which of the following quality assurance tests evaluates the generator's ability to produce consistent linearity?

A. mR/mAs

B. mA linearity

C. mA reproducibility

D. mA sphygmomanometer

118. Which of the following may be used to evaluate a focal spot for size and/or resolution?

A. Line pair test

B. Star test pattern

C. Pinhole camera

D. All of the above

119. The person designated as the radiation safety officer is responsible for evaluating the accuracy of the x-ray generator for mA linearity and mA reproducibility. How often should mA reproducibility be evaluated?

A. Monthly

B. Quarterly

C. Annually

D. Biannually

120. Which quality assurance test ensures that the x-ray production is terminated at the appropriate time?

A. Digital dosimeter

B. Spinning top test

C. Sensitometer

D. Wisconsin cassette

121. When the AEC ionization chambers reach the preset quantity of radiation, which component terminates the exposure?

A. The timer circuit

B. Step-up transformer

C. Rectifiers

D. mA filament circuit

122. A single-phase, fully rectified generator operating on 60-hertz current is used to make a radiographic exposure with 1/10 sec time set on the control panel. How many dots should be on the resultant radiograph if evaluated with a spinning top test?

A. 10 dots

B. 8 dots

C. 12 dots

D. 14 dots

123. The timer circuit should be evaluated as part of a complete performance improvement program. How often should the timer circuit be evaluated?

A. Monthly

B. Quarterly

C. Semiannually

D. Annually

124. While evaluating a single-phase generator at 1/20 sec, the resulting radiograph yields three dots. What is the most likely cause of this problem?

A. Less than four rectifiers working

B. Timer short

C. A bad photo-cell

D. Rotor did not rotate fast enough

125. Light field to radiation field can be evaluated with:

    A. Synchronous test
    B. A framing square
    C. Dosimeter
    D. Nine lead markers

126. What is the acceptable range for light to radiation field variation?

    A. $+/-2\%$ SOD
    B. $+/-2\%$ SID
    C. $+/-5\%$ SID
    D. $+/-5\%$ SOD

127. What do the initials PBL mean?

    A. Primary beam limitation
    B. Primary blockage limitation
    C. Positive beam limitation
    D. Positive blockage limitation

128. As part of a total performance improvement program, the central ray alignment should be evaluated _____ and should not vary more than _____ .

    A. Annually; $+/-1\%$ SID
    B. Annually; $+/-2\%$ SID
    C. Semiannually; 1% of the light field
    D. Annually; 1% of the light field

129. Which of the following is not a characteristic of a cassette?

    1. Radiolucent
    2. Lightproof
    3. Converts x-rays into visible light
    4. Chemically inert

    A. 1, 3, and 4
    B. 1, 2, and 3
    C. 3 only
    D. 1, 2, and 4

130. The reflective layer of the intensifying screen is primarily used for:

    A. Absorbing scatter radiation
    B. Directing light toward the radiographic film
    C. Allowing light photons to pass through to expose the radiographic film
    D. Directing the light photons toward the inside of the cassette, away from the film

131. Which of the following are important factors when considering a phosphor material?

    1. Atomic number
    2. Conversion efficiency
    3. Spectral emission
    4. Luminescence

    A. 1 and 2
    B. 1, 3, and 4
    C. 1, 2, and 4
    D. 1, 2, 3, and 4

132. What is the difference between phosphorescence and fluorescence?

    A. Fluorescence does not cease to illuminate after the exposure has ended.
    B. Phosphorescence ceases to illuminate after the exposure has ended.
    C. Fluorescence ceases to illuminate after the exposure has ended.
    D. Phosphorescence does not illuminate as intensely as fluorescence.

133. Which of the following information should be permanently recorded on the radiograph?

    A. Patient name, date, doctor's name, medical record number
    B. Date, patient name, examination, date of birth, institution name
    C. Date of birth, medical record number, institution symbol, examination
    D. Patient name, medical record number, date of birth, institution name, current date and time

134. Which of the following is critical to know when using a grid cassette?

    A. Grid ratio
    B. Focal spot
    C. Focal range
    D. More than one, but not all of the above

135. Cassettes must be ridged and strong enough to:

    A. Support 32 pounds
    B. Support an average body part
    C. Support a 350-pound patient
    D. Support the portable machine

136. If an exposure is made and the tube grid alignment is not at a 90° angle, what will the resulting radiograph demonstrate?

    A. Grid bias
    B. Overexposure
    C. Grid cut-off
    D. The grid-tube alignment does not matter.

137. Which of the following types of artifacts would be caused by a cassette that does not provide a completely lightproof environment for the radiographic film?

    A. Chemical light leak
    B. Asymmetric light field
    C. Light leak
    D. Poor film-screen contact

138. Cleaning cassettes with a cleaner not approved by the manufacturer for that purpose may lead to:

    A. Residue on the screen
    B. Changing the integrity of the screen
    C. Scratching the screen
    D. All of the above

139. Film-screen contact should be evaluated periodically as part of a total quality control program. How often should the radiation safety officer perform a film-screen contact test?

    A. Quarterly
    B. Semiannually
    C. Biannually
    D. Annually

140. Which of the following best describes radiographic screen lag?

    A. The front of the intensification screen is slower than the back.
    B. A screen speed that is below 200
    C. A film-screen combination with varying speeds
    D. A screen that continues to emit light after the exposure has ceased

141. Why is it important to check shielding material such as aprons with an image intensification unit?

    A. To ensure the integrity of the garments
    B. To ensure that the image intensification unit is working

    C. To evaluate the density of the lead used to construct the garments
    D. To evaluate the thickness of the lead used to construct the aprons and contact shields

142. Constant misuse of protective garments may lead to:

    A. Cracking of the lead lining
    B. No change in the garments
    C. Cracking of older garments
    D. Increased flexibility

143. Once a garment is identified to have a crack, it should be:

    A. Used only for portable examination
    B. Discarded or repaired
    C. Left in someone else's room
    D. Mixed in with the other garments so nobody knows which one is cracked

144. How often should the radiation safety officer evaluate protective garments?

    A. Monthly
    B. Semiannually
    C. Annually
    D. Biannually

145. The proper storage of a protective lead apron is to:

    A. Hang it on the appropriate wall holder.
    B. Fold neatly and place on the counter.
    C. Leave it crumpled up on the radiographic table.
    D. Throw it against the wall.

146. The acceptable limit for a focal spot of 0.8 to 1.5 mm is:

    A. Up to 20% larger
    B. Up to 30% larger
    C. Up to 40% larger
    D. Up to 50% larger

147. Which of the following should be evaluated during a yearly visual examination of the radiographic rooms?

    1. High voltage cables
    2. Interlock system
    3. Manual/PBL collimation
    4. Deadlock switches

A. 1 and 2
B. 2 and 4
C. 2, 3, and 4
D. 1, 2, and 4

148. The image intensification tube is constructed of Pyrex glass to enable the tube to:

    A. Withstand a large amount of heat without cracking
    B. Cost less than a crystal tube
    C. Become flexible as the tube cools
    D. Allow the tube to hold a strong negative charge

149. Where in the x-ray circuit is the primary side of the step-down transformer located?

    A. Primary side—low voltage

B. Filament circuit
C. Secondary side—low voltage
D. Secondary side—high voltage

150. Between which of the following components is the prereading KV meter located?

    1. Rectifiers
    2. Autotransformer
    3. Saturable reactor
    4. Timer

    A. 2 and 4
    B. 1 and 3
    C. 1 and 4
    D. 2 and 4

Answers appear at the end of the book.

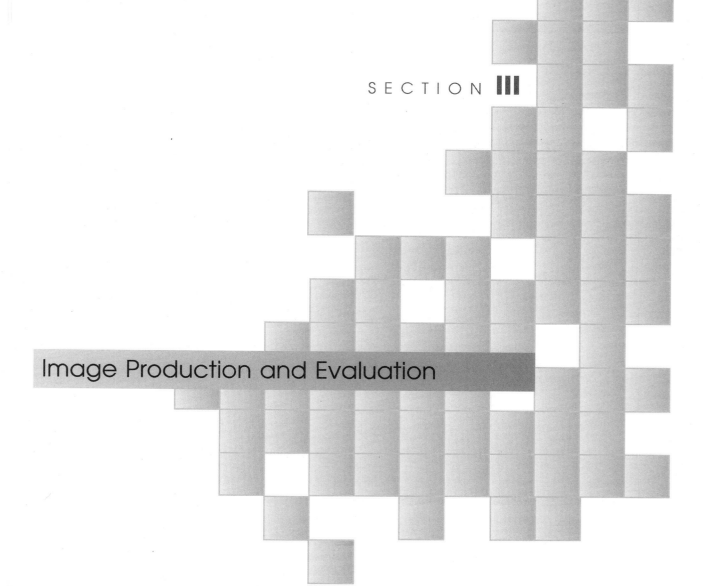

Image Production and Evaluation

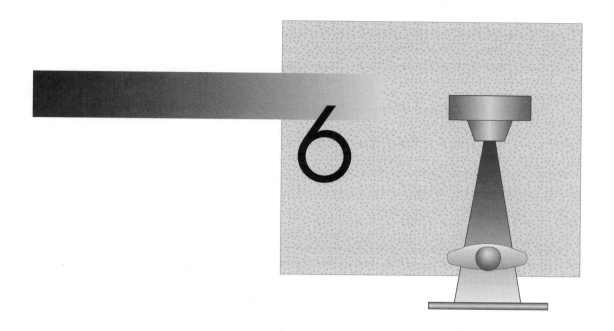

SELECTION OF TECHNICAL FACTORS

Density
 mAs
 Kilovoltage Peak
 Distance
 Film-Screen Combinations
 Grids
 Filtration
 Beam Restriction
 Anatomical and Pathologic Factors
 Anode Heel Effect

Contrast
 Kilovoltage Peak
 Beam Restriction
 Grids
 Filtration
 Anatomical and Pathologic Factors

Recorded Detail
 Object-to-Image Distance
 Source-to-Image Distance
 Focal Spot Size
 Film-Screen Combinations
 Motion

Distortion
 Size
 Shape

Film, Screen, and Grid Selection
 Film Characteristics
 Film-Screen Combinations
 Conversion Factors for Grids

Technique Charts
 Caliper Measurement
 Fixed Versus Variable kVp
 Anatomical Considerations
 Special Considerations (Casts,
  Pathology, Pediatrics, Contrast
  Media)
 Automatic Exposure Control

**Manual Versus Automatic
Exposure Control**
 Effects of Changing Exposure
  Factors on Radiographic Quality
 Selection of Ionization Chamber or
  Photocell
 Alignment of Part to Ionization
  Chamber or Photocell

DENSITY

Density is defined as a radiograph's blackness. It is measured by a densitometer. A densitometer measures the amount of light transmission through the darkened areas of the radiograph. The densities are expressed as a logarithm of the exposure used to make the density. The unit used to express the logarithms is optical density, or OD. The range of OD can vary greatly but for the diagnostic range is not less than 0.25 and not more than 3.0. It makes up the straight line portion of the H&D (Hurter and Driffield) curve. Many factors influence radiographic density, but the milliampere per-second (mAs) factor is primary in controlling density (Table 6–1).

mAs

mAs is the product of milliamperage (mA) and exposure time and is the primary controlling factor of density. Increasing the mAs value increases the quantity or number of photons produced, therefore a greater number of photons will be available to expose the radiographic film, causing it to be darker. Conversely, if the mAs value is decreased, fewer photons will be produced, resulting in a radiograph that will be lighter because fewer photons are available to expose the radiographic film either directly or via screen phosphor conversion. Changing the mAs value will change the overall tube current, but the penetrating ability of the beam remains the same. Therefore, the number of photons will increase or decrease but the penetrating ability and frequency of the photons remain the same. To see a visible difference on the radiograph, the mAs value must vary 30% or more from the original value.

Kilovoltage Peak (kVp)

The kVp can greatly influence the density on a radiograph although it is not considered a controlling factor. The penetrating ability of the photons is determined by the kVp; therefore, kVp controls the overall beam quality rather than beam quantity. With an increase in kVp, photons have an increased amount of energy demonstrated by shorter wavelength and increase of frequency and undergo less attenuation as they pass through the anatomy. This leads to an increased amount of photons reaching the radiographic film. Increasing the penetrating ability of the primary beam also increases the scatter and secondary radiation, which also contributes to an increase in density.

Distance

The source-to-image distance (SID) also influences the radiographic density. This is due partly to attenuation and scatter but mainly to the primary beam's divergence (Fig. 6–1). As the distance increases, the same number of photons is distributed over a larger area; therefore, the intensity decreases as the distance from the source increases. Distance and mAs have a direct relationship as described by the mAs-Distance formula. Since distance influences the quantity of photons available at a specific point from the source, it influences the amount of density of the resulting radiograph. The relationship is based upon the inverse square law:

$$\frac{mAs_1}{mAs_2} = \frac{(D_1)^2}{(D_2)^2}$$

Example:
A radiograph with optimal density was made using 100 mAs and a 40″ source-to-image distance. To maintain the radiographic density, what would the new mAs be if the exposure were made at 72″?

$$\frac{100}{X} = \frac{(40)^2}{(72)^2} \qquad \frac{100}{X} = \frac{1600}{5184}$$

$$X = 321.5 \text{ mAs (322 mAs)}$$

Film-Screen Combinations

Film-screen combinations will influence the density on the finished radiograph by the speed at

Table 6–1 ■ **DENSITY**		
Factors	**Change**	**Results in Density**
mAs	Increase Decrease	More density Less density
kVp	Increase Decrease	More density Less density
Distance	Increase Decrease	Less density More density
Film-screen combinations	Faster Slower	More density Less density
Filtration	Increase Decrease	Less density More density
Beam restriction	Smaller field size Larger field size	Less density More density
Pathology	Additive Destructive	Less density More density
Grids	Without a grid With a grid	More density Less density
Anode heel effect	More Less	No change

$$\frac{30 \text{ mAs}}{X \text{ mAs}} = \frac{600 \text{ RS}}{200 \text{ RS}}$$

$$X = 10 \text{ mAs}$$

Grids

Grids are devices that absorb unwanted scatter and secondary radiation minimize the unwanted energy from exposing the radiograph. Grids also absorb some primary radiation. The efficiency of the grid determines what quantity of radiation will be absorbed from the primary beam. Grid efficiency is measured by grid ratio: 8:1, 10:1, 12:1; the higher the grid ratio, the more efficient the grid. The technical adjustment that is made to compensate for grids is an adjustment in the mAs value. mAs and grid efficiency are directly proportional. How to determine grid ratio will be discussed later in this chapter.

$$\frac{\text{mAs}_1}{\text{mAs}_2} = \frac{\text{GCF}_1}{\text{GCF}_2}$$

GCF = grid conversion factors

Example:
A radiograph made with a 5:1 grid using 74 kVp at 25 mAs demonstrates good radiographic quality. The same image is going to be made with a 10:1 grid. With all other factors remaining the same, what technical factors would produce a similar radiograph? For grid conversion factors, see Table 6–7.

$$\frac{25}{X} = \frac{2}{3.5}$$

$$X = 43.75 \ (44 \text{ mAs})$$

Filtration

As the filtration increases, the density will decrease. Filtration will absorb low-energy photons from the primary beam, therefore reducing the overall radiographic density. The amount of density reduction depends upon the type of filter and the use of the filter. In certain cases an increase in technique (mAs) is not necessary to produce a quality radiograph. When a wedge filter is used in an AP projection of the foot or thoracic spine, the lower-energy photons that are filtered out are unwanted, and the use of the filter equalizes the density on the radiograph, allowing the anatomy of the upper thoracic spine or the distal phalanges to be visualized without excessive density.

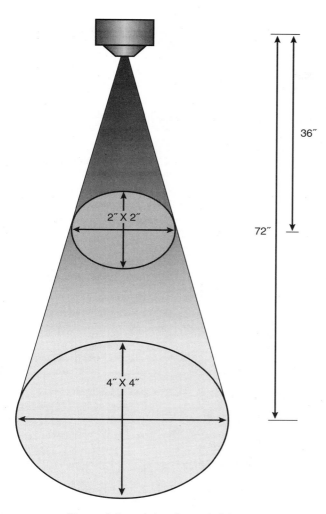

Figure 6-1 ■ Intensity and distance.

which this combination is able to respond to radiation. The faster the response time, the more density will be recorded on the radiographic film. This combination is measured by relative speed, RS. As the RS value increases, the sensitivity to radiation also increases in direct proportion. Therefore, the mAs value can be reduced to maintain the density on the radiograph. RS values are determined by the manufacturer and are usually standard from one to another. RS and mAs are inversely proportional:

$$\frac{\text{mAs}_1}{\text{mAs}_2} = \frac{\text{RS}_2}{\text{RS}_1}$$

Example:
A radiograph was made with a 200 RS system using 30 mAs. In a second radiograph, if the density was to remain the same as the first but a 600 RS system was used, what is the new mAs value for this exposure?

Beam Restriction

By restricting the primary beam, the radiation that is able to reach the film is reduced, therefore reducing the overall density of the resultant radiograph. A beam-restrictive device will decrease the overall quantity of photons that will reach the radiographic film. Beam restriction also absorbs the off-focus radiation exiting from the tube and exposing the radiograph. The amount of beam restriction can greatly affect the resultant radiograph, as can be seen in Table 6–2.

Anatomical and Pathologic Factors

These factors may change the amount of radiation that will reach the radiographic film. Bone will have a more absorptive quality than muscle or fat, because bone has a higher atomic number. But a forearm technique would be far less than a technique for an abdomen, because of the part thickness. The thicker the anatomy being radiographed, the greater the attenuation by the anatomy. If the anatomy is being adequately penetrated by the kVp, then the factor to adjust to achieve optimal density is the mAs factor. This is true for pathologic conditions as well.

Pathologic conditions can be divided into two categories: *(1) an added pathologic condition that would increase attenuation and decrease radiographic density; and (2) a destructive pathologic process that decreases attenuation and increases radiographic density.* To depict certain pathologic conditions accurately, an increase in mAs may not be enough. Under certain circumstances an adjustment in mAs or kVp, or a combination of both, may be needed to best demonstrate the anatomy along with the pathologic condition. The degree the disease has progressed also affects the radiographic density. An example is a patient with advanced COPD (chronic obstructive pulmonary disease) such as emphysema, who would require a much lower technique than a patient with asthma. When the anatomy or pathologic condition is adequately penetrated by kVp, the mAs factor is the only technical factor that would be altered to establish an optimal density on the radiograph (Table 6–3).

Table 6–2 ■ BEAM RESTRICTION

Original Film Size	New Film Size	Conversion Factor
14 × 17	10 × 12	30–35% increase in mAs
14 × 17	8 × 10	45–50% increase in mAs
14 × 17	5 × 7	55–60% increase in mAs

Table 6–3 ■ DENSITY AND CONTRAST IN PATHOLOGIC CONDITIONS

Additive	Destructive
Decrease Density and Increase Contrast	*Increase Density and Decrease Contrast*
Acromegaly	Aseptic necrosis
Kyphosis	Atrophy
Hydrocephalus	Blastomycosis
Chronic osteomyelitis	Active osteomyelitis
Osteochondroma	Ewing's sarcoma
Paget's disease	Malignancy
Proliferative arthritis	Fibrosarcoma
Sclerosis	Giant cell sarcoma
Calcified tuberculosis	Gout
Atelectasis	Degenerative arthritis
Bronchiectasis	Hemangioma
Encapsulated abscess	Active tuberculosis
Hydropneumothorax	Hodgkin's disease
Black lung	Osteolytic metastases
Ascites	Multiple myeloma
Cirrhosis	Fibrosis
Edema	Radiation necrosis
Congestive heart failure	Early lung abscess
Cardiomegaly	Pneumothorax
Empyema	Emaciation of soft tissue
Pleural effusions	Hyperparathyroidism
Pneumonia	Bowel obstruction
Pneumonectomy	Emphysema
Pulmonary edema	Osteomalacia
Calcified stones	Osteoporosis

Anode Heel Effect

Radiation produced at the anode is not monoenergetic from the cathode end of the tube to the anode end of the tube. This is due to the angle of the anode. As the electrons strike the target of the anode, they produce photons that travel down toward the tube port. The photons that travel toward the cathode end of the tube pass through less target material, therefore the photons produced in that direction will have a higher energy level. This happens because some of the energy traveling toward the anode end of the tube is absorbed by the target material.

A major factor in the anode heel effect is the *angle of the anode.* As the anode angle increases, the anode heel effect decreases (Fig. 6–2). *(The A refers to the cathode side, the B to the anode.)* Other factors affecting the anode heel effect apparent on the radiograph are *beam restriction* and *source-to-image distance (SID).* An increase in beam restriction will reduce the amount of anode heel effect apparent on the resultant radiograph (Fig. 6–3). With beam restriction, less of the lateral edges of the beam produced at the target is used in the primary beam exiting from the tube; therefore, the energy difference between the cathode side of the tube and the anode side of the tube is minimized. Also, with a longer

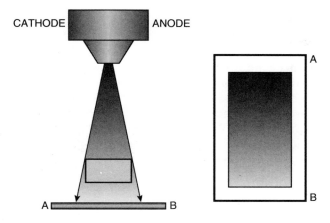

Figure 6-2 ■ Anode heel effect.

SID anode heel effect is reduced, because the primary beam has more distance to equalize the energy differences between the anode and cathode (Fig. 6–4). This occurs because the cathode end of the primary beam will lose more low-energy photons because it has more photons overall. Another result of primary beam divergence is that less of the outer edges of the field will be used to produce the radiographic image.

Anode heel effect does not always degrade the radiographic image; it can be used to the radiographer's advantage. Placing the cathode end of the radiographic tube over the thicker end of the anatomy being radiographed helps overcome the anatomical difference and allows for consistent radiographic density. Common uses of the anode heel effect:

Body Part	*Cathode End of Tube*
AP thoracic	— Lower thoracic
Lateral thoracic	— Lower thoracic
Femur	— Proximal femur
Humerus	— Proximal humerus

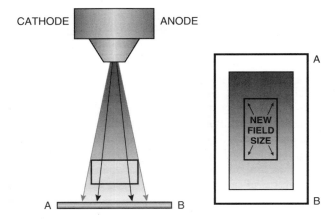

Figure 6-3 ■ Anode heel effect and beam restriction.

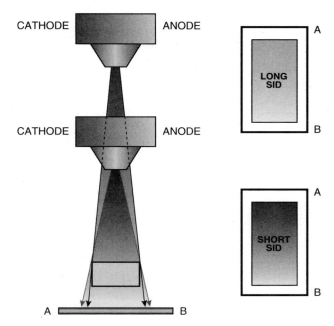

Figure 6-4 ■ Anode heel effect and source-to-image distance

CONTRAST

Contrast is the number of visible densities on the finished radiograph. A radiograph with many densities is considered low contrast, or it is said to provide a long scale of contrast. A long scale of contrast is usually produced with a high kVp technique. A radiograph with few widely varying densities is considered high or short scale contrast, and is usually produced with a low kVp.

A penetrometer or step wedge is used in evaluation of the radiographic contrast. A penetrometer consists of a radiation-absorbing range of densities arranged in a wedge. A radiograph of the penetrometer is taken, and the resultant densities are measured. This reveals the contrast available for the technical factors used (kVp, film-screen combinations, and so on).

The amount of contrast apparent on a radiograph is affected by many factors, which will be discussed later in this section. The controlling factor of radiographic contrast is kVp (Table 6–4).

Kilovoltage Peak

The kVp determines the quality or penetrating ability of the primary beam. Contrast depends directly upon the kVp used to produce the radiograph. Varying densities of adjacent structures become apparent by differential attenuation of photons passing through these structures. Correctly selected kVp can optimize the different densities of these structures, allowing them to

Table 6-4 ■ **CONTRAST**		
Factors	**Change**	**Result in Contrast**
kVp	Increase	Decrease
	Decrease	Increase
Beam restriction	Increase	Increase
	Decrease	Decrease
Grids	Without a grid	Decrease
	With a grid	Increase
Filtration	Increase	Increase
	Decrease	Decrease
Pathology	Additive	Increase
	Destructive	Decrease

have a different amount of attenuation resulting in a different radiographic density. By adjusting the kVp, the contrast can be changed while maintaining the radiographic density. This is achieved by using the kVp 15% rule, which states that if the kVp is increased by 15%, the mAs is reduced by 50%. If the kVp is decreased by 15%, the mAs value is increased by a factor of 2. Using the kVp 15% rule will result in a similar radiographic density, with a significant change in radiographic contrast.

Beam Restriction

Restricting the primary beam allows less off-focus radiation and scatter to reach the radiographic film. Although off-focus radiation will be produced in all directions, an increase in beam restriction reduces the amount of off-focus radiation that is allowed to exit from the tube port and contribute to the image. By reduction of scatter and secondary radiation the radiographic contrast will increase, creating a shorter scale of contrast. This does not increase the beam energy or quality but simply allows less radiation interaction with the patient or other matter. Beam restriction will actually reduce the amount of scatter produced.

Grids

A grid reduces the amount of radiation that is allowed to reach the film. As the primary radiation exits from the tube and interacts with the patient, scatter radiation is produced. The scatter radiation will not contribute to the diagnostic image but will degrade it and decrease contrast. A grid placed between the patient and the film will not reduce the amount of scatter produced but will reduce the amount of scatter radiation allowed to reach the film. A grid increases the radiographic contrast by absorbing scatter, re-

sulting in less fog or unwanted density. As with beam restriction, grids do not change beam quality or average beam energy; they remove unwanted photons that would expose the radiographic image. When grids are used, technical factors must be increased to compensate for the absorption, resulting in an increased patient exposure dose. These compensations are usually made with the mAs factor.

Filtration

Increasing the total filtration of the primary beam will increase radiographic contrast. As discussed previously, inherent filtration is a constant determined by the tube and tube housing construction. Added filtration is any attenuating material located between the tube part and the patient, absorbing low energy photons that do not contribute to the image. Without filtration, low-energy photons may become absorbed by the patient, increasing exposure dosage, especially to the skin, or they may scatter within the patient and contribute to increasing density or fogging on the finished radiograph. This degrades the radiograph and decreases radiographic contrast. Filtration is not used as a method of controlling or changing radiographic contrast, although filtration will influence contrast.

Anatomical and Pathologic Factors

Anatomical considerations pertaining to contrast are very similar to those pertaining to density. The type of tissue being imaged (subject contrast) determines the scale of contrast that can be recorded on the resulting radiograph. If the tissues being imaged have widely varying densities or atomic numbers, such as a forearm in which the tissues are bone, muscle, and fat, the scale of contrast will be shorter than when imaging an abdomen. The technique may influence to what degree the scale of contrast is shortened or lengthened, by kVp selection. But an anatomical area with only a few widely varying structures will always demonstrate a shorter scale of contrast.

The opposite is true for an anatomical area that has many structures with similar densities, such as the abdomen. This anatomical area has a wide variety of structures with similar attenuating capabilities, therefore when imaged, this area demonstrates a long scale of contrast. Adjustment of kVp will shorten or lengthen the degree of how long or short it will be but it will still demonstrate a long scale, if imaged to demonstrate all the anatomical structures.

Contrast as it pertains to pathologic conditions has an opposite effect as it relates to density. As stated earlier, pathologic conditions can be additive or destructive. An additive pathologic condition tends to shorten the scale of contrast. The increased anatomical density has a more absorptive quality and tends to equalize the density differences between the adjacent structures. Destructive pathologic conditions tend to lengthen the scale of contrast by decreased attenuation due to compromised tissue (see Fig. 6–3). Destructive pathology will then allow more scatter radiation to reach the image receptor.

RECORDED DETAIL

Since radiographs are two-dimensional and human anatomy is three-dimensional, there will always be some type of geometric unsharpness and overlap surrounding the image. This unsharpness is referred to as penumbra, whereas the well-defined geometric areas of sharpness are called umbra. Many factors influence the amount of recorded detail available on the finished radiograph. Recorded detail is measured in line pairs per millimeter. The more line pairs that are visible on the radiograph, the higher the resolution. One of the greatest obstacles regarding detail for the technologist to overcome is magnification. The greater the magnification of a structure, the less recorded detail. This is because the greater the magnification, the greater the amount of penumbra surrounding the structure being imaged (Table 6–5).

Object-to-Image Distance

OID describes the relationship of the anatomy to the image receptor. The shorter the distance between the anatomical part and the image receptor, the greater the recorded detail. By increasing the OID, the primary beam will pass through the structure of interest and continue to diverge before striking the image receptor. As the anatomy moves farther away from the image receptor, the magnification and penumbra increase while recorded detail decreases (Fig. 6–5).

Source-to-Image Distance

SID describes the distance between the radiation source and the image receptor. The more distance between the source and the image receptor, the more recorded detail on the radiograph. By increasing the SID, the portion of the primary beam that is used to create the image will be closer to the center of the beam. This becomes significant because that area of the primary beam will undergo less divergence, thus it will be traveling in a straighter line between the source and the image receptor. When this happens, the area of penumbra is greatly reduced, because there is less magnification (Fig. 6–6).

Focal Spot Size

The smaller the focal spot size, the more recorded detail on the radiograph. The actual focal spot size depends upon the filament size and the anode's angle. The focal track on the anode that is bombarded by the electron beam is termed the *actual focal spot*. When it strikes the anode's angle, the photons that travel off the anode become the effective focal spot (Fig. 6–7). The smaller the effective focal spot, the more detail will be recorded by the image receptor. The effective focal spot size is determined by the anode angle and the filament length. If the actual focal spot size is smaller, the primary beam will undergo less overall divergence. This will reduce the area of penumbra or geometric blurring that is created around the image, therefore increasing the recorded detail (Fig. 6–8). The formula for determining the amount of penumbra that will surround the image is

$$\text{FSS (focal spot size)} \times \frac{\text{OID}}{\text{SOD}} = \text{Penumbra}$$

When OID is object-image distance and SOD is source-object distance.

Example:
An AP projection of the abdomen was made to evaluate a renal mass located approximately 10 cm from the image receptor. The exposure was made using a focal spot size of 1.5 mm at an SID of 180 cm. How much penumbra will surround the renal mass?

Table 6–5 ■ **RECORDED DETAIL**		
Factors	Change	Result in Recorded Detail
OID	Increase Decrease	Decrease Increase
SID	Increase Decrease	Increase Decrease
Focal spot size	Larger Smaller	Decrease Increase
Film-screen combinations	Faster Slower	Decrease Increase
Motion	Increase Decrease	Decrease Increase

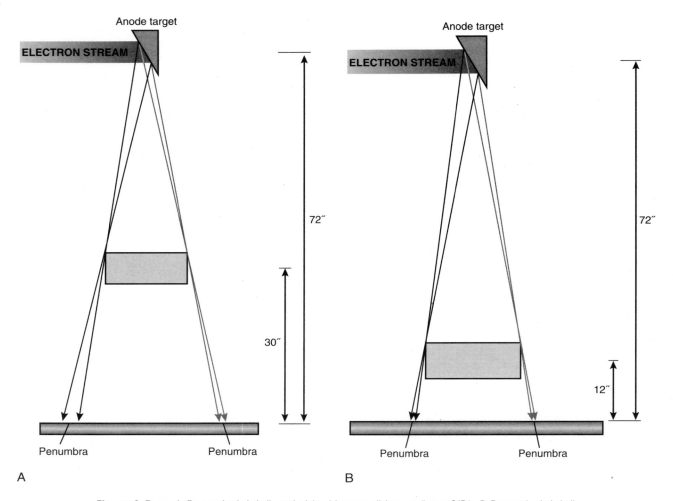

Figure 6-5 ■ *A*, Recorded detail and object image distance (long OID). *B*, Recorded detail and object image distance (short OID).

1. FSS = 1.5 mm
   OID = 10 cm
   SOD = (180 cm − 10 cm) = 170 cm

2. $1.5 \text{ mm} \times \dfrac{10 \text{ cm}}{170 \text{ cm}} = \text{penumbra}$

3. 1.5 mm × 0.0556 = penumbra
   0.834 mm = penumbra

Focal spot sizes for mammography and special procedures can be fractional focal spots that allow the image to be magnified without any loss in detail. Anode heating becomes a problem with small focal spot size because the electron beam is directed to a very small point on the anode.

Film-Screen Combinations

The way the image is recorded will greatly affect the amount of detail on the resultant image. The components of the standard imaging system are usually the film and intensifying screen. The resolving power of the film depends on the crystal size and the emulsion thickness. The smaller the crystal size, the more recorded detail on the film. Also, thinner emulsion layers are able to record more line pairs per millimeter, therefore the recorded detail will increase.

The intensifying screens also affect the resolving power of the imaging system. The smaller the phosphors and the thinner the phosphor layer, the more recorded detail on the resultant image.

Motion

This is the most influential factor concerning detail. If the patient is moving, the amount of detail is greatly reduced. Two types of motion will affect the recorded detail: voluntary and involuntary. Voluntary motion by the patient is actual physical movement and usually can be overcome by clear, concise instruction. The patient must be able to understand the instructions and be physically capable of following them. With clear in-

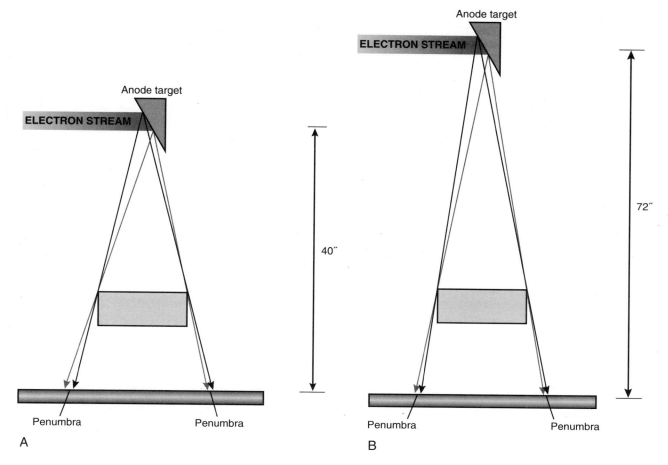

Figure 6-6 ■ *A,* Recorded detail and source-to-image distance (short SID). *B,* Recorded detail and source-to-image distance (long SID).

struction, short exposure time, and positioning aids for proper position and patient comfort, motion does not become a major problem.

Most often respiration motion needs to be suspended for many procedures. Most patients are able to suspend respiration, because respiration can be controlled voluntarily. Uncontrollable involuntary motions, such as cardiac motion and peristalsis of the abdomen, cannot be suspended. They can be minimized with very short exposure times. If the exposure time is less than the cycle of the motion, then the motion will not be recorded on the radiographic image.

Short exposure times are easily achieved with modern 3-phase or high-frequency generators but may be a problem with older, single-phase generators. When short exposure times cannot be utilized, as in fluoroscopic procedures, a medication like glucagon or Pro-Banthine can be given prior to the examination to slow down the actual motion of the structure, thus minimizing the recorded motion. Some agents, such as water-soluble contrast agents (oral Hypaque and Gastrographin), may increase peristaltic activity.

Not all motion results in a negative effect on the radiograph. Sometimes motion can be used beneficially to blur certain anatomy, allowing other anatomy to be visualized clearly. This is a very common imaging technique for the lateral thoracic spine or a transthoracic shoulder/humerus. This is commonly referred to as autotomography, that is, voluntary patient motion to blur anatomy purposely in order to visualize a specific anatomic area. Motion is also the basis for tomographic procedures. Tomography selects a particular area of interest and uses motion of the radiographic tube and film to blur all other structures.

DISTORTION

Distortion is a misrepresentation of the structures of interest by their magnification. Magnification distortion can distort the image two ways: size distortion or shape distortion (Table 6–6).

Size

Size distortion occurs because of the divergence of the primary beam. As the beam diverges, the

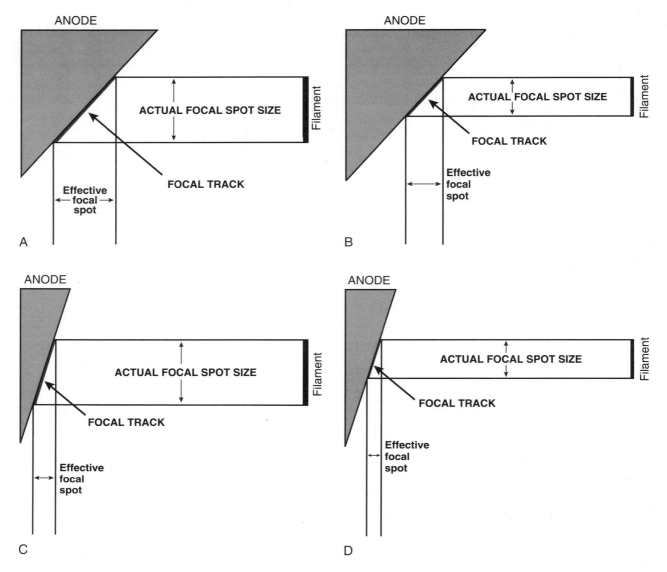

Figure 6-7 ■ *A,* Effective focal spot (large filament and large anode angle). *B,* Effective focal spot (small filament and large anode angle). *C,* Effective focal spot (large filament and small anode angle). *D,* Effective focal spot (small filament and small anode angle).

area that the radiation covers increases. The SID, position of the part, and position of the film will greatly affect the amount of magnification recorded on the radiographic image. The formula used to determine the amount of magnification is

$$\text{Magnification} = \frac{\text{SID}}{\text{SOD}}$$

Example 1:
If the SID is 72″ and the SOD is 12″, what is the magnification factor?

$$\text{M} = \frac{72}{12}$$

$$\text{M} = 6$$

Example 2:
What is the magnification factor for the following: A structure that is located 4″ from the image receptor and a SID of 40″?

1. Solve for SOD first:
   SID = 40″
   OID = 4″ − (object image distance)
   SOD = SID − OID
   SOD = 40″ − 4″
   SOD = 36″
2. Solve for magnification:

$$\text{M} = \frac{40\ (\text{SID})}{36\ (\text{SOD})}$$

Magnification factor = 1.11

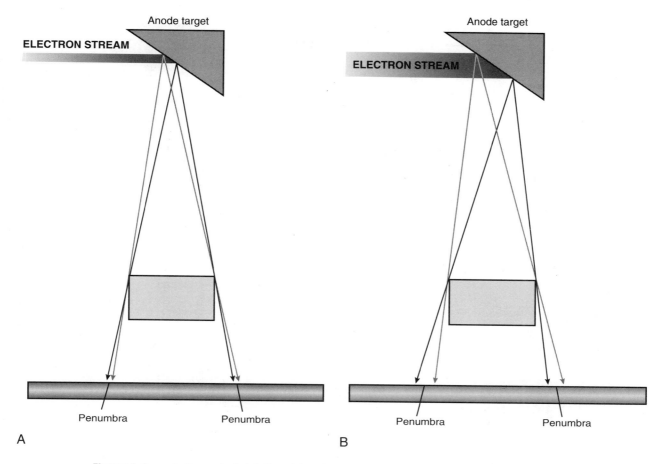

Figure 6–8 ■ *A,* Recorded detail and focal spot size (small focal spot). *B,* Recorded detail and focal spot size (large focal spot).

The amount of size distortion is controlled by the following two factors:

Source-to-Image Distance

The farther the source (tube) is from the image receptor, the less size distortion will be recorded on the radiograph. As the SID is reduced, the size distortion will increase; they are inversely proportional. If the SID is increased, the photons that are located in the center of the beam are used to produce the image. Because less divergence occurs with this portion of the beam, less magnification will occur (Fig. 6–9).

Object-to-Image Distance

The farther the object of interest from the image receptor, the more size distortion there will be. As the OID decreases, the size distortion will decrease; they are directly proportional. Magnification occurs because after the primary beam exits from the structure of interest, the distance between the patient and the film will allow the photons to continue to diverge before striking the image receptor (Fig. 6–10).

Shape

Shape distortion occurs when the structures imaged are magnified unequally, causing one area of the structure to be larger than another area.

Table 6–6 ■ **DISTORTION**		
Factors	**Change**	**Result in Distortion**
Size		
SID	Increase	Decrease
	Decrease	Increase
OID	Increase	Increase
	Decrease	Decrease
Shape		
Tube alignment	Proper alignment	Decrease
	Misalignment	Increase
Film alignment	Proper alignment	Decrease
	Misalignment	Increase
Anatomical part alignment	Proper alignment	Decrease
	Misalignment	Increase

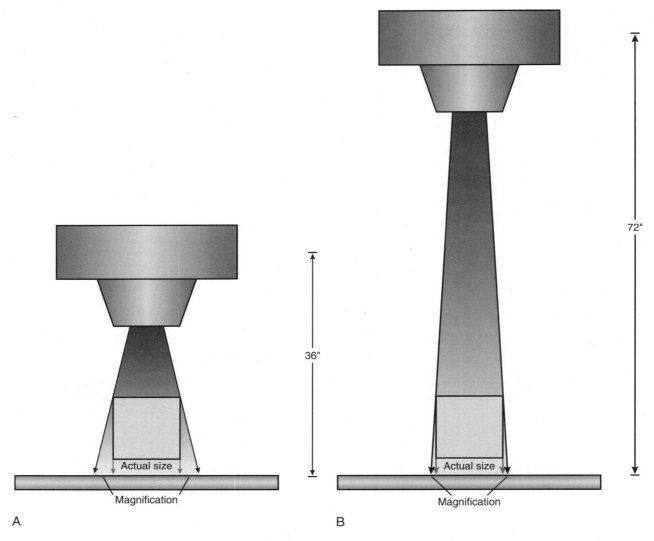

Figure 6-9 ■ *A*, Size distortion and source-to-image distance (short SID). *B*, Size distortion and source-to-image distance (long SID).

In certain situations shape distortion is desirable, by distorting one structure it may help visualize another structure, such as the AP axial skull for occipital bone review. This type of distortion is classified as *elongation,* or *foreshortening.* Elongation occurs when the tube or film is angled or misaligned. Foreshortening will occur only when the actual structure is misaligned. Three factors control shape distortion. In a perfect scenario, the primary beam will pass through the structure of interest perpendicularly, and the film alignment will be parallel to the structure of interest (Fig. 6–11).

Tube Alignment

Imaged structures depend greatly upon proper alignment of the tube to minimize the amount of distortion recorded. The radiation source (primary beam) should be aligned perpendicular to the anatomical structure of interest and the image receptor. When tube angulation is employed, either intentionally or unintentionally, elongation distortion of the anatomical structures will be recorded on the image (Fig. 6–12).

Film Alignment

Film alignment is critical in minimizing shape distortion. The radiographic film should be positioned parallel to the structure of interest and perpendicular to the radiation source (primary beam). If not, elongation distortion of the anatomical area will be recorded on the radiographic image (Fig. 6–13).

Anatomical Part Alignment

Anatomical part alignment is imperative if structures are to be radiographed accurately. Ideally,

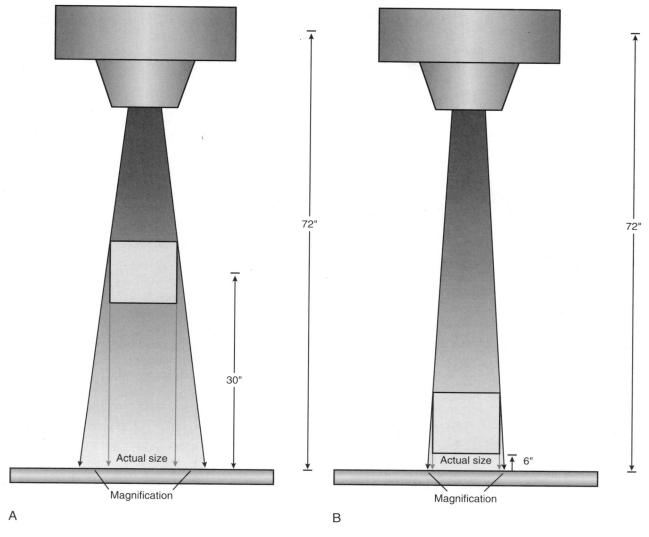

72"

30"

Actual size

Magnification

A

72"

Actual size

6"

Magnification

B

Figure 6-10 ■ *A,* Size distortion and object image distance (long OID). *B,* Size distortion and object image distance (short OID).

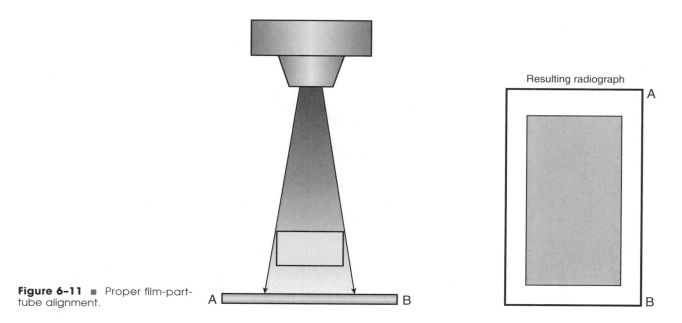

Figure 6-11 ■ Proper film-part-tube alignment.

A   B

Resulting radiograph

A

B

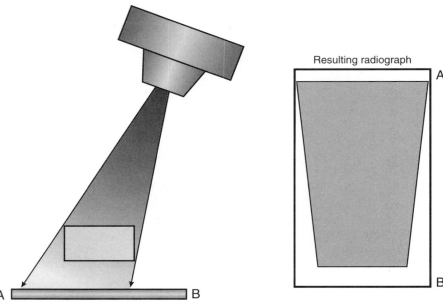

Resulting radiograph

Figure 6-12 ■ Improper tube alignment.

anatomy should be positioned perpendicular to the primary beam and parallel image receptor. Because of the design of the human body, it is nearly impossible to do this for all structures. Many radiographic examinations require tube angulation as a method of overcoming anatomical location within the human body. Tube angulation and patient position reduce shape distortion by aligning structures in a specific way to the primary beam path and the radiographic film. When anatomy is misaligned or improperly positioned, the resulting radiograph will demonstrate foreshortening distortion. It is important to remember that improper part position will produce foreshortening distortion only, never elongation distortion, whereas tube angulation or film misalignment results in elongation distortion only and never foreshortening distortion (Fig. 6–14).

FILM, SCREEN, AND GRID SELECTION

Film Characteristics

Film characteristics will determine how sensitive the film is to radiation and the type of radiation the film is sensitive to. Film can be sensitive to

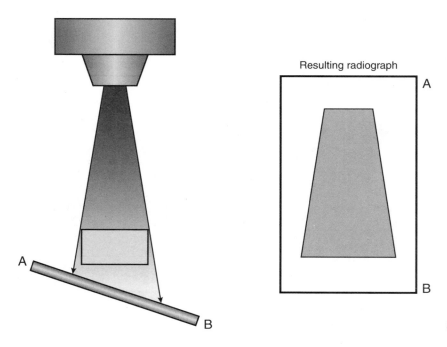

Resulting radiograph

Figure 6-13 ■ Improper film alignment.

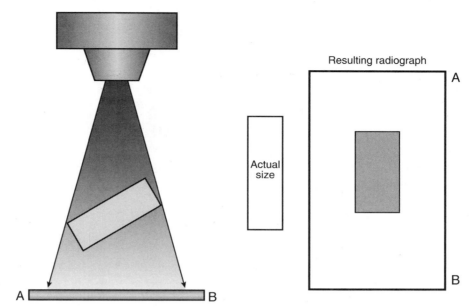

Figure 6-14 ■ Improper part alignment.

a specific type of light—blue light sensitive or green light sensitive. Film can be either *panchromatic*—sensitive to all visible light wavelengths, or *orthochromatic*—sensitive to all visible light wavelengths except red. Thus a red light can be used in the darkroom without changing the quality of the film.

Film Characteristic Curve

The *film's characteristic curve* is also known as the H&D (Hurter & Driffield) curve or D/Log E (Density/Log Exposure) curve (see Fig. A–6). A film's characteristic curve is the method by which film speed is measured, or how it responds to radiation. This factor determines the film contrast and exposure latitude (Fig. 6–15). A slower speed film will demonstrate low contrast and wide exposure latitude. A faster speed film will demonstrate high contrast with narrow exposure latitude. Exposure latitude and contrast are inversely proportional. Two factors that control latitude and speed are

- The *emulsion thickness* is directly proportional to the film speed. The thicker the emulsion layer, the faster the film's response to radiation. But it will result in a film that has longer scale (low) of contrast with a wide exposure latitude. Thinner emulsion layers will result in a film with decreased speed and a shorter (high) scale of contrast.
- The *crystal size* is also proportional to the film speed. The larger the crystals, the faster the film will respond to radiation,

resulting in a longer (low) scale of contrast radiograph with wide exposure latitude. But smaller crystals will result in a shorter (high) contrast radiograph with less exposure latitude.

Film Construction

How the film is constructed plays a major role in radiographic contrast and density (Fig. 6–16). Most radiographic films that are used for diagnostic procedures have an emulsion layer on either side of the base material (double emulsion). This means that both sides of the film are sensitive to radiation or light photons. This type of film is used with a cassette that has two intensifying screens, allowing the light emitted from each side of the screen to expose the radiographic film and produce the radiographic image. The overall radiographic exposure necessary to form the radiographic image is thereby reduced. The layers of the film are:

1. *Supercoat*—a protective coating that ensures the protection of the emulsion layer and makes the radiograph almost impossible to tear or rip.
2. *Emulsion*—composed of a gelatin containing photosensitive silver halide crystals. The gelatin is a clear, porous material that allows for both light and chemical transmission. It also aids in the suspension of the crystals in a lattice formation, holding them evenly over the surface of the film to ensure an even radiographic density.
3. *Adhesive*—a specialized glue that adheres the

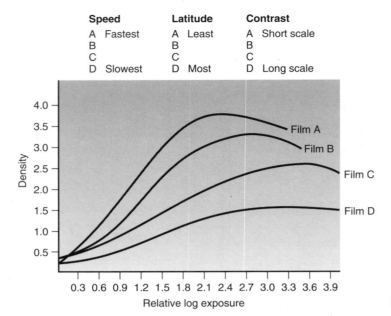

Speed	Latitude	Contrast
A Fastest	A Least	A Short scale
B	B	B
C	C	C
D Slowest	D Most	D Long scale

Figure 6-15 ■ Characteristic film curve.

emulsion to the base and prevents it from pulling apart during handling and processing.
4. *Base*—a polyester plastic gives the film its structure, strength, and form. Polyester is the material of choice because it allows for good light transmission and is dimensionally

stable (retaining its size and shape without shrinking or stretching, even postprocessing). This characteristic is sometimes referred to as the film's memory. The base material is tinted with a colored dye, usually blue, to minimize glare and allow the viewer greater visual acuity by preventing some light

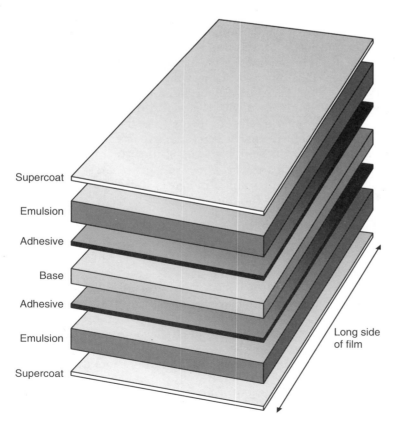

Figure 6-16 ■ Cross-section of radiographic film construction, enlarged to demonstrate detail.

transmission through the film. The dye also helps prevent cross-talk, a condition that occurs when light transmission from one intensifying screen exposes the emulsion layer on the opposite side of the film.

Relative Speed

This determines how quickly the intensifying screen responds to radiation. There are three ways to measure the screen speed:

1. Use of an intensification factor. This measures the actual x-ray–to–visible light photon conversion.
2. Use of a descriptive system in which par is a medium-speed screen, high-speed is faster than par, and fine-detail or high-resolution screens are slower than par.
3. The relative speed system. This is the most common system in use today. The screen manufacturers assign the par or medium screen an arbitrary number, usually 100. Faster screens are assigned a number higher than the par screen 100. These values range between 200 and 1200, depending upon the actual speed of the screen and are proportional to the par screen. High-resolution or-detail screens are assigned numerical values proportionally lower than the par screen of 100, ranging from 20 to 80.

Because the values are proportional, different speed screens can be used interchangeably. The formula used to maintain density between different screen speeds is

$$\frac{mAs_1}{mAs_2} = \frac{RS_2}{RS_1}$$

Example:
If 80 mAs and a 200 RS imaging system were used to produce an acceptable radiograph and the screen speed was changed to 400 RS, what mAs is needed to maintain the radiographic density?

$$\frac{80}{X} = \frac{400}{200} \qquad 80 \times 200 = 400\,(X)$$

$$400X = 16,000$$

$$X = 40$$

Single- Versus Double-Emulsion Films

Single-emulsion film has only one layer of emulsion on one side of the film, appearing as the dull side of the film in the darkroom. The emulsion side of the film is the only side capable of re-cording an image and must be placed toward the imaging device. Single emulsion film must be loaded toward the intensifying screen because it has a special layer of antihalation to prevent back scatter and minimize blurring of the image.

Double-emulsion film has two layers of emulsion, one on each side of the base material. These films are sometimes called duplitized film. This type of film can record an image on either side regardless of which way it is loaded in the cassette. It must be used with two intensifying screens, one on either side of the film, although it doesn't matter which side of the film is against which side of the intensifying screen.

Special Applications

Most special application films have been developed for a specific need, and most of these films are single emulsion. These types of films are usually fine-grain, high-resolution, such as mammography or surgical films. They do require an increased patient exposure dose, but as advancements are made in technology the doses are decreasing while resolution is increasing.

Another type of special application single-emulsion film is laser film, such as computed tomography (CT), magnetic resonance imaging (MRI), nuclear medicine (NM), and ultrasound (US) film. This film is used to record a digital image and has an extremely high resolving power. Because the laser can be adjusted to a variety of intensities, the laser film can be a very slow speed without increasing the patient exposure dosage. It is usually sensitive to red laser light and therefore is not safe in a red-light darkroom. Specialty films that are usually double emulsion are 9 × 9 spot films used for fluoroscopy and 70- or 105-chip film or 35-mm roll film.

Subtraction Film. The two types of subtraction film are *subtraction mask* and *subtraction film*. This type of film is used in angiographic procedures to enhance the visibility of the vascular structures. They have clear base materials and are fine detail with high resolution. Once a scout film is made, the mask film is used to make a reversed polarity copy, black bone image. Then the subtraction film copies the masked image and literally subtracts the anatomy away, leaving only the angiographic procedure. With advancements in technology, this can be done with computer software rather than manually copying the scout films and subtracting the image.

Duplication Film. This type of film makes an exact copy of a radiograph. Since radiographs are negative (black bone images), a special type of film is needed for this process to work properly.

If we used regular film to copy the radiograph, we would get an image similar to a subtraction mask, black bone image. The film used to copy a radiograph is solarized. This means the film is pre-exposed and is at D Max (maximum density). The duplication film is placed on top of the radiograph to be copied and briefly exposed to ultraviolet light. This allows the radiograph to be copied exactly as it is, white bone. The longer the ultraviolet light is allowed to expose the duplication film, the lighter the copy will be. The ultraviolet light decreases the density of the duplication film because the film is already at D Max. Duplication film can be used to copy an overexposed radiograph in order to decrease the density on the copy and allow more anatomy to become visible, but this is not a recommended method of density control.

Film-Screen Combinations

The radiographic film and the intensifying screens must be correctly matched to produce a high-quality radiograph.

Phosphor Type

Spectral matching is an integral part of the film-screen combination. The color of the visible light emitted by the intensifying screen must match the film to optimize the exposure and in order to keep patient doses to a minimum. Two types of intensifying screens are widely used today:

1. Calcium tungstate. These intensifying screens emit visible light in the violet to blue wavelength. An average of only 5% of x-ray energy will be converted into visible light energy. These screens are considered slow, with an RS of 200 to 800. These slow screens provide excellent recorded detail.
2. Rare earth (gadolinium, lanthanum, yttrium). The major advantage of rare earth screens is the increased speed, requiring less radiation to produce a similar-quality image. The conversion of radiation to visible light for a rare earth screen is 15% to 20%. Another advantage of rare earth screens is that they may operate at a wide range of speeds, RS 200 to 1200. Rare earth screens emit light visible in the green-light spectrum. As the screen speed increases, the recorded detail decreases.

Conversion Factors for Grids

To alter the technique used to produce a quality radiograph with or without a grid requires math-

Table 6–7 ■ **GRID CONVERSION FACTORS**			
	60–70 kVp	**80–95 kVp**	**100–120 kVp**
5:1 grid	2 times the mAs	2.5 times the mAs	3 times the mAs
8:1 grid	3 times the mAs	3.5 times the mAs	4 times the mAs
10:1 grid	3.5 times the mAs	3.75 times the mAs	4 times the mAs
12:1 grid	4 times the mAs	4.5 times the mAs	5 times the mAs
16:1 grid	4 times the mAs	5 times the mAs	6 times the mAs

ematical calculation. Generally it is not practical to use these mathematical formulas to convert a technique between different grid ratios or grid to nongrid, although the radiographer should be aware that many factors are affected by changing the grid ratio. Table 6–7 lists some common grid conversion factors.

Grid Construction

Grids are constructed with alternating materials. One material is radiopaque and one material is radiolucent. The radiopaque material, usually lead, has a high atomic number and attenuates excess scatter radiation. The radiolucent material, usually aluminum, allows the photons to pass through with a minimal amount of absorption.

Grid Ratio (Fig. 6–17)

This is a mathematical relationship between the height of the lead strips and the distance between the lead strips, described by the following formula:

$$\text{Grid ratio} = \frac{\text{Height}}{\text{Distance}}$$

Example:
In a grid that has an interspace of 0.25 mm and lead strips that are 6 mm high, what is the grid ratio?

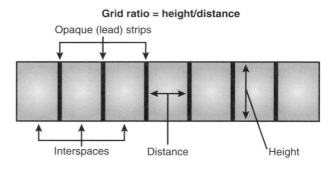

Figure 6–17 ■ Grid ratio.

Cross-hatched grid

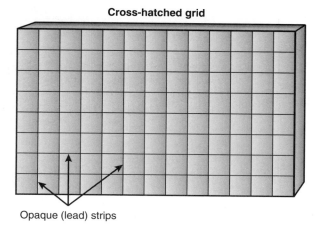

Opaque (lead) strips

Figure 6-18 ■ Cross-hatched grid.

$$GR = \frac{6 \text{ mm}}{0.25 \text{ mm}}$$

$$GR = 24:1$$

Grid Frequency

This deals with the number of lead strips in a given length, measured in inches or centimeters. Increasing the grid frequency without changing the grid ratio will in effect make the lead strips thinner to enable a greater number of lead strips to fit within a given length.

Types of Grids

There are basically two types of grids:

Criss-Cross or Cross-Hatched Grid (Fig. 6–18). This grid has vertical and horizonal lead strips that form squares throughout the grid. With this type of grid, it is imperative that the primary beam is directed perpendicular to the grid (Fig. 6–18).

Linear Grid (Fig. 6–19). In this grid, lead strips run the length of the grid along the grid's long axis. This allows the primary beam to be angled along the long axis without grid cut-off. There are two types linear grids:

Linear Parallel Grid. In this type, all the lead strips are aligned parallel to one another throughout the grid. Generally these grids are not widely used as stationary grids because they allow a large amount of primary radiation to become absorbed. For this reason parallel grids are not available in high-grid ratios, therefore minimizing the grid cut-off but also not providing good scatter reduction.

A special use of the parallel grid is in a Potter-Bucky or Bucky. The Bucky is located under the radiographic tabletop and above the radiographic cassette. During the prep stage of the exposure, the Bucky is set in motion and reciprocates or oscillates, causing the grid lines to be blurred. The grid motion must be perpendicular to the long axis of the lead strips of the grid, otherwise the lead strips will be imaged (Fig. 6–20). The grid motion must also be faster than the exposure time; this will also prevent the lead strips within the grid from being recorded.

Linear Focused Grid. In this type, the lead strips are slightly angled, with a greater degree of angulation toward the lateral edges of the grid. Therefore, if an imaginary line were drawn from each strip of lead, there would be a point at which they would converge (Fig. 6–21). The height of this convergence from the grid is known as the grid radius. The point at which they meet for the entire length of the grid is the grid convergence line (Fig. 6–22). All focused grids are designed to have a specific convergence line that allows use in a narrow range of distances such as 36″ to 44″ or 48″ to 72″, without major grid cut-off, referred to as the grid focal range. This information is available on the grid.

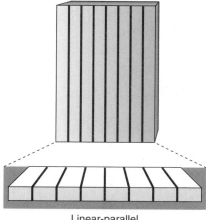

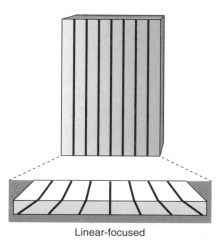

Figure 6-19 ■ Linear grid (parallel and focused).

Linear-parallel

Linear-focused

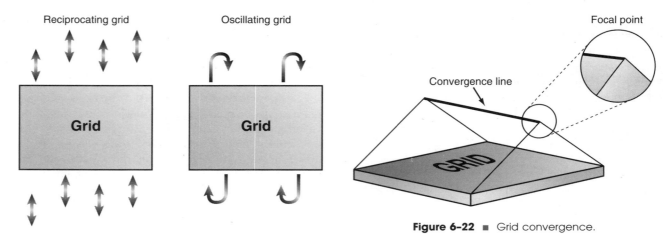

Figure 6-20 ■ Bucky grid motion.

Figure 6-22 ■ Grid convergence.

Grid Problems

Grids are designed to minimize scatter radiation from reaching the radiographic image. Problems occur when the grid is used in a way that it was not designed to be used.

Off-Level Grid. When the primary radiation and the grid are not perpendicular to one another, major grid cut-off will occur, with all types of grid. This can occur two ways: (1) angling the radiographic tube across the grid, against the long axis of the lead strips within the grid, or (2) angling the actual grid. The finished radiograph will demonstrate grid cut-off as an underexposed area on the lateral edge of one side of the film.

Off-Focus. This occurs when the exposure is made and the radiographic tube is well outside the focal range of a focused grid. This will not happen with a linear parallel grid. The finished radiograph will demonstrate an underexposed area on both lateral edges of the film.

Off-Centered Grid. This occurs when the radiographic tube is not directed toward the center of a focused grid to coincide with the divergence of the beam. This will cause increased absorption of the image-forming radiation. This will not happen with a linear parallel grid. The finished radiograph will demonstrate an underexposed area on the lateral edge of one side of the film.

Upside-Down Grid. This happens to a focused grid when the grid is placed upside down and the primary beam is directed toward the back of the grid (will not occur with a linear parallel grid). A huge increase in the absorption of the image-forming radiation will result. This occurs because the x-ray beam is diverging one way and the lead strips within the grid are angled in the opposite way. The angulation of the lead strips toward the middle of the grid is minimum, therefore this area will allow most of the image-forming radiation to pass through and expose the film. The finished radiograph will demonstrate a minimum decrease in exposure in

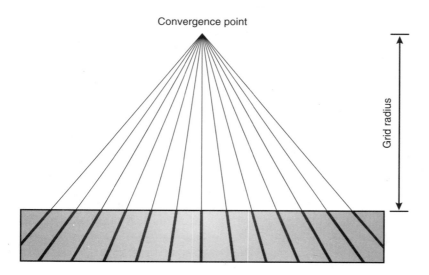

Figure 6-21 ■ Grid radius.

the center of the radiograph, with severe under-exposure to both lateral edges of the radiograph.

Bucky. Reciprocating or oscillating grids are linear parallel grids that rarely produce problems. One concern is when the grid does not move fast enough to blur the grid lines so that they are not visible. If the grid is not reciprocating or oscillating faster than the exposure time, then the grid lines will be recorded on the radiographic image. The finished radiograph will demonstrate blurry lines throughout.

There are three common causes of grid lines with moving grids. (1) If the exposure time selected is faster than the grid is able to move; the grid is visualized. (2) A jammed grid prevents free motion. This problem is usually caused by something, such as a marker, stuck in the Bucky tray. (3) The third type of problem with Bucky grids occurs when the central ray is angled across the long axis of the grid. This results in grid lines.

TECHNIQUE CHARTS

A technique chart is a methodical way to produce consistently high-quality radiographs. A good technique chart will equalize or compensate for a variety of variables, including the number one variable, the patient.

Caliper Measurement

A caliper is an instrument that measures an anatomical part thickness. The measurement is displayed in centimeters and then used to formulate an adequate technique. Caliper measurement can be made two different ways:

Central Ray Measurement. This simply states that the caliper will measure the anatomical thickness that is in the path of the central ray. If the central ray is angled, the caliper will be angled to follow the central ray.

Measurement Through the Thickest Part. This measures the thickest anatomical part regardless of the entrance and exit point of the central ray, or even whether the central ray is angled.

Fixed Versus Variable kVp

Fixed kVp Technique Charts. This type of technique chart determines the kVp range that will best depict an area of anatomy. When kVp is constant, any technical changes will be in mAs. The kVp is matched to specific anatomy, such as 45 kVp for a hand.

Variable Technique Charts. This type of technique chart determines a minimum kVp required for adequate penetration and then adds or subtracts kVp as part thickness increases or decreases. Changes are usually in increments of 2 kVp/cm.

Anatomical Considerations

Tissue Density. The great variations in anatomy are hardest for the technologist to overcome. Elderly patients with bone demineralization and pediatric patients with immature or growing anatomy will attenuate the primary beam differently than will a young or middle-aged adult. Technical changes must be made to compensate for these variations.

Part Thickness. To adjust for the thickness of the parts of interest, increases in kVp and mAs or a combination of both factors must be made.

Special Considerations

Eliminating variables from the many factors that determine a radiographic technique will help keep results constant. Knowing your patient is extremely helpful when formulating a technique. An elderly patient or a pediatric patient requires a much different technique from that of a healthy, middle-aged patient. In addition pathologic conditions require different amounts of radiation to depict the anatomy and pathology adequately.

Contrast medium (plural: media) is a radiopaque material that enhances certain structures that do not have good contrast naturally. The medium may be positive, such as barium or an iodine-based contrast, or negative contrast, such as air or a combination of both. The technical factors used for these procedures will vary greatly from one examination to another. It is important to know which type of contrast is being used to prevent overpenetration by using excessive kVp. Generally, for barium studies the kVp range is between 90 and 120, and for iodine-based contrast agents, between 65 and 75.

Casting materials also require special considerations. The thickness and type of material used are very important when selecting technical factors. Plaster casting material absorbs radiation much more than a fiberglass cast. Also, whether the material is wet or dry will greatly affect the attenuating quality of the cast. Generally for fiberglass casts the technique is increased as though the anatomical part with the cast was actually that thick. A general guideline for adjusting technical factors for part thickness is

2 kVp per cm or 1/2 or ×2 mAs per 5 cm

Both wet and dry plaster casts require a greater increase in technical factors. A general guideline for this increase is

> Dry cast: 10 kVp or × 2 mAs increase
> Wet cast: 15 kVp or × 3 mAs increase

In certain cases, a "sugar tong" or a split cast application may be used, in which casting material is placed on either side of the extremity and is held together by an Ace bandage or tape. This application can be fiberglass or plaster. It is generally used only temporarily for the evaluation of the fracture and immobilization of the site until the final reduction is done. In this case, the technique is increased for the projections that travel through the casting material but should not be increased for the projections that do not pass through the casting material. *Example:* in a comminuted wrist fracture, the orthopedist may elect to use a split cast and place the cast material on the anterior and posterior aspect of the wrist. The technique would be increased for the PA and oblique projection, but the lateral projection would not require an increase in technique.

Automatic Exposure Control

AEC can produce a quality radiograph with consistent results. Much of the consistency lies with the technologist's positioning. A patient not positioned properly greatly affects the radiographic density. Proper selection of the ion chambers is also a crucial aspect of AEC to maintain consistent results. The body part must correspond to the selected chamber for optimal results. With all other variables eliminated, AEC will select the range of mA (falling load generators) and determine the exposure time. The technologist is still responsible for the selection of the kVp, although some modern radiographic units provide the technologist with an average kVp.

When the exposure is made, the radiation passes through the patient and strikes the ion chambers. When the ion chambers detect a preset amount of radiation, the timer circuit is terminated. If an excessive amount of kVp is used, the timer circuit will terminate prematurely, resulting in a radiograph that has insufficient density. This is due to an increased amount of scatter radiation that is detected by the ion chambers. The ion chambers cannot differentiate between primary and scatter radiation and therefore terminate prematurely. If the kVp selected is too low, the timer circuit will remain on longer but the radiograph will not be adequately penetrated.

MANUAL VERSUS AUTOMATIC EXPOSURE CONTROL

Effects of Changing Exposure Factors on Radiographic Quality

Exposure factors are the most important components of radiographic quality. A change in kVp will affect many factors that might result in a change in density and contrast on the radiograph. A radiographer's perception of what the radiograph will look like when it is finished will determine how and when technical factors are changed. When changing technical factors to achieve optimum contrast and density, only one factor should be altered at a time.

Selection of Ionization Chamber or Photocell

In an automatic exposure system, care must be taken when the ionization chambers are selected. The wrong cells may result in a radiograph that will not depict the anatomy required. In a PA chest x-ray, if the center cell is turned on and the other two are turned off, the machine will read the spine and exposure will continue until adequate density is made over the spine. This leads to overpenetration of the lungs—they will be overexposed and unable to provide a diagnosis of possible lung pathology. The radiographer should be aware of the position of the photocells or ionization chambers (Fig. 6–23).

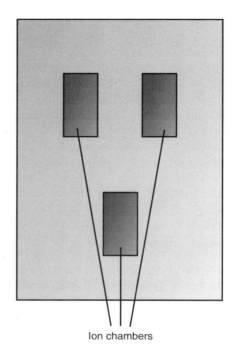

Ion chambers

Figure 6-23 ■ Location ion chambers.

Alignment of Part to Ionization Chamber or Photocell

If the anatomy of interest is positioned in any area other than over the ion chamber and an automatic exposure system is used, the resulting radiograph will be light or dark. The machine will read only the area that is selected. When using an AEC system, it is important to position the anatomy correctly. If the desired anatomy is not centered over the selected photocell or ioniza- tion chamber, it will not have the appropriate radiographic density.

Bibliography

Burns EF: Radiographic Imaging; A Guide for Producing Quality Radiographs. Philadelphia, WB Saunders, 1992

Bushong S: Radiographic Science for Technologists. 5th ed. St. Louis, Mosby–Year Book, 1993

Carlton R, Adler A: Principles of Radiographic Imaging. Albany, NY, Delmar Publishers, 1992

Thompson T: Cahoon's Formulating X-ray Techniques. 9th ed. Durham, NC, Duke University Press, 1979

Chapter 6 Questions

1. The black areas on a radiograph are called density. Which of the following instruments is used to measure the density recorded on a radiograph?

   A. Sensitometer
   B. Galvanometer
   C. Densitometer
   D. Dynamiter

2. The unit of measure for density is optical density. Which of the following range of optical densities best represents the diagnostic range?

   A. 1.0 to 10.0
   B. 2.5 to 3.0
   C. 0.10 to 0.35
   D. 0.25 to 3.0

3. Which of the primary radiologic factors controls density?

   A. kVp
   B. mA
   C. mAs
   D. kVp and mAs equally

4. The radiographic factor that controls the number of photons that are produced is:

   A. kVp
   B. mA
   C. Distance
   D. mAs

5. How much must the mAs factor be varied to have a visible effect on the radiographic density seen on the radiograph?

   A. ×2 or 1/2 of the original value
   B. 15% of the original value
   C. 30% of the original value
   D. 50% of the original value

6. How does kVp influence the radiographic density?

   A. Increases the radiographic density
   B. Increases the penetrating ability of the photons
   C. Decreases the number of photons produced
   D. Controls the radiographic quantity

7. Reducing the distance by two will cause:

   A. Twice as many photons available to expose the film
   B. Four times as many photons available to expose the film
   C. The same number of photons to expose the film
   D. None of the above

8. What is the mathematical relationship between mAs and distance?

   A. $\dfrac{I_1}{I_2} = \dfrac{(D_2)^2}{(D_1)^2}$
   B. Directly proportional
   C. Inversely proportional
   D. More than one but not all of the above

9. A radiograph is made at 36″. If another radiograph is made at 72″, what factor would be altered to maintain the radiographic density?

   A. Increase the mAs by 50%
   B. Increase the mAs by 2×
   C. Increase the film speed by 2
   D. Increase the mAs by 4×

10. Using 35 mAs, a radiograph was made at 72″. A repeat exposure is made changing the distance to 40″. What new mAs factor is used to maintain the radiographic density?

    A. 9 mAs
    B. 114 mAs
    C. 70 mAs
    D. 6.3 mAs

11. A radiographic exposure with optimal density was made at 30″ using 300 mA at 0.10 sec. If another is to be made with twice as much distance, what new technical factors will produce a radiograph with similar density?

    A. 30 mAs
    B. 60 mAs
    C. 120 mAs
    D. 240 mAs

12. What effect will a high-speed imaging system have on density?

    A. Increase density
    B. Decrease density

C. Maintain density

D. Have no effect on density

13. What is the relationship between density and RS?

A. Increases mAs

B. Directly proportional

C. Inversely proportional

D. These factors are unrelated.

14. The RS is increased from 200 to 600. What would the new mAs factor be if the original mAs were 150 mAs?

A. 300 mAs

B. 50 mAs

C. 600 mAs

D. 37.5 mAs

15. What effect will the use of a grid have on radiographic density?

A. Increased density

B. Decreased density

C. Has little effect on density

D. More than one but not all of the above

16. Which of the following types of radiation are not absorbed by grids?

A. Primary radiation

B. Secondary radiation

C. Scatter radiation

D. All of the above

17. The efficiency or absorptive quality of the grid is determined by:

A. Grid radius

B. Length and width of the grid

C. Grid ratio

D. Height of the grid convergence

18. A radiograph is made with 70 kVp at 5 mAs without a grid. If another exposure is made with an 8:1 grid, what are the new exposure factors?

A. 70 kVp at 15 mAs

B. 70 kVp at 20 mAs

C. 70 kVp at 12.5 mAs

D. 70 kVp at 19.5 mAs

19. What effect will additional filtration have in regard to density on the radiograph?

A. Filtration will not affect density.

B. Filtration will increase the overall beam energy by filtering out low-energy photons.

C. Filtration will decrease density by attenuating low-energy photons.

D. Filtration does not affect density; it only affects contrast.

20. With an increased beam restriction, why will the overall density decrease?

A. Beam restriction will allow fewer photons to exit from the tube port.

B. Beam restriction has little to no effect on radiographic density.

C. Beam restriction will increase density rather than decrease density.

D. Beam restriction will lower the tube current, preventing excess scatter production and therefore reducing density.

21. Which of the following tissue types will attenuate the least amount of radiation?

A. Bone

B. Muscle

C. Fat

D. Air

22. An added pathologic process would:

A. Increase density

B. Decrease density

C. Leave density unchanged

D. Cause the radiograph to be overexposed

23. A radiograph of the lumbar spine was made using an average spine technique. The technologist later became aware that the patient has advanced osteoporosis, a progressive demineralizing bone disease. How would this affect the radiographic quality?

A. The radiograph would be underexposed owing to overpenetration.

B. The radiograph would be overexposed.

C. The radiograph would have insufficient density.

D. This condition would not affect radiographic quality.

24. If the exposure factors were altered to compensate for a patient with pneumonia, how would they be changed?

A. Increase the mAs factor by 50%
B. Double the mAs and reduce the kVp by 15%
C. Increase the mAs
D. Double the kVp

25. Osteomalacia would be considered which of the following?

    A. A destructive pathology
    B. An added pathology
    C. A disease that causes bones to become soft
    D. More than one but not all of the above

26. In regard to the anode heel effect, which end of the radiographic tube has a decreased quantity of x-radiation?

    A. Anode
    B. Cathode
    C. The side toward the patient
    D. The side away from the patient

27. Which of the following affect the amount of anode heel effect on the radiograph?

    A. Beam restriction
    B. SID
    C. Anode angle
    D. All of the above

28. If anode heel effect is to be used to the technologist's advantage, which end of the radiographic tube would be positioned over the thicker anatomical area?

    A. It does not matter.
    B. Cathode end of the tube
    C. Anode end of the tube
    D. Anode end if a large filament is used and cathode if a small filament is used

29. Which of the following anatomical areas is/are able to use anode heel effect to increase visibility?

    A. Femur
    B. Thoracic spine
    C. Forearm
    D. More than one but not all of the above

30. Contrast can be defined as:

    A. The number of densities available on the finished radiograph
    B. The overall darkening of various structures throughout the radiograph

C. The latitude of the radiographic film
D. A long or low contrast radiograph

31. Of the primary radiographic factors, which of the following control the radiographic contrast?

    A. Distance
    B. mAs
    C. kVp
    D. Tube current

32. A radiograph that is made with a high kVp technique will yield a film that is considered to have:

    A. High contrast
    B. Low contrast
    C. Excessive scatter
    D. None of the above

33. What effect will increasing beam restriction have on radiographic contrast?

    A. Decrease contrast
    B. Increase contrast
    C. No effect on contrast
    D. Doubles the amount of densities visible

34. What effect will the use of a grid have on radiographic contrast?

    A. Increase contrast
    B. Decrease contrast
    C. Increases radiographic contrast but decreases tissue contrast
    D. Does not affect radiographic contrast but will increase tissue contrast

35. Beam restriction limits the primary beam that exits from the radiographic tube. How does a grid work?

    A. Decreases the amount of scatter that is produced
    B. Increases the tube efficiency to allow a higher-quality radiograph to be produced
    C. Allows less radiation to interact with the patient
    D. Allows less radiation to interact with the radiographic film by absorbing scatter radiation

36. Added filtration will have which of the following effects on radiographic contrast?

    A. Increases contrast

B. Decreases contrast
C. Minimizes contrast
D. Little to no effect on radiographic contrast

37. An added pathology such as Paget's disease will increase contrast. Why?

A. An added pathology will cause more attenuation, making a bigger difference between adjacent anatomy.
B. An added pathology causes anatomy to change in atomic number, structure, and function.
C. An added pathology will cause adjacent structures to attenuate radiation similarly, causing an increase in radiographic contrast.
D. The contrast difference is minimal and considered of no concern.

38. Which of the following factors would cause an increase in scatter radiation?

1. Increased kVp
2. Increase mAs
3. Advanced osteoporosis
4. Empyema

A. 1, 2, 3, and 4
B. 1 only
C. 2 and 4 only
D. 1 and 3 only

39. Which of the following tissue type(s) attenuate(s) the greatest quantity of radiation?

A. Bone
B. Fat
C. Muscle
D. Cortex of the kidney

40. How is recorded detail measured?

A. By a sophisticated measuring device
B. By the quality assurance personnel
C. Line pairs per millimeter
D. Recorded detail is unmeasurable.

41. Why is recorded detail an issue in radiography?

A. Because modern imaging systems are very slow and do not provide a high degree of detail

B. Because radiologists have such high standards
C. The only films that need a high degree of detail are pediatric films, because they are the most important.
D. Because anatomy is three-dimensional and the film records only images that are two-dimensional

42. What is the relationship between recorded detail and magnification?

A. None
B. Inversely proportional
C. Directly proportional
D. Inversely proportional to the square of the distance

43. The area of unsharpness that surrounds the image is referred to as:

A. Magnification
B. Umbra
C. Distortion
D. Penumbra

44. Why is magnification minimized with the use of a long SID?

A. Magnification is not minimized with a long SID, but a long SID will reduce the overall area of unsharpness.
B. Because with a long SID less overall umbra will surround the radiographic image
C. The area of the beam used to produce the image is traveling with less divergence compared with the lateral edges of the beam.
D. A long SID can be used only with a long OID to minimize magnification.

45. A small focal spot will provide the radiographic image with a higher degree of detail. What is also true in regard to small focal spots?

A. They are not able to image large objects because they are too small.
B. Photons bombard a narrow track on the anode, creating extreme heat in a relatively small area.
C. There is no disadvantage to the use of a small focal spot.
D. More than one but not all of the above

46. In regard to radiographic film, the smaller the crystal size:

    A. The greater the penumbra
    B. The greater the density
    C. The greater the detail
    D. The thicker the emulsion layer

47. Which of the following would help reduce the amount of motion recorded on a finished radiograph?

    1. Patient instructions
    2. Shortest exposure time
    3. Highest effective milliamperage
    4. Positioning aids, including restraining devices

    A. 1, 2, and 4
    B. 1, 3, and 4
    C. 1, 2, 3, and 4
    D. 1 only

48. Radiographic distortion can be separated into two categories. What are they?

    A. Magnification and blur
    B. Size and shape
    C. Umbra and penumbra
    D. Minification and magnification

49. Which of the following will minimize the amount of size distortion that is recorded on the finished radiograph?

    1. Long SID
    2. Short SID
    3. Long OID
    4. Short OID

    A. 1 and 4 only
    B. 2 and 3 only
    C. 1 and 3 only
    D. 3 and 4 only

50. Calculate the magnification for the following: A structure that is located 3.5″ from the image receptor at an SID of 72″.

    A. 1.05
    B. 0.95
    C. 0.06
    D. 0.05

51. Which of the following contributes to the greatest amount of size distortion:

    A. SID

    B. OID
    C. Tube angulation
    D. Focal spot size

52. Shape distortion can be defined as:

    A. Magnification of the structure of interest
    B. The structure of interest is elongated.
    C. Unequal magnification of the structures of interest
    D. None of the above

53. Tube misalignment will result in which of the following?

    A. Foreshortening
    B. Magnification
    C. Elongation
    D. More than one but not all of the above

54. Which of the following will result in foreshortening distortion?

    A. Tube alignment
    B. Film alignment
    C. Part alignment
    D. More than one, but not all of the above

55. A radiographic film that is sensitive to all types of light except red light is referred to as:

    A. Panchromatic
    B. Orthochromatic
    C. Double emulsion
    D. Single emulsion

56. Which of the following will produce a radiographic film that will provide the highest degree of exposure latitude?

    A. Large film crystals
    B. Small film crystals
    C. Thin emulsion layer
    D. Single emulsion layer

57. The relative speed of the intensifying screen and the mAs needed to provide adequate density have which type of relationship?

    A. Inversely proportional
    B. Directly proportional
    C. Relative speed squared equals the mAs.
    D. The relationship is not able to be quantified.

58. Locate emulsion layers for a double emulsion film:

    A. One on each side of the base material
    B. Two on one side of the base material
    C. It is special film that really has only one emulsion layer.
    D. Two emulsion layers on adjacent sides of the base material

59. Solarization of duplication film is achieved by:

    A. Reversing the emulsion
    B. Pre-exposing to visible light and sensitive to ultraviolet light
    C. Pre-exposing to visible light and sensitive to infrared light
    D. Using special silver salts in the emulsion

60. Which of the following phosphor types are the most sensitive to radiation?

    A. Calcium tungstate
    B. Gadolinium
    C. Isovue
    D. Silver halide

61. What is a grid conversion factor used for?

    A. To convert a technique from grid to nongrid
    B. To compensate for part thickness and scatter production
    C. To compensate for a nongrid technique when a grid is to be used
    D. More than one but not all of the above

62. Calculate the following for grid ratio:

    Lead strip thickness = 0.25 mm
    Lead strip height = 3 mm
    Distance between lead strips = 0.15 mm

    A. 20:1
    B. 30:1
    C. 10:1
    D. 8:1

63. Which of the following is used to determine grid ratio?

    A. Interspace distance divided by the height of the lead strip
    B. The amount of lead strips per inch or centimeter

    C. The thickness of the lead strips divided by the height of the lead strips
    D. The height of the lead strip divided by the space between the lead strips

64. Which of the following will increase grid efficiency and maximize scatter absorption while minimizing primary radiation absorption?

    A. Grid ratio
    B. Grid frequency
    C. Focused grid
    D. All of the above

65. Which type of grid has a convergence point?

    A. Cross-hatched grid
    B. Linear parallel grid
    C. Linear focused grid
    D. Potter-Bucky grid

66. What would result from using a linear parallel grid upside down?

    A. Nothing
    B. Grid cut-off on the lateral edges of the radiograph
    C. Grid cut-off toward the middle of the radiograph
    D. Grid cut-off equally throughout the radiograph

67. A Potter-Bucky grid uses motion to blur grid lines so they are not recorded on the radiograph. What is the most common motion used to achieve this effectively?

    A. Up and down
    B. Parallel to the long axis of the grid
    C. Perpendicular to the long axis of the grid
    D. Back and forth

68. A patient is scheduled for a wrist radiograph as a follow-up postreduction. The patient arrives at the department with a wet plaster cast. How would the technologist compensate for the cast material?

    A. Measure the part and increase 2 kVp per cm
    B. Double the mAs
    C. Increase the kVp by 15
    D. Halve the kVp and increase the mAs × 3

69. Which of the following are important considerations when using AEC?

    A. Selection of the appropriate ion chambers
    B. The kVp selection
    C. The patient position
    D. All of the above

70. An AEC unit will determine which of the following factors?

    A. Exposure time mAs
    B. mAs
    C. kVp
    D. More than one but not all of the above

Answers appear at the end of the book.

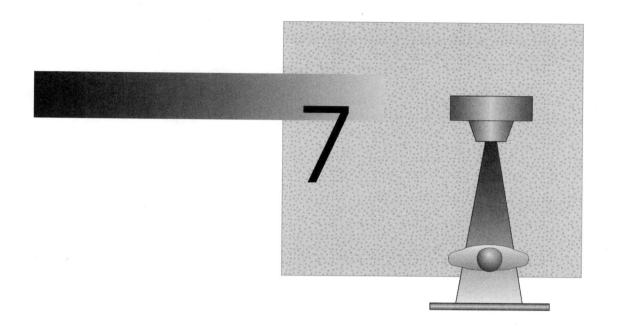

FILM PROCESSING AND QUALITY ASSURANCE

Film Storage
Pressure Artifacts
Radiographic Fog (Age, Chemical,
Radiation, Temperature, Safelight)

Cassette Loading
Matching Film and Screens
Film-Handling Artifacts (Static,
Crinkle Marks, Fog)

Radiographic Identification
Methods (Photographic,
Radiographic)
Legal Considerations (Patient Data,
Examination Data)

Automatic Film Processor
Processor Chemistry
Components and Systems
Maintenance
System Malfunctions

FILM STORAGE

Radiographic film should be stored in a cool dry place, on edge. Film is packaged in a lightproof foil or paper wrapper, which is hermetically sealed, then packaged in a cardboard box. There are usually 100 sheets per box, and some manufacturers include a chemically inert sheet of paper between each film to prevent sticking. Storing the films on edge also helps prevent the films from sticking to one another. The temperature of the film storage should be between 60° and 70° at a relative humidity of between 40% and 60%. Any variation outside of this range will result in artifacts/fog on the film.

Pressure Artifacts

Radiographic film is pressure sensitive; therefore, if a heavy object is placed on the film or if the film is folded, there will be a fogged area on the radiograph, an increased density. This artifact can be localized lines, smudge marks, or a widespread fog across the film. This is why radiographic film should be stored on edge even when loaded into a radiographic cassette. Pressure artifacts can also be caused by rough handling during loading and unloading, resulting in finger smudges, a fingernail mark, or a crinkle line from folding the radiograph.

Radiographic Fog

This is defined as increased radiographic density recorded on the radiographic film that does not contribute to the diagnostic image. Fog decreases the radiographic contrast and degrades the quality of the overall radiographic image. Radiographic fog has several categories:

Age Fog

All radiographic film has an expiration date on the box it is shipped in. Expired film will demonstrate an increased amount of fog and a decreased amount of radiographic contrast. In general, film is usually stored for only 45 days at a time, but it may be stored for up to a year if refrigerated or frozen. To avoid this problem, film stock should be rotated.

Chemical Fog

This type of fog is usually related to processing chemicals but may be caused by a variety of other chemicals. Processor chemical fog is discussed later in this chapter. Other chemical fog could result from anything that may come in direct contact with the film or by chemical fumes. Film should always be stored in a clean, chemical-free area, and the darkroom should be free of all chemicals as well. Chemical exposure fog decreases the contrast and speed of the film.

Radiation Fog

This type of fog is the result of improper storage. Radiographic film is very sensitive to radiation exposure. Whether in the shipping package or loaded into radiographic cassettes, film responds to minimum amounts of radiation. Therefore this protection is a major issue, for once the film is exposed to radiation it becomes twice as sensitive to radiation. Film must be stored in a nonradiation area, and the darkroom must be designed to provide adequate radiation protection. Any exposure to radiation that does not contribute to the diagnostic image will increase the amount of fog and decrease the contrast of the radiographic film.

Temperature Fog

The radiographic film is temperature and humidity sensitive and should be stored in a cool (60° to 70°), dry (40% to 60% humidity) place. It should never be stored next to heating units or steam pipes, or in boiler rooms. Storing film in a area with an average temperature of more than 70° will result in increased fog and decreased contrast. Frozen or refrigerated radiographic film will respond to radiation much slower than normal. Radiographic film stored in a place with less than 40% humidity will show a greater increase in static discharge artifacts. A high humidity of 60% or more will cause condensation to form on the inside of unopened packages and soften the emulsion layer. This may lead to films sticking together or increasing the fog on the radiograph. Too much or too little humidity will decrease the radiographic contrast.

Safelight Fog

The light in the darkroom serves no other purpose than as an aid to the personnel. This safelight in the darkroom can greatly affect the amount of fog on radiographs. Panchromatic film, usually digital film, is sensitive to all wavelengths of visible light. Therefore, the darkroom must be completely black to prevent light fog on the film. Orthochromatic film, used for most diagnostic studies, is sensitive to all wavelengths of light except red. Therefore the safelight in the darkroom is red. This provides good illumination of the darkroom while protecting from fog. Darkroom safelight tests are performed to ensure that the lighting used is not fogging the radiographs. The color of the darkroom also aids in protection of the radiographic film. It is usually painted a light color, which allows for the light to be reflected, so that the least amount of light can be efficient.

CASSETTE LOADING

Matching Film and Screens

The spectral matching of the films and intensifying screen is a crucial aspect to providing quality radiographs and patient protection. The sensitivity of the radiographic film must match the spectral emission of light by the intensification screen. This is discussed in detail in Chapter 6.

Film-Handling Artifacts

These types of artifacts are by far the most common problem. Rough handling of films increases when the radiology department becomes busy. Radiographic films should be handled with clean hands without lotion or cream, which might lead to smudge marks on the radiographs. The radiograph should be handled only by the edges and never bent or folded, as this would lead to fold or crinkle artifacts on the film. Gloves increase the chance of having a static discharge, resulting in a static artifact on the film, and wet hands will damage the emulsion layer, causing it to have an odor.

RADIOGRAPHIC IDENTIFICATION

Several types of identification are normally recorded on a radiograph in addition to the image. Most often, radiographic identification is thought to be only items such as patient's name, medical record number, institution, and so on. But radiographic identification includes any identifying markers that appear on the film. These include right and left markers, patient position markers (upright, supine, prone), time markers for timed studies such as small bowel studies or intravenous pyelograms, and for studies performed outside the radiology department, such as portable or operating room procedures. It is important to understand that any type of identification that is intentionally placed permanently onto the radiograph, along with the radiographic image, is considered legal radiographic identification.

Methods

There are two basic methods of radiographic identification.

Photographic Identification

This involves the use of a specially designed machine, a flash machine, to photographically record data onto the film. This is done by printing or writing the information on a card and inserting the card onto the machine with the radiographic film under it. A bright white light is used to record permanently the data on the radiograph. This is the most widely used system for recorded patient information. Most radiographic cassettes have a built-in window to allow this information to be recorded without removing the film from the cassette. The minimum information that should be included in this type of identification is patient's name, institution's name, medical or radiology number, and date.

Radiographic Identification

This type of identification is made by placing a radiopaque marker between the radiation source and the radiographic film. This records the information of the marker permanently. At the time of exposure, the high density of the markers attenuates the radiation that strikes them, leaving a decreased area of density where it is placed. Such information is usually the patient's side (RT or LT), patient position, time the radiograph was taken, and so on. Patient name and institution identification can also be recorded with opaque markers, but this method is awkward and is generally not used in modern departments. This type of information is usually recorded photographically with a flash machine.

Legal Considerations

Legal considerations of radiographic marking are fully discussed in Chapter 11. Basically, it is the technologist's responsibility to identify the radiograph accurately with the patient's name, the date, the medical record or radiology number, and the institution's name. The technologist is also responsible for marking the radiograph with any and all markers deemed necessary or pertinent to the identification or diagnosis of that radiograph: RT and LT markers, erect or supine, AP or PA, lateral or oblique, and so on. Markers that are not permanently recorded into the film's emulsion are not considered legal. These types of markers include stickers, china markers, and any marking scratched into the emulsion.

AUTOMATIC FILM PROCESSOR

This machine develops the latent radiographic image into the finished radiograph or visible image by a complex system of rollers and chemicals that bathe and transport the film. This whole process is generally done in about 90 sec, but some processors are able to perform the entire process in 45 sec or less (Fig. 7–1).

Processor Chemistry

Three types of solutions are used in the processor: developer, fixer, and water.

Developer

This is the first solution the film is exposed to. The developer is also responsible for making the latent image visible. The latent image is formed photographically in the film's emulsion when the exposure is made but is completely invisible until the film is exposed to the developer chemicals. The developer softens the emulsion layer chemically and changes the exposed silver halide crystals into black metallic silver. This process is responsible for all densities, ranging from fine-detail grays to the dark-black areas. The developer chemicals also prevent the unexposed silver crystals from being chemically processed. The last action of the developer is to begin hardening the emulsion layer, sealing the image within it. The developer is composed of many different chemicals, each having an individual part in the development process (Table 7–1). The temperature of the developer is the key in achieving optimal density on the radiograph: it should be maintained at 95°. The film is exposed to the developer chemicals for 20 to 25 sec, based upon a 90-sec processing time.

Fixer

This is the second chemical solution the radiograph is submerged in. The fixer stops the devel-

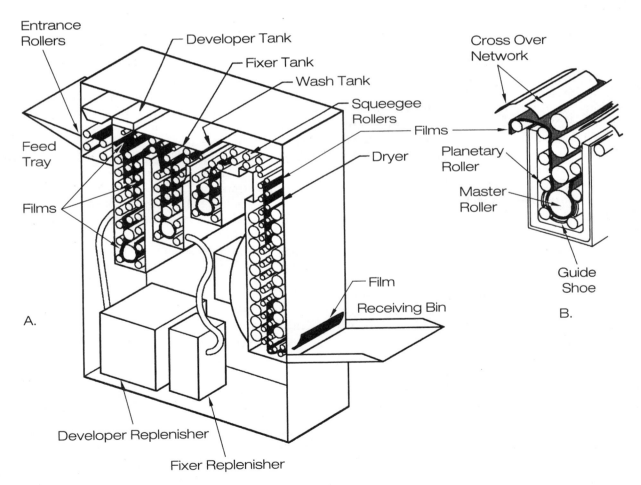

Figure 7-1 ▪ *A*, A modern automatic x-ray film processor. *B*, A transport rack and cross-over networks in a single tank. Reprinted with permission from Carlton R, Adler A: Principles of Radiographic Imaging; An Art and Science. 2nd ed. Albany, NY, Delmar Publishers, 1996, p. 298. Copyright 1996.

Table 7-1 ■ DEVELOPERS (ALKALINE)

Phenidone	Reducing or developing agent	Rapidly builds gray tones and gives fine detail *Makes the toe portion of H&D curve (see Fig. A–6)*
Hydroquinone	Reducing or developing agent	Slowly builds heavy densities, black tones *Makes the shoulder portion of the H&D curve*
Sodium carbonate	Activator	Allows the gelatin to swell and produces an alkaline pH
Potassium bromide	Restrainer	Prevents unexposed crystals from becoming chemically developed; decreases reducing or developing agents and antifogging agent
Sodium sulfite	Preservative	Controls oxidation and maintains balance among developer components
Glutaraldehyde	Hardener	Reduces gelatin swelling and hardens emulsion
Water	Universal solvent	Dissolves chemicals for use

oper action and removes the unexposed silver halide crystals from the emulsion layer. The fixer also continues to harden the emulsion layer. This process will actually stiffen and shrink the emulsion, fixing the image onto the film and making it permanent. The film is in the fixer for about 20 sec based upon a 90-sec processing time (Table 7–2).

Wash

The wash solution is simply water, a universal solvent, which serves to remove any excess chem-

Table 7-2 ■ FIXERS (ACIDIC)

Acetic acid	Activator	Provides an acidic pH and stops the reducing by the developer components
Ammonia thiosulfate	Clearing agent	Clears away the unexposed silver crystals
Potassium alum	Hardener	Stiffens, shrinks, and hardens the emulsion layer
Sodium sulfite	Preservative	Maintains chemical balance and prevents deterioration of chemicals
Water	Solvent	Dissolves chemicals for use

ical residue left by the developer and fixer. The temperature of the wash should be 5° below that of the developer, about 90°. The temperature is maintained by a heating element. The wash bath is about 20 sec long, based upon a 90-sec processing time.

Once the wash bath is over, the film is transported to the dryer where forced hot air is used to dry the emulsion layer of the film. The drying time is about 25 to 30 sec, based upon a 90-sec processing time. When the film is completely dry, it falls into a receiving bin as a finished product.

Components and Systems

The basic components of an automatic processor are

1. Feed tray
2. Microswitch
3. Developing tank
4. Fixing tank
5. Drying chamber
6. Receiving bin

One important aspect of processing is the darkroom, which is discussed in this section. Descriptions of the various systems associated with the automatic processor follow.

Transport System

This will move the film throughout the processor from the feed tray to the receiving bin. The entire transport system is made up of rollers. They are arranged onto racks and direct the film into each tank, allowing the chemicals to process the latent image. The rollers take the film to the bottom of the tank, turn it around, then carry it up and into the next tank. A special roller assembly, called a turnaround assembly, turns the film at the bottom of the tank. It consists of one large roller, called a master roller, and several planetary rollers and guide shoes to prevent jamming and kinking of the film. The roller assembly that transports films between tanks is called the cross-over rack. These rollers are generally smaller, they also use guide shoe assemblies to aid in the transition. These rollers are unique in that they act as squeegees to keep the chemicals in their respective tanks. The entire transport system is driven by an electric motor using a gear, pulley, or chain. The speed of the processor is governed by the speed of the transport system and should not vary from more than 2% of the manufacturer's specifications.

Temperature Control System

Of the three baths (developer, fixer, wash), the developer is the most temperature sensitive. The temperature must be maintained at a certain level, usually 95°. Reading above 95° will result in a radiograph that is overdeveloped and a reading below 95° will result in an underdeveloped radiograph. The wash is also temperature dependent and needs to be maintained at 90° (or 5° below the developer) to properly wash off the chemical residue. The temperature within these tanks is thermostatically controlled and maintained by a heating element.

Circulation System

This is a vital part of the processing of radiographs. The developer, fixer, and wash all require constant agitation to ensure that the chemicals are mixed evenly and that the temperature is maintained throughout the entire tank. This is achieved by a recirculation pump. Each tank has its own pump although they may all be driven by a common motor. The developer and fixer circulation systems also have special built-in filters to trap any small particles and prevent them from adhering to the rollers. This is especially important in the developer tank. The fixer and developer tanks are on closed systems, which means that the same chemicals recirculate back into the tank. The wash tank, however, is an open system; it continuously pumps fresh water over the film and disposes of the used water.

Replenishment System

During the process of developing, the chemicals lose their effectiveness and must be replenished. Chemicals within each tank lose their potency through oxidation, evaporation, and use (processing). The replenishment system keeps the chemicals fresh and provides a chemical balance within each tank. There are two types of replenishment:

- *Volume*—Replenishes per inch of film fed into the feed tray by use of a microswitch
- *Flood*—Replenishes at specific intervals regardless of use

Silver Recovery Systems

The chemicals that process the radiographic film cannot be drained into the public sewer because of their toxic nature. Also, the silver that is not used in the radiograph can be reclaimed and sold. This recycling can supply up to 10% of the total film budget in some institutions. The largest concentration of silver is in the fixer, which can make the fixer worth more after processing than

before. When the fixer is replenished the bath goes into a special receiving tank so that the silver can be separated from the other chemicals. Among many, three common ways of silver recovery are metallic replacement, electrolytic, and chemical perception. The principle is basically the same for all these methods: they provide a surplus of electrons that attract the positive charge of the silver.

The factors that determine the efficiency of any of these systems include the dwelling time of the recovery system and the agitation within the recovery tank. Longer dwelling times allow more silver to find the electrons, and with more agitation within the tank, the more silver comes in contact with the electrons.

Darkroom

The darkroom is an integral part of the film-processing system. This is a lighttight room that facilitates the removal of the radiographic film from the cassette and its development or placement into an automatic processor. After the radiograph is made, the film becomes twice as sensitive to light. Care is needed when handling the film in the darkroom to prevent handling artifacts and light fog.

Lighting within the darkroom may greatly affect the quality of the radiograph. Safelights are used to ensure that additional density is not allowed to be recorded on the radiograph once the exposure is made. The safelights are very low-wattage bulbs with filters used to illuminate the darkroom. Safelights usually have a dark red filter (Wratten B) placed over a 7- to 15-watt bulb, hung 4' or more from the work surface to provide a safe environment for film handling.

If brighter illumination is going to be used, the lights may be used indirectly rather than directly. This means that the lights would be directed toward the ceiling and only reflected light would be striking the film, as reflected light loses a substantial amount of its intensity.

A safelight test is performed to determine the length of time the film can be exposed to the safelight without increasing fog.

Maintenance

This is an important aspect of quality assurance in today's modern radiology department. If consistent results are expected from the processor, then regular maintenance must be performed. As the demand on the processor increases, the chance of a malfunction will also increase; therefore, maintenance must be done weekly or monthly to minimize processor problems.

Maintenance includes a visual inspection and lubrication of all moving parts and early identification of any potential problems within the processor. A regular schedule of preventive maintenance (PM) facilitates a time when parts can be replaced and a full inspection of the processor can be done, including any mechanical calibrations that may be needed. This type of maintenance helps reduce any sudden processor breakdowns.

Sensitometric Measurement

A major aspect in constant processor results is sensitometric measurement. This should be performed daily with a sensitometer and densitometer. A *sensitometer* is an electrical unit that exposes a radiographic film to a range of light intensities, resulting in a film similar to a step wedge. The film is then processed, and densitometer readings are taken from the film and recorded on a daily log. The log will reveal any widely varying differences from day to day and any trends that may be occurring over time. Appropriate corrective measures can be taken consistent with high-quality radiographs. This test should be performed on every processor in the institution, every day.

System Malfunctions

Because of the amount of systems and moving parts associated with the automatic processor, a wide variety of malfunctions can occur. It would be far beyond the scope of this text to include all the potential problems, but the most common one are described briefly:

Film Jams. These can be caused by transport rollers not seated properly, because of broken or faulty gear mechanisms. Films may become bent and stick within the processor.

Chemical Fog. This fog may resemble light fog on the radiograph. It can be caused by any number of problems, including improper replenishment rates, cross-contamination of fixer and developer, excess chemical residue caused by cross-over rollers not squeezing the chemistry out completely, or insufficient wash. If the film comes out with a yellowish brown tint, it probably results from a developer problem; if the film comes out with a white crystal-like film, it is probably a fixer problem.

Guide Shoe Marks. These are caused by the guide shoes being in improper position and scratching the emulsion of the radiograph. Also, the transport rollers may not be seated properly.

Pi Lines. These are caused by a dirty or stained roller marking the emulsion of the radiograph in a specific pattern, each mark being 3.14″ apart. This occurs because the diameter of the roller is 1″, making the circumference of the roller 3.14″, or pi.

Pick-Off or Build-Up. This can be caused by dirty rollers that mark the emulsion or pull pieces of it off the radiograph, showing round areas of increased or decreased density in a nonspecific pattern on the surface of the radiograph. This is a special problem in mammography, as emulsion pick-off resembles calcification and/or screen artifacts.

Bibliography

Burns EF: Radiographic Imaging; A Guide for Producing Quality Radiographs. Philadelphia, WB Saunders, 1992

Bushong S: Radiographic Science for Technologists. 5th ed. St. Louis, Mosby–Year Book, 1993

Carlton R, Adler A: Principles of Radiographic Imaging 2nd ed. Albany, NY, Delmar Publishers, 1996

Thompson T: Cahoon's Formulating X-ray Techniques. 9th ed. Durham, Duke University Press, 1979

Chapter 7 **Questions**

1. Why is it important to store radiographic film on edge?

    A. To prevent films from sticking together
    B. To prevent pressure artifacts
    C. To save space in small radiology departments
    D. More than one but not all of the above

2. What type of effect will radiographic fog have on film contrast regardless of the origin of the fog?

    A. As the fog increases, the contrast will also increase.
    B. As the contrast increases, the radiographic fog will also increase.
    C. Radiographic fog and contrast are directly proportional to one another.
    D. As the radiographic fog increases, the radiographic contrast will decrease.

3. Which of the following best describes chemical fog?

    A. A radiograph that has been exposed to an unstable isotope such as iodine-131
    B. Chemical fog results only from exposure to the processing chemicals.
    C. A contrast agent that comes in contact with the radiographic film after it has been processed
    D. Any chemical substance that may affect the radiographic emulsion, causing an unwanted density to be recorded on the radiographic film

4. Which of the following is not true regarding radiographic film?

    A. Storage temperature should be between 60° and 70°.
    B. Storing film in a refrigerator will increase its shelf life.
    C. Radiographic film should be stored at a relative humidity of 60% to 70%.
    D. Should not be stored in a radiation area

5. What determines the color of the light used to illuminate the darkroom?

    A. The sensitivity of the film that is going to be processed
    B. The taste of the administrator managing the department

    C. The color of the light used is not as important as the number of lights used.
    D. Any color may be used with panchromatic film.

6. What color should the radiographic darkroom be painted?

    A. Black or a very dark color, hence "darkroom"
    B. There is no significance to the darkroom's color.
    C. A very light color to allow the maximum reflection of light within the room
    D. The same shade of red as the red safelight; this will make it seem brighter than it really is

7. Which of the following may lead to film-handling artifacts?

    A. Dirty hands
    B. Wet or lotion-covered hands
    C. Rough handling
    D. All of the above

8. How are radiographic markers recorded on a radiograph?

    A. Photographically or radiographically
    B. Scratching it into the emulsion
    C. Flashed into the emulsion and stickers or permanent markers
    D. All of the above

9. Radiographic identification refers to:

    A. Recording information on a radiograph
    B. Using radiation to record identification markers into the emulsion of the radiograph
    C. Being able to identify a radiograph
    D. Using a special machine to record pertinent information into the emulsion of the radiograph

10. Legally, which of the following need to be included in the identification of a radiograph?

    A. The patient's phone number
    B. The institution's address
    C. The patient's medical or radiology number
    D. The examination type

11. In an automatic processor, the developer is responsible for:

    A. Giving the radiograph its stiffness and indestructible quality
    B. The dark areas
    C. Removing the unexposed silver crystals
    D. Removing the supercoat to speed up the developing process

12. Which of the processor chemicals is the most sensitive to temperature?

    A. Developer
    B. Fixer
    C. Wash
    D. All the chemicals are equally temperature dependent.

13. Which of the following are functions of the fixer?

    A. Stops the developer action
    B. Removes the unexposed silver crystals
    C. Shrinks and stiffens the emulsion
    D. All of the above

14. Which of the following systems are responsible for keeping the processing chemicals fresh?

    A. Temperature control system
    B. Circulation system
    C. Replenishment system
    D. Silver recovery system

15. After processing, which of the processor chemicals has the highest silver concentration?

    A. The developer
    B. The fixer
    C. The wash
    D. All the chemicals have an equal amount of silver.

16. What method is used to ensure that safelight fog does not become a problem?

    A. Using only half the lights that are in the darkroom
    B. Doing annual sensitometric tests
    C. Doing annual light bulb checks, usually done by the darkroom technologist
    D. Safelight testing will ensure that the safelights do not fog the radiographic film.

17. A safelight test determines which of the following?

    A. The distance of safelights from work area
    B. The type of filter necessary
    C. The necessary wattage of the bulb
    D. All of the above

18. The tool used to perform the test to determine whether any processor fog is present on the radiographic film is:

    A. Densitometer
    B. Sensitometer
    C. Processor PM
    D. Any one of the above

19. What type of artifact would result from improper roller seating?

    A. Pick-off
    B. Guide shoe marks
    C. Pi lines
    D. All of the above

20. A film comes out of an automatic processor with a brownish yellow tint over the entire surface of the film. What could be a cause of this problem?

    A. A fixer problem
    B. A developer problem
    C. A wash problem
    D. Insufficient replenishment system

Answers appear at the end of the book.

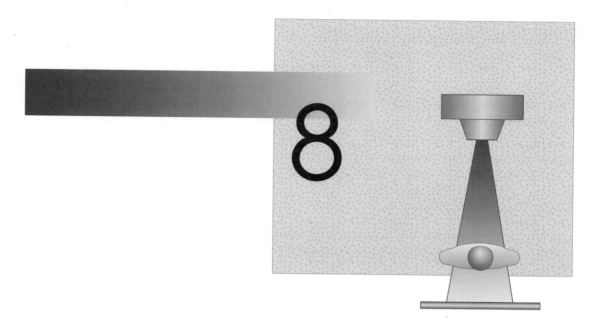

EVALUATION of RADIOGRAPHS

This chapter must be prefaced with the following information: We will attempt to provide an overview of radiographic film evaluation, but should you require more in-depth information, please refer to *Radiographic Critique* by Kathy McQuillen-Martensen, published by W. B. Saunders, Philadelphia, Pennsylvania. This is the most comprehensive radiographic evaluation book currently on the market. Also refer to Chapter 6 of this text for more detail of technical factors.

CRITERIA FOR DIAGNOSTIC QUALITY RADIOGRAPHS

If you are or ever were a radiography student, you must have been involved in Film Critique class, be it formal or informal. A radiograph is displayed for viewing and evaluating. A form may accompany this process to document the evaluation's criteria and findings. If you are or plan to be a competent technologist, you must perform this film evaluation process mentally each time you review a radiograph. All the criteria must be reviewed in your own mind and applied through honest observation. It is always the case, when you are in a hurry or cutting corners and you pass a suboptimal radiograph, that it will return to haunt you. It is really much easier for you and more beneficial to the patient to repeat the radiograph in question at the time of the procedure.

The Film Evaluation Process

The following is a model of what should go on inside your brain every time you review a radiograph. Ask yourself: *Is it optimal?*

Demographics? Patient, facility, date, and further information accurate and visible?
Is the radiograph marked properly with lead markers; are they visible?
Is the requested anatomy visualized and centered appropriately?
Positioning considerations:
    Tube, part, film alignment?
    Cassette size and orientation?
Exposure factor selection:
    Density. Is there adequate density?
    Contrast. Is the anatomy penetrated?

If these factors have been selected properly and there is a problem with the resultant exposure, look to these other, less obvious, causes:

Processor malfunctioning?
Improper screen-film combo?
Improper source-to-image distance (SID) utilized?
Disease process active within patient?

Equipment malfunctioning?
Improper grid alignment?
How good is the resolution?
    Motion? (usually the culprit)
    Distortion, magnification—SID, object-to-image distance (OID)?
    Film-screen combo?
    Focal spot size (FSS)—correct selection?
    Artifacts present?
    Film-screen contact?
    Grid alignment and use?
Patient considerations?
    Pathology—affect the outcome?
    Preparation—level of compliance?
Radiation protection demonstrated?
    Evidence of collimation?
    Patient shielding? (when applicable)
    Cassette size not larger than required?
Is the requisition/order or electronic order completed properly?

That sums it up. If you are truly answering these questions every time you review a radiograph, you'll be aware of whether or not the film needs to be repeated.

CAUSES OF POOR RADIOGRAPHIC QUALITY AND CORRECTIVE ACTION

Now let's examine each one of our evaluation criteria and determine how to correct a suboptimal radiograph.

Demographic Information

This is important permanent legal information that becomes the patient's medical record. It is best if this information is flashed onto the film at the time of the procedure or preprocessing. Adhesive label information is unsightly, can eventually peel off and get lost or thrown away, and renders the radiograph questionable in a court of law.

If the information did not flash properly, check the position of your flash card; perhaps it was placed in the flashing mechanism upside down or tilted. Sometimes, if the flasher is used more than once on the same film, the information will be too dark to read. Obviously, if this information is illegible, you will not repeat the film for that correction alone. This would not make sense for radiation protection requirements. If you must add this information onto the film postprocedure, use the standard label for such purposes available at your facility. Use black or blue ink and print the information clearly and accurately.

Film Markers

Is the radiograph marked properly with lead markers?

It is critical that the right or left marker be placed within the field of view on each exposure, at the time of the exposure. This also is a legal requirement. We all realize that this doesn't happen 100% of the time, but we should all strive for that result. Placing the right marker on the cassette for a lumbar spine radiograph and then collimating it out of the field of view is not acceptable. Neither is it acceptable to place the marker over anatomy that is necessary to visualize. Clip-on markers can be awkward for certain examinations. It is good to have two different types of marker styles to insure placement accuracy regardless of the positioning requirements.

Any other current substitute for lead marker placement is not considered legal in a court of law and ultimately can have an entire case thrown out of court on that count alone. When you must use a replacement, labels are probably the best alternative. Scratching into the emulsion and using china markers are not good choices. Again, repeating the film to satisfy this requirement is not acceptable due to radiation protection requirements.

Positioning Considerations

Is the requested anatomy visualized and centered appropriately?

When positioning, the patient's area of interest must be centered properly to the film, either directly or on top of the upright Bucky or table. If you are radiographing an area that requires a horizontal or vertical beam, center the anatomy of interest as close to the center of your film as possible. The central ray should be centered directly through that particular anatomy. For an example: Center the wrist to the center of the cassette and direct the vertical central ray through the carpals, and they will appear in the center of the film.

When radiographing anatomy that requires angulation, it is actually *the exit point of the central ray* that is most critical to the correct placement of your film. Let's imagine something simple as an example. If you are radiographing a calcaneus, you would not center the part to the center of your cassette. Due to the steep angulation of the central ray, the anatomy will be directed to where the central ray exits. It is at *that* exit point that the calcaneus will appear. If you center the anatomy to the center of the cassette, it will be thrown off the film entirely. These concepts apply to all radiographic examinations.

Use your facility's protocol to determine desired cassette size and orientation per procedure. Evaluate the radiograph with these concepts in mind. Adjust accordingly.

Exposure Factors

Density

Milliampere-second (mAs) is the *primary* control over the density that appears on the resultant radiograph. If insufficient exposure occurs, the radiograph will appear washed-out, appear heavy with soft tissue visualization, but demonstrate limited bony trabeculae. A 30% increase/decrease in mAs is required to obtain a *visible* difference in density.

Contrast

Kilovoltage peak (kVp) is the *primary* controlling factor for contrast on the resultant radiograph. This gives the radiation its penetrable force. Adequate visualization of the cortical structures of the bone determine whether the radiograph is overpenetrated or underpenetrated. It is important to know the kVp recommendations per body part to assist in the proper selection. An underpenetrated antero-posterior (AP) lumbar spine would not afford viewing of the spinous processes. The radiation, due to its low energy, would attenuate in the spine's body and not provide enough penetration to afford visualization of the processes. An overpenetrated radiograph would demonstrate all cortical structures but with a decrease in viewing contrast. Because of the high energy level of the radiation, attenuation would be limited and scatter radiation production would occur, creating low contrast and visible fog, obscuring visible detail. A 15% increase/decrease in kVp will create a visible density difference on the radiograph.

Other Causes

If you are certain that all of your selected exposure factors are correct and your radiograph is less than optimal, you must look elsewhere for the answer. These are just a few options: Processor temperature can create havoc with radiographic density, as can contaminated or oxidized chemistry, so check your processor and sensitometry outcomes. Is the proper film-screen combination being used? If there are multiple film-screen variations to choose from in your department, check to be sure you have the correct combination. You may have substituted a 200-speed film and detail cassette system for a 400-speed system. Someone may have loaded the incorrect film into the darkroom bin. Stranger things have happened. Was the tube at the correct SID? Even a few inches will make quite a visible difference because of the effects of the inverse square law. Does your patient have pathology that is affecting the outcome of your examination? Emphysema will render the usual chest exposure factors worthless, resulting in an overexposed radiograph because of the bronchial hyperinflation. Another problem may be the equipment's calibration. When was the last recorded calibration? Perhaps it needs adjusting—consult the physicist or radiologic engineer. Are you using a grid? Are you using it correctly? Grid cut-off will wash out your film's density and contrast. Prior to exposure, always check for grid and central ray alignment, as well as correct SID range for focused grids.

Resolution

How good is the resolution?

When there is a problem with resolution, it is most frequently motion. Motion can be voluntary or involuntary. In either case, it is time reduction and/or a faster film-screen combination that will help solve the problem. Precise patient instruction is also a valuable corrective tool. Motion will blur all the sharp edges of the radiograph's image. It is the same as if someone moves while you are attempting to photograph him. The greater the movement, the greater the blurriness. If you can increase the selected mA and, in turn, decrease the selected time to maintain mAs, this will aid in the reduction of motion. A faster speed film-screen system requires less radiation for exposure, so time, once again, may be reduced. Making certain that your patient is complying with your instructions is also important. Do a trial run for the breathing to be sure the patient is following your directions. Sometimes, if motion is a severe problem and you are limited in your corrective actions, reducing the lengthy breathing instruction will help. Just tell the patient to "stop breathing."

Distortion by magnification can sometimes be a problem. SID and OID control the magnification factors on the radiograph. Most magnification is minimal and therefore inconsequential. Once in a while, a problem will arise. It takes creative technology to minimize the magnification. Many men or older women with kyphosis who require skull radiographs have trouble tucking their chins down far enough to obtain the correct skull placement for an AP axial. A lot of sponges are placed under their heads and before long, the OID is extreme. Remember that the anatomy farthest from the film will be projected farthest with angulation. In this case, the anatomy of interest will also be magnified and projected out of place by not being placed properly to begin with. The answer here is to reverse the position. Do a PA axial, reversing the central ray angulation to cephalic and limiting the OID considerably. Occasionally, grossly obese patients will need to be radiographed. If you attempt to radiograph a shoulder at 40″ with an upright Bucky, a magnified version of a shoulder will result. Increase your SID to 72″ and the OID is compensated, resulting in a better-detailed radiograph.

Film-screen combination is critical for resolution. The slower the system, the greater the resolution, as well as the patient dose. If the clinical history involves a foreign body, fine-detail systems should be used. A sea urchin spine embedded in a finger, for example, would be missed completely using a high-speed system. Focal spot size is also a consideration for detail. The small focal spot will afford the greatest detail. Most x-ray generators have this set up automatically to correspond to the mA settings. Some older equipment will allow you, as the operator, to select it manually. The lower mA stations will accommodate small focal spot settings. The trade-off with selecting low mA stations is that you must use more time. More time will give way to motion. Motion completely obliterates any increased resolution gained by using the small focal spot. Your patient's condition and ability to hold still will dictate which choice would be more beneficial.

Artifacts are any undesirable structures or substances that appear on a radiograph. Sometimes they are difficult to track down and identify. They may fall into any one of these categories:

Anatomical	A patient's arm not fully extended for a lateral chest radiograph
External	Earrings not removed for a skull radiograph
Internal	An intrauterine device (IUD) on a pelvic radiograph
Equipment-related	Cables from the x-ray tube in between the tube and the patient during an exposure
Processing-related	Crease marks in the emulsion from improper film handling

Most processor artifacts are easily recognized. Static, roller marks, pi lines are all possible. Humidifying the darkroom and processor preventive maintenance generally correct those artifacts. It is essential to have an identification system in place for your cassettes. Most facilities number them. If an artifact appears, it can be traced back to the cassette used. Always check the cassette, the table, and the patient's gown or coverings. Sometimes the artifact will be inside the patient. After a thorough investigation without success, you may wish to question the patient discreetly. Many excellent articles and books have been devoted to this subject alone. They are interesting and sometimes very humorous. Try reading some of them in your free time.

Film-screen contact can create areas of distortion on the radiograph. If the film and screen breach contact with one another, blurry areas will be seen. The cassette may be tested to see whether the screen is warped. Wire screen/mesh is placed on top of the cassette and radiographed. Areas of screen warp will be easily identified on the resultant radiograph. Grid alignment is also important in resolution. A radiograph that is full of grid lines or grid cut-off destroys detail. As mentioned previously, always check the grid's alignment and its alignment with the central ray, as well as the SID recommendations for focused grids, prior to the exposure.

Patient Considerations

As mentioned earlier in this chapter, pathology can create problems with the resultant radiographs. Refer to Chapter 6, Table 6–3, to see how specific diseases must be compensated for by adjusting the exposure factors to produce optimal results. It is always in everyone's best interest to identify the pathology prior to the procedure. Obtaining a complete and accurate clinical history before radiographing the patient is critical to obtaining the best results. Exposure factors can then be adjusted before, rather than after, the study. This results in decreased repeats.

Patient preparation has been mentioned continuously throughout this book. It is so essential for a successful procedure. If the patient has been educated and understands what is expected of him or her, the odds for a successful examination increase tremendously. Even if the department is hectic, this portion of the procedure must not be eliminated. The time that is spent in preparation of the patient cannot be minimized. If you choose not to prepare the patient or provide comprehensive instruction, do not be surprised to be repeating the entire procedure. If patients cannot comply after comprehensive instruction, you must communicate with them to attempt to gain their cooperation. There will be rare occasions when the compliance of the patient is so poor

that the procedure must be canceled. This is an obvious loss to everyone.

Radiation Protection Factors

There are several factors to check. Is there evidence of collimation? Four-sided collimation is the zenith, but most of us are happy with a nicely two-sided or three-sided collimated image. Collimation takes practice. Years ago, cylinder cones were utilized for many procedures. Technologists tried to outdo one another with their tightly collimated images. Granted, these radiographs were challenging to obtain and lovely to behold. Unfortunately, many radiographic interpretations were inaccurate, due to the loss of the surrounding information.

Today, the standards have changed. Most emergency department physicians, as well as radiologists, would be displeased if you submitted an ankle radiograph demonstrating ONLY the ankle joint, no distal tibia or fibula. You would most likely have to repeat the examination. Liability and misdiagnosis turned the collimation tide. The patient also receives far less radiation than was received 30 years ago, due to high-speed, rare earth film-screen systems, as well as more efficient equipment. If your radiograph does not demonstrate four-sided collimation, do not repeat it for that reason. It defeats the purpose. It is best not to overdo it. Better to collimate conservatively than to have to repeat an examination because of overcollimation.

Some tissues are more sensitive to radiation than others. They are the *eyes, thyroid, breasts* and *gonads.* Because of their sensitivity, they should be shielded if they are in close proximity to the primary beam (2.5″). Use a lead contact shield or a shield designed specifically for this purpose. These sensitive tissues should also be collimated out of the field of exposure when possible. Odontoid radiographs are the perfect example. Reduce the field of exposure to exclude the eyes. Become familiar with the anatomical location of these radiosensitive organs and shield them prior to exposure.

Requisitions and Electronic Orders

Is the requisition order or electronic order complete?

Always review the order to insure that the proper procedure was completed. Obtain the clinical history and document it for the radiologists. Fill in other pertinent information, such as how many and what size films were used, repeat film number, the time the case was begun and ended, initials of those involved in the procedure. These items will vary from facility to facility. Many times, this information must be used to track procedures that involve litigation, billing problems, or physician's requests. It is essential information.

As you can see, radiography is a technology composed of numerous variables. If only one of those variables is not met, the case is not considered optimum quality. No one factor is any more or less important than the next. They must all be evaluated separately and together to measure the level of success.

FUTURE CONSIDERATIONS

With the advent of PACS (**P**icture **A**rchiving and **C**ommunications **S**ystem) or electronic imaging, *filmless* evaluation will take on a very different approach. As long as sufficient radiation (based upon predetermined exposure values) is used to obtain the digital image, the electronic image can be manipulated for gray scale or subtraction capabilities (bone window) on the monitor prior to or at the time of soft copy interpretation.

Patient and facility demographics will be accessed through the system and will be visible on the image. The importance of the accuracy of this information will not be any less valuable, however, because inaccuracy will create "broken or lost" studies within the system that become very burdensome to track down and correct.

Artifacts will now include ghostlike images that will appear along with the ordered image, if the digitized computed radiography (CR) plates are not discharged properly. Quality assurance standards and acceptance testing must be developed and maintained for optimal imaging. These may include signal-to-noise ratio, signal linearity, system plate travel speed, and the consistency of the laser's sweeping motion across the plate. Scatter of radiation affects the signal-to-noise ratio of the digitized image. Tight collimation practice may very well be implemented again optimally to enhance the electronic image.

Electronic imaging will change the way in which radiology, as we now know it, will function. The impact of computerized image management is yet to be realized. The technology is here, expanding on a daily basis with new software and hardware innovation. The turn of the century will manifest a growth in computer technology that may be likened to the industrial age of the last century. These advancements are sure to streamline and simplify complex technology, including our own radiologic technology. It will be critical to stay abreast of these advancements within our technology and expand our role contemporaneously.

Bibliography

Ballinger PW: Merrill's Atlas of Radiographic Positions and Radiologic Procedures. 7th ed. St. Louis, CV Mosby, 1991

Lobick J: Image Optimization for Computed Radiography: Decisions in Imaging. Economics Supplement. Marina del Ray, CA, Allied Health Care Publications, May/June 1997

McQuillen-Martensen K: Radiographic Technique. Philadelphia, WB Saunders, 1996

Statkiewicz MA, Vieconte PJ, Ritenour RE: Radiation Protection in Medical Radiography. 2nd ed. St. Louis, CV Mosby, 1993

Chapter 8 **Questions**

1. Film evaluation is done:

   A. Only by the radiologist
   B. Only by the QA supervisor
   C. To determine whether the radiograph is optimal
   D. Only by students in class

2. What is a frequent contributor to loss of resolution?

   A. Motion
   B. SID
   C. OID
   D. Artifacts

3. Patient/facility demographics are:

   A. Unnecessary for an optimum study
   B. Only entered into the computer
   C. Important permanent information that becomes part of the patient's medical record
   D. Used exclusively in admitting

4. The only replacement for legally marking radiographic films for right and left orientation:

   A. Is a china marker
   B. Is right and left stickers that can be placed on the film after exposure
   C. Consists of etching the radiograph's emulsion, as right or left
   D. There is no legal replacement.

5. The primary controlling factor for density is:

   A. mAs
   B. SID
   C. OID
   D. Film-screen system

6. You choose 10 mAs, 60 kVp for a shoulder examination. The resultant radiograph is penetrated but requires additional density. Your exposure factors for the repeat examination would be:

   A. 20 mAs, 60 kVp
   B. 10 mAs, 70 kVp
   C. 8 mAs, 60 kVp
   D. 13 mAs, 60 kVp

7. What bony feature depends on kVp for its optimal visualization?

   A. The trabeculae
   B. The coracoid
   C. The cortical structures
   D. The spinous process

8. SID is an important factor in film density due to the:

   A. Tube current
   B. Inverse square law
   C. Photoelectric effect
   D. kVp

9. One of the best methods to control unwanted motion on the radiograph is to:

   A. Raise the kVp
   B. Lower the time
   C. Admonish the patient
   D. Lower the mAs

10. SID and OID directly affect:

    A. The magnification on the radiograph
    B. Density
    C. The anode heel effect
    D. Contrast

11. To reduce magnification due to increased OID:

    A. Reduce kVp
    B. Use a large focal spot
    C. Increase SID
    D. Increase mAs

12. Radiographic artifacts are:

    A. Old relics
    B. Earrings
    C. IUDs
    D. Any undesirable structures or substances that appear on the radiograph.

13. It is important to be knowledgeable regarding disease processes in evaluating films because:

    A. You can better diagnose the patient
    B. You can select the appropriate exposure factors
    C. You can counsel the patient regarding the disease

D. You can tell your friends about the patient

14. Which of the following is not a radiosensitive tissue?

A. Eye
B. Thyroid
C. Brain
D. Breast

15. The patient's correctly completed requisition is:

A. Unimportant in film evaluation
B. Used only for billing
C. Used only by the film librarians
D. An essential factor of an optimal study

Answers appear at the end of the book.

Section III Questions

1. The unit used to express logarithmic density is called:

   A. Density
   B. Contrast
   C. Hounsfield
   D. Optical density

2. The primary factor that controls density is:

   A. Distance
   B. Time
   C. mAs
   D. kVp

3. The mAs factor controls which of the following?

   A. The amount of radiation produced
   B. The energy frequency of the radiation produced
   C. The resultant radiographic contrast
   D. The penetrating power of the radiation produced

4. Increasing the kVp will do which of the following?

   A. Increase the radiographic density
   B. Increase the penetrating ability of the primary beam
   C. Increase the frequency of the photons produced
   D. All of the above

5. kVp is primarily responsible for controlling:

   A. Density
   B. Quantity of radiation produced
   C. Quality of radiation produced
   D. Quantity of photons produced

6. kVp can influence the radiographic density by:

   A. Increasing the secondary and scatter radiation production
   B. Limiting the focal spot size
   C. kVp has no effect on density.
   D. Controlling the quantity of radiation produced

7. Attenuation is another term for:

   A. Molecular collision
   B. Absorption
   C. Crystal interaction
   D. Penetration

8. Which of the following formulas describes the mathematical relationship between mAs and distance?

   A. $\dfrac{mAs_1}{mAs_2} = \dfrac{(D_1)^2}{(D_2)^2}$

   B. $\dfrac{(D_1)^2}{mAs_2} = \dfrac{(D_2)^2}{mAs_1}$

   C. $\dfrac{mAs_2}{mAs_1} = \dfrac{(D_1)^2}{(D_2)^2}$

   D. $\dfrac{(D_1)^2}{(D_2)^2} = \dfrac{(mAs_1)^2}{(mAs_2)^2}$

9. An exposure of an abdomen is made using 200 mAs at 75 kVp with a 400 RS imaging system. If the RS of the imaging system is changed to 800 RS, how does this alter the technical factors?

   A. Increase the mAs by a factor of 4
   B. Decrease the mAs by a factor of 2
   C. Increase the kVp by 15% and decrease the mAs by a factor of 2
   D. Increase the kVp by a factor of 4

10. As the relative speed of an imaging system increases, the mAs will:

    A. Increase
    B. Decrease
    C. Be directly proportional
    D. Be squared

11. If all exposure factors remain constant, which grid would provide the maximum efficiency of scatter absorption?

    A. 5:1
    B. 8:1
    C. 10:1
    D. 12:1

12. The primary function of a filter is to:

    A. Absorb low-energy radiation
    B. Absorb all energy levels of radiation
    C. Produce a monoenergetic beam
    D. Reduce scatter radiation

13. The origin of off-focus radiation is:

    A. The patient
    B. The table

C. The grid

D. The tube

14. You have radiographed an AP abdomen of your patient. The radiologist requests an AP spot view of L4–L5 on an 8 × 10. If all the exposure factors remain the same, the resultant spot film will:

    A. Have an increased density

    B. Have a decrease in resolution

    C. Appear to have a decrease in density

    D. Have a longer scale of contrast

15. Additive and destructive pathology may require an alteration of:

    A. kVp and/or mAs

    B. SID

    C. Focal spot size

    D. mA

16. You are radiographing a patient's femur. If the anode heel effect is to be used, the _____ should be placed over the _____.

    A. Anode; hip joint

    B. Cathode; hip joint

    C. Anode; knee joint

    D. More than one but not all of the above

17. A soft tissue neck is an example of:

    A. Short-scale, high-contrast radiograph

    B. High-kVp, low-contrast radiograph

    C. Low-kVp, high-contrast

    D. Long scale, low-contrast

18. The quality of the primary radiation is directly affected by:

    A. kVp

    B. Film-screen combinations

    C. Grids

    D. SID

19. Selecting 80 kVp ensures that the resultant radiation will be:

    A. 80 keV

    B. Polyenergetic

    C. Monoenergetic

    D. Homogeneous

20. Increasing the collimation will result in:

    A. A shorter scale of contrast

    B. Increased primary beam radiation

    C. A longer scale of contrast

    D. An increase in secondary radiation

21. Radiographic grids will reduce scatter radiation between:

    A. The anode and the tube housing

    B. The tube and the patient

    C. The patient and the radiographic film

    D. Radiographic grids do not affect scatter.

22. Filtration that is placed between the patient and the primary beam will affect the resultant:

    1. Contrast

    2. Patient dosage

    3. Detail

    A. 1 only

    B. 2 only

    C. 1 and 2

    D. 1, 2, and 3

23. Two exposures were taken with a step wedge. Number 1 was with an abdomen phantom at 70 kVp and Number 2 with a skull phantom at 65 kVp. Which of the following statements are true?

    1. Exposure Number 1 will demonstrate short scale; high-contrast.

    2. Exposure Number 2 will demonstrate short scale; high-contrast.

    3. Exposure Number 1 will demonstrate long scale; low-contrast.

    4. Exposure Number 2 will demonstrate long scale; low-contrast.

    A. 1 only

    B. 2 only

    C. 2 and 3 only

    D. All are correct.

24. A patient diagnosed with gout and ascites requires a radiograph of the great toe and abdomen. You would:

    A. Increase exposure factors for the abdomen and decrease for the toe

    B. Decrease exposure factors for the abdomen and increase for the toe

    C. Increase the exposure for the abdomen only

    D. No adjustment in exposure factors is necessary.

25. Calculate the amount of penumbra that will be imaged for the following:

100 cm—SID	75—kVp
5 cm—OID	350—mAs
300—RS	12:1 grid
1.0 mm—focal spot size	

    A. 0.413 cm
    B. 0.134 mm
    C. 0.0413 mm
    D. 1.341 mm

26. Which of the following combinations will produce the least amount of magnification?

    A. Short SID and long OID
    B. Long SID and short OID
    C. Short SID and short OID
    D. Long SID and long OID

27. A radiograph is taken with a large amount of object-to-image distance. Which of the following will help minimize the magnification of the structure being imaged and maximize the resolution?

    A. Decrease the SID and use a large focal spot.
    B. Increase the SID and use a small focal spot.
    C. Maintain the SID and use a small focal spot.
    D. SID and focal spot size will affect only the magnification but have no effect on the resolution.

28. Film and intensifying screens that will provide the greatest line pairs per millimeter have the following:

    A. Thick emulsion layer and large crystals
    B. Thin emulsion layer and small crystals
    C. Thick emulsion layer and small crystals
    D. Thin emulsion layer and large crystals

29. Peristalsis is considered:

    A. Involuntary motion
    B. Voluntary motion
    C. Spontaneous motion
    D. Indiscriminate motion

30. Which of the following pharmaceutical agents can be used to decrease peristalsis?

    1. Glucagon
    2. Pro-Banthīne
    3. Gastrographin

    A. 1 only
    B. 3 only
    C. 1 and 2
    D. 1 and 3

31. Automography utilizes:

    A. CT scanners to optimize visualization
    B. The patient's own breathing pattern to optimize visualization
    C. The patient's own peristalsis to optimize visualization
    D. Hypocycloidal tomographic patterns to optimize visualization

32. Automography is not used for which of the following radiologic procedures?

    A. Sternum
    B. Nephrotomography
    C. Lateral thoracic spine
    D. Transthoracic humerus

33. A chest lesion is located 2″ from the image receptor at a SID of 72″. What is the magnification factor?

    A. 0.2″
    B. 1.5″
    C. 1.2″
    D. 1.7″

34. Calculate the magnification factor for the following:

75 kVp	45 mAs
FFS—1.5 mm	150 cm
5 cm—OID	10:1 grid
RS—200	
3-phase, 12-pulse generator	

    A. 1.034 cm
    B. 0.103 mm
    C. 2.356 mm
    D. 3.005 cm

35. Using Figure 6–15 in Chapter 6 (see also Fig. A–6), which H&D curve depicts the film that has the thickest emulsion with the largest crystals?

    A. Film A
    B. Film B
    C. Film C
    D. Film D

36. The blue tint that is used in the base material of the radiographic film serves to:

    1. Prevent the cross-talk
    2. Provide greater visual acuity
    3. Decrease the base plus fog

    A. 1 only
    B. 3 only
    C. 1 and 2
    D. 1 and 3

37. Which radiographic film type provides the maximum amount of radiographic detail?

    A. Duplicating
    B. Subtraction
    C. Single emulsion
    D. Duplitized

38. Which of the following is true regarding solarization of radiographic film?

    A. The film is at D Max.
    B. The film is at D Min.
    C. The film used is duplitized
    D. The film is used only in digital substraction

39. Solarized film is:

    A. Dental film
    B. Mammographic film
    C. Duplitized film
    D. Duplicating film

40. You are duplicating a radiograph and use an exposure time of 4 sec in the copy machine. The resultant film is darker than the original radiograph. What could you use to correct this problem?

    A. 8 sec of exposure time
    B. 2 sec of exposure time
    C. 3 sec of exposure time
    D. 1 sec of exposure time

41. Which image receptor provides the greatest resolution?

    A. A calcium tungstate screen cassette and film
    B. A rare earth cassette and film
    C. A VDT (visual display terminal)
    D. A cardboard holder and film

42. A technologist uses a focused grid (48″ to 72″) for a portable abdomen examination, with a SID of 36″. The resulting radiograph will exhibit which of the following?

    A. Underexposed in the center of the film
    B. Underexposed at one edge of the film
    C. Underexposed at both edges of the film
    D. Underexposed evenly over the entire radiograph

43. Technique charts may be:

    A. Fixed kVp
    B. Fixed anatomically
    C. Variable kVp
    D. More than one, but not all of the above

44. A PA chest radiograph, exposed using automatic exposure control, results in an overexposed image. The most likely cause of this is:

    A. Only the center ion chamber was selected
    B. Only the outer ion chambers were selected
    C. There was insufficient backup time.
    D. A large focal spot was used.

45. To prevent films from sticking to each other, the films should be stored:

    A. Between 40° and 60° at 60% to 70% humidity
    B. Between 60° and 70° at 40% to 60% humidity
    C. Between 70° and 80° at 40% to 60% humidity
    D. In a cool and moist environment

46. Which is not a type of radiographic film fog?

    A. Chemical fog
    B. Age fog
    C. Temperature fog
    D. Freezer fog

47. Radiographic film that is exposed to radiation is _____ more sensitive to radiation than unexposed radiographic film.

    A. $1\times$
    B. $2\times$
    C. $3\times$
    D. $4\times$

48. If the technologist's hands are wet while handling the film, which of the following may be demonstrated?

    A. Emulsion artifacts
    B. Static discharge artifacts
    C. Smudge artifacts
    D. More than one but not all of the above

49. Lead radiopaque markers, indicating right and left disposition, placed prior to the exposure are:

    A. One of the many ways to mark a radiograph
    B. The only recognized legal method of marking a radiograph
    C. Not acceptable for tightly collimated projections; use stickers
    D. Sometimes unable to be used due to equipment limitations; use another method

50. Which of the following is known as a universal solvent?

    A. Potassium bromide
    B. Acetic acid
    C. Sodium carbonate
    D. Water

51. Which reducing agent is responsible for the toe portion of the H&D curve?

    A. Phenidone
    B. Hydroquinone
    C. Glutaraldehyde
    D. Sodium sulfide

52. Which of the following developer processing agents hardens the emulsion of the radiographic film?

    A. Phenidone
    B. Potassium bromide
    C. Sodium sulfite
    D. Glutaraldehyde

53. Which of the following processing chemicals are alkaline in nature?

    A. Developer
    B. Fixer
    C. Stop bath
    D. Water bath

54. Which of the following is true regarding the fixer solution?

    A. Removes unexposed silver halide crystals
    B. Softens the emulsion
    C. Neutralizes the acidic developer
    D. Regulates the temperature of the emulsion

55. How long will the wash process take in a 90-sec processor?

    A. 20 sec
    B. 30 sec
    C. 45 sec
    D. 60 sec

56. The cross-over rollers are:

    A. Large and numerous
    B. Small and act as squeegees
    C. Found only between the fixer and the wash
    D. The reason for pi line artifacts

57. The chemical responsible for unexposed silver halide removal is:

    A. Phenidone
    B. Acetic acid
    C. Ammonia thiosulfate
    D. Water

58. Which of the following is the hardening agent in the fixer solution?

    A. Glutaraldehyde
    B. Sodium sulfite
    C. Potassium alum
    D. Acetic acid

59. The circulation system is:

    A. An open system
    B. A closed system
    C. Not part of the wash
    D. More than one but not all of the above

60. The silver reclaiming process occurs at which point in the processing system?

    A. Developer
    B. Fixer
    C. Stop bath
    D. Wash

61. The darkroom safelight has an average wattage of:

    A. 7 to 15 watts
    B. 10 to 15 watts
    C. 15 to 25 watts
    D. 30 watts

62. Processing quality assurance requires the use of:

    A. A sensitometer and penetrometer
    B. A densitometer and penetrometer
    C. A sensitometer and densitiometer
    D. A sensitometer and the H&D curve

63. Pi line artifacts are usually associated with:

    A. Faulty gears
    B. Guide shoes
    C. Transport rollers
    D. Cross-contamination

64. Dirty rollers may cause:

    A. Cross-contamination
    B. Pick-off
    C. Pi lines
    D. More than one but not all of the above

65. A processed radiograph comes out of the processor with a white crystal-like coating on it. What is a likely cause of this problem?

    A. Exhausted developer solution
    B. Exhausted fixer solution
    C. Insufficient wash bath
    D. Low temperature

66. Which of the following contributes to increased magnification?

    A. Increased SOD
    B. Increased SID
    C. Decreased OID
    D. Decreased SOD

67. The only legal method of radiographic identification of patient data is:

    A. Lead opaque markers
    B. Flashing the radiograph or electronic capture
    C. Labeling the radiograph with a sticker
    D. More than one, but not all of the above

68. The radiographic exposure factor that controls the radiographic quality is:

    A. mAs
    B. kVp
    C. Quality assurance
    D. Focal spot size

69. Under which of the following circumstances will patient motion not degrade the radiographic quality?

    A. Involuntary motion during an AP abdominal radiograph
    B. Voluntary motion during a lateral chest radiograph
    C. Breathing motion during a lateral thoracic spine radiograph
    D. Any motion degrades the radiographic quality.

70. Which of the following factors will affect the recorded detail on the radiograph?

    A. Film-screen combinations
    B. SID
    C. Focal spot size
    D. All of the above

71. Which of the following factors will increase the amount of distortion that will be recorded on the radiograph?

    A. Increased tube angulation
    B. Increased SID
    C. Decreased OID
    D. Increased SOD

72. The selection of technical factors is directly dependent upon:

    A. The age of the patient
    B. The size of the patient
    C. The pathologic disease the patient is diagnosed with
    D. All of the above

73. If the mAs factor is to be altered, what change will make a visible difference on the radiograph?

    A. Doubling the mAs
    B. 20% of the original mAs value
    C. 50% of the new mAs value
    D. 30% of the original mAs value

74. Gonadal shielding should be employed:
    A. Every time a pediatric patient is radiographed
    B. Any time the shield does not interfere with the area being imaged
    C. Only on women who are within their reproductive age
    D. Only on pregnant women

75. The main purpose of the radiologic requisition is:
    A. To bill the patient
    B. To allow for the patient's films to be filed properly
    C. To allow all caregivers pertinent information about the patient
    D. None of the above

Answers appear at the back of the book.

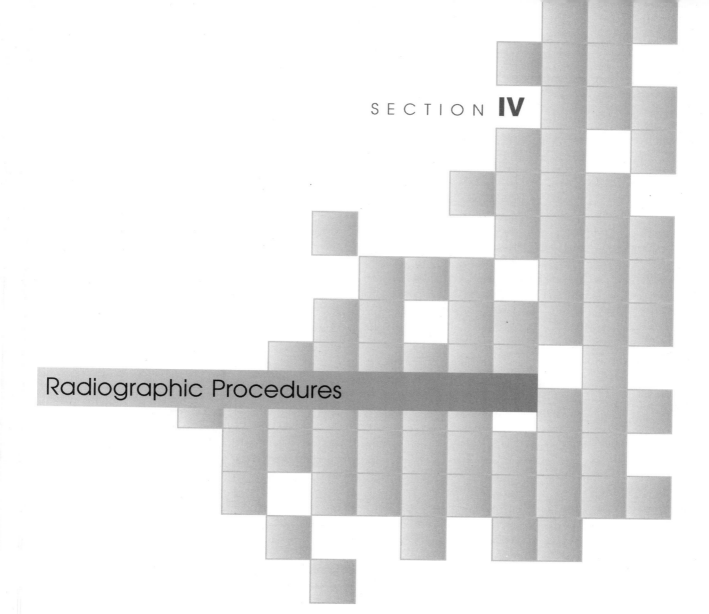

Radiographic Procedures

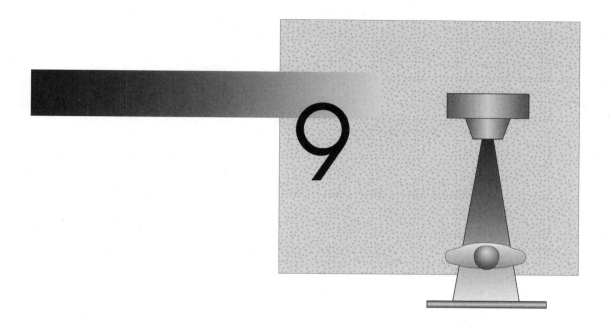

GENERAL PROCEDURAL CONSIDERATIONS

Every one of us has, at some point in our lives, either been a patient or known someone close to us who was. It is never an easy time. Fear seems to surround the occasion. When people are afraid, they may exhibit a variety of emotions, not always pleasant. The primary step that a radiographer can take to ensure a successful procedure is winning the patient's confidence, and the best way to do it is to be professional and friendly.

- Attempt to pronounce the patient's name correctly and clearly.
- Identify the patient by a secondary means (check the patient's name band, date of birth, address, and so on).
- Introduce yourself and anyone else involved in the procedure.

PATIENT PREPARATION

Patient education is a hot topic these days. The Joint Commission on Accreditation of Healthcare Organizations (JCAHO) and other accrediting agencies are declaring it our duty to duly inform the patient and/or the patient's caregiver regarding the procedure and any postprocedural follow-up. This means you must understand the procedure well enough to explain it to someone else. You must also be able to ascertain how well your audience will comprehend your explanation.

- Assess your patient or check the chart for any nursing evaluations previously documented.
- Determine whether you will require additional support to prepare and educate properly (foreign language interpreters, sign language interpreters, nurses, doctors, and so on).
- Document, if necessary, that you have fully informed your patient and/or the caregiver.
- Provide time for questions. Don't assume that the patient understands you the first time around.
- Provide written instructions for postprocedural recommendations, if necessary.
- Provide a telephone number so that the patient may contact the facility with questions and concerns.

Educating your patient is not the only requirement for a successful procedure. Patients who require special instruction must be identified before the examination begins. A 6 year old having a voiding cystourethrogram (VCU) needs reassurance before, during, and after the procedure that it is all right to void on the table. This is especially difficult when it is realized that half of a child's life has been focused on specifically not doing what you are asking him or her to do!

Patients receiving lower gastrointestinal tract examinations have to understand that if they cannot retain the barium, the examination will be repeated. If this is presented with concern and dignity, most patients oblige. It is especially helpful to have intravenous pyelogram (IVP) patients void prior to the procedure. If their bladders are empty to begin with, there is less likelihood that they will ask to void prior to the anticipated time. It also presents well on the scout or preliminary radiograph, neither obscuring nor falsely presenting pathology or anatomical variation. These are just a few examples of the importance of precise instruction.

Patients should be informed about changing out of their street clothing whenever necessary before specific examinations. It seems that today very few radiographers interpret this as necessary. Radiographic journals are full of artifact articles that demonstrate just what can happen if the patient is not properly attired for a study. Pathology is missed or misinterpreted by the radiologist because the tee shirt that the patient wore had some type of decal that created an artifact. Hair braids, dentures, denim jeans, toupees, bandages, dressings, and earrings, which can pierce just about any spot on or in the human body, can also have deleterious effects on the radiographic outcome.

In summary:

- Change your patient properly.
- Determine whether your patient is wearing or harboring any type of device, decorative or otherwise, that may obscure or distort detail on the resultant radiograph.
- Provide a safe, secure location for your patient's belongings.
- Provide a gown, or if necessary, two gowns, to cover your patient fully for modesty. Use a sheet to cover exposed body areas not being radiographed.
- Allow your patients to keep their shoes on or provide disposable slippers if they are expected to walk around.
- Remove bandages/dressings only when necessary and with permission of the physician and/or nurse. Bloody, gaping wounds or burns are best left dressed, despite artifact production. Use common sense.

EQUIPMENT CAPABILITIES

Room preparation is equally important for a successful examination. First, selecting the correct room for the procedure is a consideration. You must know your equipment and its capabilities. For example, if your patient's study requires weight-bearing feet, you will appear rather foolish if you begin the examination and realize that the tube doesn't go down far enough. The patient's confidence in you is now in question, as you hunt around the department, patient in tow, hoping to find another room. Another example is in the examination of a baby or toddler. Would you prefer to use a room that has a generator providing 300 mA or one with 600 mA capability? Let's hope you know the answer. If not, read on.

Setting up the room ahead of time is a great concept. Just knowing that you have everything necessary at your fingertips to complete the examination is comforting. The patient will think you are well organized—and you are! Radiologists who normally breeze in and out of the room so quickly that you are uncertain if they've noticed anything will notice. It is something to strive toward.

While preparing the room, be especially careful to notice any residual contrast medium retained on sponges, tables, or mats. This too will provide some mysterious artifacts. Crumpled sheets and blankets can also add unwanted artifacts to a radiograph. Use them as necessary, just make sure they are clean and smooth. Obviously, maintaining a clean and orderly environment for your patients is paramount. Take the time to clean and refresh the room after every case. Maintain order throughout the examination as well. Sort the exposed cassettes from the unexposed to eliminate double exposures. Properly discard used syringes promptly; this eliminates any unintentional needle sticks. Urinals and bedpans are best disposed of immediately.

- Know your equipment's capability and compatibility for each procedure.
- Prepare your room prior to each procedure.
- Keep your room organized throughout each procedure.
- Keep your room clean and stocked postprocedure.

POSITIONING TERMINOLOGY

Nothing seems to confuse first-year radiography students more than radiographic positioning terminology. Basically, there are three different ways to describe what may appear to be the same thing. No wonder there's confusion!

Projection

Imagine that you are the x-ray beam. How do you enter and exit from the patient's body? Do you go in from the back (posterior) and leave from the front (anterior) to expose the film? That would be considered a PA projection. Let's get more difficult now. Let's remember that you are the x-ray beam. Only this time you enter under the chin (submental) and exit at the topmost portion of the skull (vertex). What is the projection?

It would be a submentovertical projection. It defines the direction and entrance and exit points of the actual x-ray beam. This is extremely important in positioning because the anatomy that is located in the path where your x-ray beam is exiting will be in the center of your radiograph under optimum conditions.

View

Now we get to pretend we are the cassette or any other type of image receptor. Imagine that the patient is having a standard chest radiograph. You have become the cassette. You are looking at the patient. What do you see? You see the front (anterior) portion of the patient's body first, then the posterior. We would then refer to this as an AP view. Even though the projection in this case would be PA, the view is AP. Another way of looking at it is that every time radiologists look at a radiograph on a view box, they are pretending that they are the image receptor, and that becomes their vantage point of viewing the patient.

A lot of people seem to be confused regarding the word "view." It gets used synonymously with projection by some of the best-respected medical personnel. Philip Ballinger has eliminated view from his positioning texts, leaving only its definition. Just stick to projection and you'll be fine.

Position

Position refers to bodily placement of the patient, nothing more, nothing less. Our technology embraces the correct positioning skills required to demonstrate particular anatomy. How else would we know how to place a patient's body unless we used positioning terminology? For example: The order is for a Chest, Four View (there's that word again!). How do you position the body? Decubitus? Oblique? These words were invented for a reason. Lateromedial wouldn't cut it. But if you are told that the patient must be erect for an AP lordotic, left lateral, right anterior oblique, and left anterior oblique, now you would know exactly what is required to position that patient.

How many projections are noted in the previous scenario? Hopefully, you've answered "AP." That's it. All the rest refer to patient position.

A lot of wonderful people developed radiographic methodology throughout the years by regarding how to visualize the required anatomy by different means. Some of their names are Law, Waters, Mayer, Neer, Jones. The Registry used to use the proper names of specific methods of positioning, but the problem was that these people didn't dream up just one method, they thought of several. How do you differentiate between one Waters and another? Fortunately, in the early 1980s there began a trend to refer to these methods more accurately, so there would be less confusion. So by today's standards, a Towne's projection of the skull is now referred to as an AP axial. The reverse, a Haas, is now a PA axial. This naming process includes the projection and tube alignment. We will explore this further in the positioning chapter. KUB and flatplate are two words used to describe an AP projection of a supine abdomen. Flatplate is an outdated term and should be eliminated. KUB refers to visualization of the kidneys, ureters, and bladder all on one radiograph. A complete list of positioning terminology may be found by referring to the references' glossaries.

PATIENT RESPIRATION AND MOTOR CONTROL

Patient Instructions

Unwanted motion destroys the radiographic image. It is imperative for you to discuss this with the patient before taking an exposure. How familiar are you with this scenario? The radiographer has scrupulously positioned the patient for a chest procedure. Everything is perfect. The radiographer begins the breathing instructions from the control booth: "Take a deep breath in and hold it," while "rotaring" and exposing almost simultaneously. Just as the exposure button clicks in, the patient turns toward the booth and asks, "Now?" It is probably all too familiar.

Radiographers need to remember that although this might be the tenth chest examination that they have done today, their present patients may be on their first chest examination experience. It really doesn't require an inordinate amount of dialogue to express to the patient the importance of correct breathing or lack of it. Instructions may be incorporated while you are positioning the patient. Always ask whether the patient understands.

Exposure factors also help control motion. The best way to eliminate unwanted motion is to use the shortest time possible. That means selection of a high mA setting. What good is a small focal spot selection via low mA setting in order to achieve the best detail, if the resultant radiograph is full of motion? You must know your patients. Assess them to see whether they will be able to hold still and suspend respiration for the time required to obtain the necessary exposures.

Age-specific competencies are also being required by accrediting agencies. You must demonstrate that you are competent to radiograph a neonate, infant, toddler, child, adolescent, adult, and mature adult in order to continue to do so. Certain factors are required and measured. Immobilization techniques and selection of appropriate exposure factors are just some that apply in this portion of the text. If an area is deemed weak, inservicing must take place with a measured improvement demonstrated.

Proper immobilization requires specific accessories in order to obtain the desired results. Compression bands, sponges, sandbags, specially designed immobilizers, sheets, tape, Ace bandages—all these contribute to eliminating unwanted motion. Restraining infants and children is of concern to most parents. A full explanation is required so that they understand the ramifications if it is not done. Most parents would prefer that you restrain their child to refrain from additional exposures.

Increasing the source-to-image distance (SID), minimizing the object-to-image distance (OID), and using a small focal spot, as long as a high mA can also be used, will provide the maximum detail when used with proper patient instruction and immobilization techniques. It is also important to remember that using a higher-speed film-screen combination will also reduce your exposure factors. If normally you use a detail system for extremities and you have a young child who will not hold still, even with immobilization, go to a faster speed system and sacrifice some detail for elimination of motion.

Involuntary motions, such as peristalsis and generalized muscle spasm, are greater problems. Some injectable medications will limit involuntary motion. Glucagon and Pro-Banthīne are two that are used to relax the GI tract, reducing peristalsis, allowing the patient greater retention, and also providing the radiologist more time for fluoroscopic evaluation of the anatomy. Always ask a nurse or physician if the patient can receive a muscle-relaxing medication either prior to or during the procedure, if necessary. To attempt to radiograph a patient writhing in pain from spasm produced by a kidney stone without some type of pharmaceutical relaxant is next to impossible, even for the most highly educated radiographer.

Try to keep these ideas in mind to limit motion:

■ Assess your patient.
■ Provide complete patient instruction.
■ Select proper exposure factors (lowest exposure time possible).
■ Use immobilization when necessary.
■ Increase SID, minimize OID.
■ Increase the speed of your screen-film.
■ Request medication for the uncooperative patient in pain.

TECHNIQUE AND POSITIONING VARIATIONS

It would be a wonderful thing if a standard were established that would apply to every patient, no matter what. You would be able to learn just the standard positions with their associated exposure factors, and that would be it. Unfortunately, a multitude of variables is associated with this professional field of study. There is no easy way around it.

Certain situations call for modifications. You will require modifications, as a rule, for the following categories of patients:

■ Pediatric patients
■ Mature adult patients
■ Severely ill patients
■ Trauma patients
■ Pregnant patients

Let's approach each of these individually.

Pediatric Patients

Several factors must be assessed when performing radiographic procedures on pediatric patients:

■ Pediatric competency level of radiographer
■ Immobilization technique application
■ Radiation protection for patient, assistants, and medical personnel
■ Infection control practice (standard precautions)
■ Knowledge of positioning variations
　Translateral applications
　AP, rather than some standard PA projections
　Deviation from standard positioning angles, due to immature bone development and body habitus
　Specialty positions used primarily in pediatric cases

■ Exposure factor selection (minimal time must be used to limit motion)

Mature Adults

Mature adults are similar to pediatric patients in some regard, so that some of the variables are the same:

■ Mature adult level of competency for radiographer
■ Immobilization/restraint application
■ Infection control practice (standard precautions)
■ Positioning variations, (translaterals, reverse positioning so that the patient doesn't have to turn)
■ Comfort considerations (table mats, blankets, sponges, and so on)
■ Exposure factor selection (short time to limit motion, low kVp to maximize contrast)

Severely Ill Patients

It is important to limit the amount of time that this type of patient is in the radiology department. Many facilities are now involved with patient focus care plans, and many examinations are done at the bedside. Some additional considerations are:

■ Limiting transfer and movement of the patient
■ Obtaining sufficient help when moving the patient for any reason
■ Comfort considerations (use of table mats, sponges, and so on)
■ Infection control practice (standard precautions)
■ Positioning variations (limit routine positions; when necessary, use translaterals, reverse positioning to limit patient turns)
■ Exposure factor selection (know the various disease processes and how they present in radiography; select the appropriate factors)

Trauma Patients

This is perhaps the most challenging patient population for the radiographer. In one respect you are limited immediately by what can actually be obtained on a trauma patient, just by the nature of the injuries. But this is where the challenge begins. If you are a knowledgeable radiographer, you may now employ all of the unusual positions that can't be routinely used. It is this creativity that will provide the radiologist with all of the necessary information to dictate an accurate report. Consider the following:

- Limiting transfer and movement of the patient
- Obtaining sufficient help for any patient activity
- Infection control practice (standard precautions)
- Positioning variations (translaterals and reverse positioning become necessary, variant positions and limited studies become acceptable)
- Exposure factor selection (short time to limit motion)

Pregnant Patients

Every facility should have an established written policy for imaging the pregnant patient. Refer to the specific policy and procedure of your facility. There are generalities that may be referred to, however, if necessary.

- Establish that your patient may be pregnant (doctor's note, 10-day rule, and/or laboratory results).
- Recognize the patient's ultimate right to give consent for the procedure.

- Shield, and document the fact that you have done so.
- Limit positions, when necessary.
- Select appropriate exposure factor (use high kVp if you are radiating the fetal region).
- Be prepared to answer basic radiation protection/biology questions or at least be able to refer the patient to the proper professional (radiation safety officer, physicist).

This summarizes the specific categories of patients, but the radiographer should be prepared to deviate from the standard whenever it is beneficial to the patient. Being familiar with various positions so that they may be substituted at will is the goal of the competent radiographer. These variations must always be documented for the radiologist so that he or she understands the reference point of the position and reports accordingly.

Bibliography

Ballinger PW: Merrill's Atlas of Radiographic Positions and Radiologic Procedures. 7th ed. St. Louis, Mosby–Year Book, 1991
Bontrager KL: Textbook of Radiographic Positioning and Related Anatomy. 3rd ed. St. Louis, Mosby–Year Book, 1993
Joint Commission on Accreditation of Healthcare Organizations. Essentials 1997. Oakbrook Terrace, IL, JCAHO, 1996

Chapter 9 Questions

1. Which method should be used to identify your patient?

   A. Ask for first and last name.
   B. Request date of birth.
   C. Check name bracelet.
   D. All of the above

2. Your patient speaks and comprehends only Spanish.

   A. There is no need to explain the procedure, because you can't speak Spanish.
   B. You assume the nurse explained the examination.
   C. You provide an interpreter for the patient, so that the patient fully understands what is being done.
   D. You hope that the radiologist can explain the procedure.

3. Your patient requires a knee examination. The department is very busy. You decide it is best to:

   A. Not change the patient
   B. Ask the patient to roll up his jeans
   C. Ask the patient to remove his pants
   D. Refuse to radiograph the patient until the physician removes the bandage

4. Age-specific competencies ensure that the:

   A. Geriatric patient is able to withstand the radiographic procedure.
   B. The technologist possesses the skills required to radiograph patients of different ages.
   C. The radiologist is old enough to interpret the images.
   D. The pediatric patient is radiographed with parental consent.

5. The most appropriate exposure factors for a pediatric case are:

   A. 50 mA/1.0 sec
   B. 100 mA/0.5 sec
   C. 200 mA/0.25 sec
   D. 500 mA/0.10 sec

6. An x-ray beam enters the parietal bone and exits through the orbit. This would be termed a(n):

   A. Rhese position
   B. Parieto-orbital projection
   C. Orbitoparietal projection
   D. Oblique view

7–10. Match the following:
   The patient requires an abdominal radiograph. The patient is supine.(7)
   The central ray is entering the anterior aspect and exiting from the posterior aspect of the body.(8)
   The resultant radiograph will provide a(n)_____view.(9)
   The final radiograph will demonstrate the kidneys, ureters, and bladder.(10)

   7. ____   a. KUB   e. AP projection
   8. ____   b. AP view   f. Position
   9. ____   c. PA view   g. Flatplate
   10. ____ d. PA   h. Superior-inferior
                projection   projection

11. The most important factor in eliminating motion is:

    A. Exposure time
    B. kVp selection
    C. Use of a grid
    D. Focal spot size

12. Factors affecting detail are:

    A. SID
    B. OID
    C. FSS (focal spot size)
    D. All of the above

13. A high-speed film-screen system provides:

    A. Less detail, less exposure, less motion
    B. More detail, more exposure, more motion
    C. Less detail, more exposure, less motion
    D. More detail, less exposure, more motion

14. Certain diseases require changes in the following:

    A. Standard precautions
    B. Patient shielding practice
    C. Exposure factor selection
    D. All of the above

15. Variations in positioning are most often applied to:

    A. Neonates
    B. Bowel cancer patients
    C. Women expecting twins
    D. Motor vehicle accident patients

Answers appear at the end of the book.

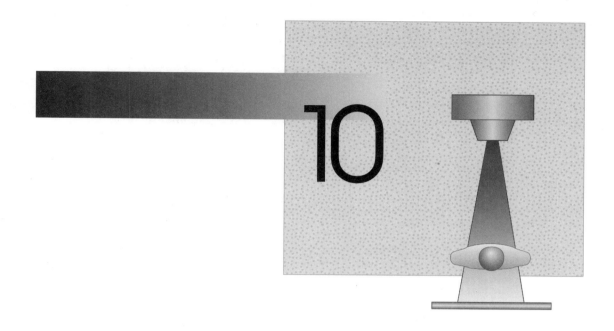

SPECIFIC IMAGING PROCEDURES

Charts
Upper Extremity
Lower Extremity
Hips and Pelvis
Vertebral Column
Cranium
Thorax
Abdomen

Skeletal Surveys
Scoliosis Series
Long Bone Measurement
Bone Age
Bone Survey

Contrast
Arthrography
Myelography
Hysterosalpingography
Venography
Esophagogram
Upper Gastrointestinal Series
Small Bowel Series
Lower Gastrointestinal Series
Urologic Studies
Cholecystography
Tomography

This chapter is designed for ease in reviewing radiographic positioning and the associated anatomy. Only the most current and frequently used positions are included. (Greater detail or information about unusual positions may be obtained from the Bibliography for this chapter.)

The positions are placed in anatomically categorized charts per projection, central ray placement, structures demonstrated, and evaluation criteria utilized. All positioning is done at 40″ SID unless otherwise specified. Directly following each major positioning section, you will find anatomy references correlating to the previous positions.

The following abbreviations appear in the charts:

AP– anteroposterior
ASIS– anterior superior iliac spine
CT– computed tomography
EAM– external auditory meatus
fib– fibula
LAO– left anterior oblique
LPO– left posterior oblique
PA– posteroanterior
RAO– right anterior oblique
RPO– right posterior oblique
SC– sternoclavicular
SMV– submentovertical
tib– tibia
TMJ– temporomandibular joint

Chart 10–1 ▪ **UPPER EXTREMITY**				
	PROJECTION	**CENTRAL RAY**	**STRUCTURES SHOWN**	**EVALUATION CRITERIA**
FIRST DIGIT (Thumb) *(See Figures 10–1, 10–2)*	AP	Directed perpendicular to the metacarpophalangeal joint	AP projected of the entire 1st digit to include the 1st metacarpal and carpal (scaphoid)	• Visualization of phalanges, first metacarpal, and scaphoid • Interphalangeal and metacarpophalangeal joints should be open • True AP projection free of rotation
	PA oblique (45°)	Directed perpendicular to the metacarpophalangeal joint	Oblique projection of the entire 1st digit to include the 1st metacarpal and carpal (scaphoid)	• First metacarpal and phalanges should appear at a 45° oblique • Visualization from distal phalanx to scaphoid • Interphalangeal and metacarpophalangeal joints should be open
	Lateral	Directed perpendicular to the metacarpophalangeal joint	Lateral projection of the entire 1st digit to include the 1st metacarpal and carpal (scaphoid)	• Visualization from distal phalanx to scaphoid • Interphalangeal and metacarpophalangeal joints should be open • Position of the fingernail shows a true lateral position
DIGITS 2–5 *(See Figures 10–1, 10–2)*	PA	Directed perpendicular to the proximal interphalangeal joint	PA projection of the fully extended digit	• Distal metacarpal to distal phalanx visualized without overlap from adjacent digits • Interphalangeal and metacarpophalangeal joint spaces should be open and free of rotation
	PA oblique (45°)	Directed perpendicular to the proximal interphalangeal joint	Oblique projection of the fully extended digit Medial oblique is done for 2nd digit to decrease OID	• Entire digit projected at a 45° oblique without overlap from adjacent digits • Interphalangeal and metacarpophalangeal joint spaces should be open • Distal metacarpal to distal phalanx should be included
	Lateral	Directed perpendicular to the proximal interphalangeal joint	Lateral projection of the fully extended digit Mediolateral for the 2nd digit is done to decrease OID	• Interphalangeal and metacarpophalangeal joint spaces should be open • Proximal metacarpophalangeal joint should not be overlapped by the other digits • Distal metacarpals to distal phalanx should be included

Chart continued on following page

Chart 10–1 ■ **UPPER EXTREMITY** *Continued*				
	PROJECTION	*CENTRAL RAY*	*STRUCTURES SHOWN*	*EVALUATION CRITERIA*
HAND *(See Figures 10–1, 10–2)*	*PA*	Directed perpendicular to the 3rd metacarpophalangeal joint	PA projection of the entire hand (oblique thumb) to include the wrist and distal radius/ulna	• Metacarpophalangeal and interphalangeal joints should be open • All anatomy distal to the radius and ulna should be included • Palmar surface should be flat against the film and free of rotation
	PA oblique (45°)	Directed perpendicular to the 3rd metacarpophalangeal joint	Oblique projection of the entire hand to include the wrist and distal radius/ulna AP oblique (semisupination) when 4th or 5th digit is of interest to avoid overlap of metacarpals	• Minimal of the 3rd-4th and 4th-5th metacarpal shafts • Slight overlap of the metacarpal bases and heads; separation of 2nd and 3rd metacarpals • Metacarpophalangeal and interphalangeal joints should be open • All anatomy distal to the radius and ulna should be included
	Lateral	Directed perpendicular to the 3rd metacarpophalangeal joint	Lateral projection of the entire hand to include the wrist and distal radius/ulna	• Superimposed phalanges, metacarpals, and distal radius and ulna (digits are visualized separately if fan lateral is done) • Thumb should be free of overlap of the other digits • All digits should be fully extended
WRIST *(See Figures 10–1, 10–2)*	*PA*	Directed perpendicular to midcarpal area	PA position of the proximal metacarpals, carpals, and distal radius and ulna	• Include proximal metacarpals and distal radius-ulna • Carpals should be without rotation and without superimposition of metacarpals or radius-ulna • Styloid process of ulna should be visualized
	PA oblique (45°)	Directed perpendicular to mid-carpal	Oblique position of the proximal metacarpals, carpals, and distal radius-ulna	• Include proximal metacarpals, carpals, and distal radius-ulna • Distal radius-ulna should have slight overlap • Visualization of lateral carpal bones, especially the scaphoid and trapezium, with minimum superimposition • Distal ulna superimposed over the radius
	Lateral	Directed perpendicular to mid-carpal area	Lateral position of the distal radius-ulna, carpals, and proximal metacarpals	• Include proximal metacarpals, carpals, and distal radius-ulna • Radius-ulna are directly superimposed • Metacarpals should be superimposed

		Chart 10–1 ■ **UPPER EXTREMITY** *Continued*		
	PROJECTION	**CENTRAL RAY**	**STRUCTURES SHOWN**	**EVALUATION CRITERIA**
	Ulnar flexion (radial deviation)	Directed perpendicular to the scaphoid. May also be performed with a 15°–20° angulation (proximal or distal)	PA projection of the scaphoid and adjacent carpals with open joint spaces	• Wrist should be free of rotation • Scaphoid should be demonstrated with mimimal foreshortening • The degree of flexion is evident by the anatomical position on the radiograph
	Radial flexion (ulnar deviation)	Directed perpendicular to the midcarpal area	Carpal joint spaces on the medial side of the wrist should appear open	• Wrist should be free of rotation • Carpals on the medial side of the wrist should be demonstrated with open joint spaces • The degree of flexion is evident by the anatomical position on the radiograph
FOREARM *(See Figures 10–1, 10–2, 10–3)*	*AP*	Directed perpendicular to the midforearm area	AP projection of the forearm, including the proximal carpals and the elbow joint	• Wrist and elbow joint should be included • Radial head, neck, tuberosity slightly superimposed over the proximal ulna • Supinate hand to avoid crossing of radius and ulna at their proximal end • Humeral epicondyles should not be rotated or elongated or foreshortened • Lower shoulder to place forearm parallel to the film's surface
	Lateral	Directed perpendicular to the midforearm area	Lateral position of the elbow, forearm, and wrist with 90° flexion of the elbow joint	• Wrist and elbow should be included with 90° flexion • Radius-ulna should be superimposed at their distal third • Radial head superimposed over the coronoid process
ELBOW *(See Figures 10–1, 10–3 B & C)*	*AP*	Perpendicular to the midelbow joint; 3/4″ distal to the epicondyles	AP projection of the elbow, including the distal humerus and proximal forearm	• Radial head, neck, and tuberosity should be slightly superimposed over the proximal ulna • Elbow joint should be open, with the epicondyles in a true AP position free of elongation or foreshortening
	AP internal oblique (medial) (hand pronated)	Perpendicular to the midelbow joint; 3/4″ distal to the epicondyles	Oblique position of the elbow joint; coronoid process free of superimposition	• Coronoid process well demonstrated and in profile • Medial epicondyle and trochlea elongated • Olecranon process within its fossa

Chart continued on following page

	Chart 10–1 ▪ **UPPER EXTREMITY** *Continued*			
	PROJECTION	**CENTRAL RAY**	**STRUCTURES SHOWN**	**EVALUATION CRITERIA**
	AP external oblique (lateral) (hand supinated and obliqued 45°)	Perpendicular to the midelbow joint; 3/4″ distal to the epicondyles	Oblique position of the elbow joint; radial head free of superimposition	• Proximal radius free of superimposition of the ulna, including the head, neck, and tuberosity • Lateral epicondyle and capitulum elongated
	Lateral	Perpendicular to the midelbow joint; 3/4″ distal to the epicondyles	Lateral position of the elbow joint in 90° flexion to include the proximal forearm and distal humerus	• Elbow should be flexed at 90° and the joint should be open with epicondyles superimposed • Olecranon visualized in profile • Radial head will slightly superimpose the coronoid process, and the radial tuberosity will face anteriorly
HUMERUS *(See Figures 10–1, 10–4, 10–5)*	*AP*	Directed perpendicular to the midshaft of the humerus	AP projection of the entire length of the humerus, with the maximum visualization of the epicondyles	• Entire humerus to include shoulder and elbow joint • Epicondyles are seen in profile • Humeral head and greater tubercle in profile • Lesser tubercle superimposed between the greater tubercle and humeral head
	Lateral	Directed perpendicular to the midshaft of the humerus	Lateral projection of the entire length of the humerus, with superimposition of the epicondyles	• Entire humerus to include shoulder and elbow joint • Epicondyles superimposed • Lesser tubercle in profile • Greater tubercle superimposed over humeral head
	Transthoracic lateral (proximal humerus)	Directed perpendicular to the surgical neck. (If the patient is unable to elevate the unaffected shoulder, direct the central ray 10° to 15° cephalic) Use breathing technique: low mA, long time exposure	Lateral projection of the proximal two thirds of the humerus seen through the lateral thoracic spine	• Humerus in a true lateral position • Lesser tubercle in profile • A well-defined outline of the proximal humerus • Unaffected side should not superimpose the affected side • Affected side free from superimposition of the thoracic vertebrae
SHOULDER *(See Figures 10–1, 10–5)*	*AP Neutral rotation*	Directed perpendicular to the coracoid process	AP projection of the shoulder joint to include the superior scapula, lateral clavicle, and proximal humerus	• Greater tubercle partially superimposed over the humeral head • Humeral head in partial profile • Slight overlap of the humeral head on the glenoid fossa

	Chart 10–1 ■ **UPPER EXTREMITY** *Continued*			
	PROJECTION	*CENTRAL RAY*	*STRUCTURES SHOWN*	*EVALUATION CRITERIA*
	AP *Internal rotation*	Directed perpendicular to the coracoid process	AP projection of the shoulder joint to include the superior scapula, lateral clavicle, and proximal humerus	• Lesser tubercle in profile medially • Greater tubercle superimposed on the humeral head • Significant overlap of the humeral head on the glenoid fossa
	AP *External rotation*	Directed perpendicular to the coracoid process	AP projection of the shoulder joint to include the superior scapula, lateral clavicle, and proximal humerus	• Humeral head in profile • Glenohumeral joint visualized with minimum overlap of humeral head • Lesser tubercle superimposed on the humeral head • Greater tubercle in profile laterally
	Transthoracic shoulder	Directed perpendicular to the surgical neck. (If the patient is unable to elevate the unaffected shoulder, direct the central ray 10° to 15° cephalic) Use breathing technique: low mA, long time exposure	Lateral projection of the shoulder and proximal humerus	• Scapula, clavicle, and humerus visualized within the lung field, free of superimposition of the thoracic spine • A well-defined outline of the proximal humerus • Unaffected side should not superimpose the affected side
	PA oblique scapular Y	Directed perpendicular to the glenohumeral joint	The humeral head is superimposed over the Y of the scapula placed between the acromion and coracoid processes (for evaluation of dislocation)	• Scapular body is free of the thoracic anatomy • Acromion is projected laterally free from superimposition • Coracoid superimposed or projected above the clavicle • Acromion, coracoid, and scapular body form the letter Y
SCAPULA *(See Figures 10–1, 10–5)*	*AP* *(with arm abducted 90°)*	Directed perpendicular 2″ inferior to the coracoid process	A true AP projection of the scapula	• Axillary border of the scapula free of superimposition • Entire scapula should be included, with most projected through the lung field • Scapular body should not show rotation
	Lateral *(with hand of affected side placed on opposite shoulder, to remove humerus from scapula)*	Directed perpendicular to the midvertebral border of the scapula	A lateral projection of the scapula	• Axillary and vertebral border should be superimposed • Free from superimposition of the thorax and humerus

Chart continued on following page

		PROJECTION	CENTRAL RAY	STRUCTURES SHOWN	EVALUATION CRITERIA
	Chart 10–1 ■ **UPPER EXTREMITY** *Continued*				
CLAVICLE *(See Figures 10–1, 10–5)*		*PA or AP*	Directed perpendicular to the midshaft of the affected clavicle	A true frontal projection of the clavicle (PA will afford a decreased part-film distance)	• Demonstrate the entire clavicle without excessive density • Lateral aspect of the clavicle projected above the scapula • Medial aspect of the clavicle superimposed over the thorax • Must include medial and lateal articulations
		PA or AP axial	PA—Directed 25° to 30° caudad to the supraclavicular fossa (25° to 30° cephalic for AP)	An axial projection of the affected clavicle (PA will afford a decreased part-film distance)	• Most of the clavicle projected above the scapula • Clavicle in a more horizontal position • Entire clavicle should be included without excessive density • Must include medial and lateral articulations
ACROMIOCLAVICULAR ARTICULATIONS *(See Figures 10–1, 10–5)*		*AP* (with and without weights)	Directed perpendicular to the midline at the level of the acromioclavicular joints; 1.5″ above jugular notch	True frontal projection of the acromioclavicular joints (bilaterally) to demonstrate joint separation	• Acromioclavicular joint should be visualized without excessive density or rotation • Should always be done bilaterally with the appropriate markers (RT, LT, w/weights, and w/o weights) at 72″ SID • Performed erect with weights to demonstrate joint separation or dislocation

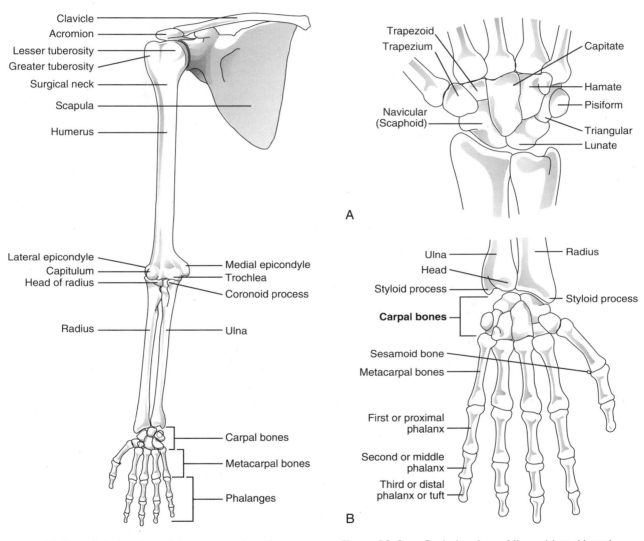

Figure 10-1 ■ Anterior view of the upper extremity.

Figure 10-2 ■ Posterior view of the wrist and hand.

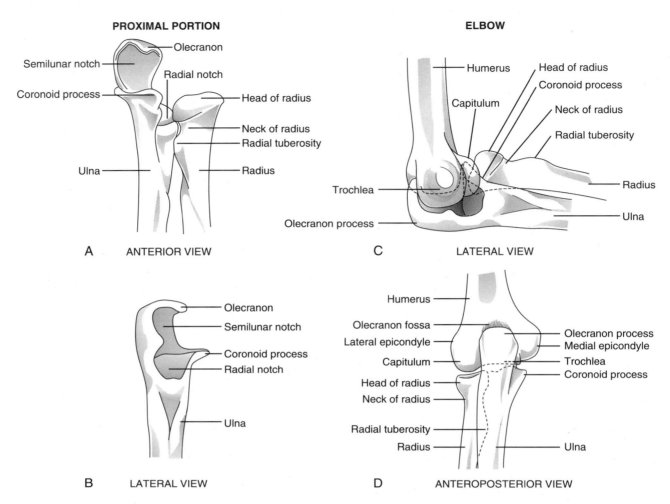

PROXIMAL PORTION

Semilunar notch
Coronoid process
Olecranon
Radial notch
Head of radius
Neck of radius
Radial tuberosity
Ulna
Radius

A ANTERIOR VIEW

Olecranon
Semilunar notch
Coronoid process
Radial notch
Ulna

B LATERAL VIEW

ELBOW

Humerus
Head of radius
Coronoid process
Neck of radius
Radial tuberosity
Capitulum
Radius
Trochlea
Ulna
Olecranon process

C LATERAL VIEW

Humerus
Olecranon fossa
Lateral epicondyle
Capitulum
Head of radius
Neck of radius
Radial tuberosity
Radius
Olecranon process
Medial epicondyle
Trochlea
Coronoid process
Ulna

D ANTEROPOSTERIOR VIEW

Figure 10-3 ■ AP and lateral views of the elbow joint.

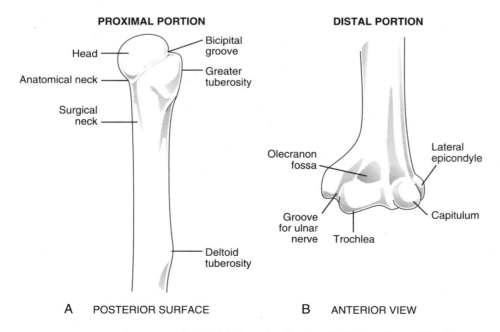

PROXIMAL PORTION

Head
Anatomical neck
Surgical neck
Bicipital groove
Greater tuberosity
Deltoid tuberosity

A POSTERIOR SURFACE

DISTAL PORTION

Olecranon fossa
Groove for ulnar nerve
Trochlea
Lateral epicondyle
Capitulum

B ANTERIOR VIEW

Figure 10-4 ■ Proximal and distal portions of the humerus.

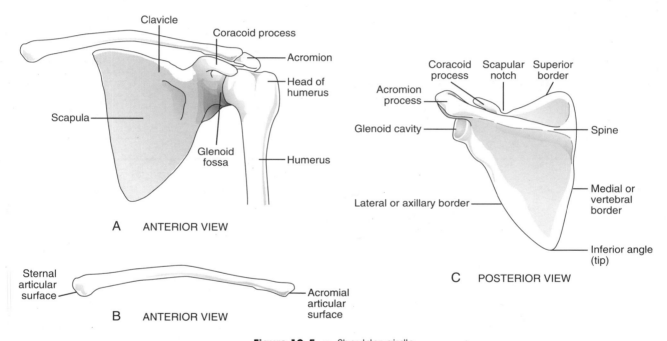

Figure 10-5 ■ Shoulder girdle.

<table>
<tr><td colspan="5" align="center">Chart 10–2 ■ **LOWER EXTREMITY**</td></tr>
<tr><td></td><td>*PROJECTION*</td><td>*CENTRAL RAY*</td><td>*STRUCTURES SHOWN*</td><td>*EVALUATION CRITERIA*</td></tr>
<tr>
<td>**TOES**
(See Figures 10–6, 10–7)</td>
<td>*AP*</td>
<td>Directed perpendicular to the proximal metatarsophalangeal joint
Use 10° to 15° cephalic if interest is metatarsals</td>
<td>Anterior projection of the phalanges and distal metatarsals</td>
<td>• Interphalangeal and metatarsophalangeal joints open
• All phalanges and distal metatarsals demonstrated without rotation
• All anatomy should be included without excessive density</td>
</tr>
<tr>
<td></td>
<td>*Medial oblique* (30°–45°)</td>
<td>Directed perpendicular to the proximal metatarsophalangeal joint</td>
<td>Oblique projection of the distal metatarsals and phalanges</td>
<td>• Interphalangeal joints 2 through 5 should be open
• Digits should not overlap
• Metatarsals to distal phalanges should be included
• All anatomy should be included without excessive density</td>
</tr>
<tr>
<td></td>
<td>*Lateral*</td>
<td>Directed perpendicular to the proximal interphalangeal joint</td>
<td>Lateral projection of the affected digit free of superimposition of adjacent structures</td>
<td>• Interphalangeal and metatarsophalangeal joint should be open
• Phalanges should be in a true lateral
• Affected digit should be free from superimposition on the other digits</td>
</tr>
<tr>
<td>**FEET**
(See Figures 10–6, 10–7)</td>
<td>*AP*</td>
<td>Directed perpendicular or with a 10° to 15° angle toward the heel at the base of the 3rd metatarsal (angle to open the joint spaces)</td>
<td>AP projection of the foot, including the tarsals anterior to the talus to the distal phalanges</td>
<td>• A true AP projection free of rotation
• Overlap of the 2nd to 5th metatarsal bases
• Adequate density of proximal tarsals to distal phalanges
• Metatarsophalangeal joint spaces should be open</td>
</tr>
<tr>
<td></td>
<td>*Medial oblique*
The plantar surface forms a 30° angle with the plane of the film</td>
<td>Directed perpendicular to the base of the 3rd metatarsal</td>
<td>Oblique projection of the entire foot, demonstrating the joint spaces of the lateral tarsals</td>
<td>• 3rd through 5th metatarsal free of superimposition
• Demonstration of most of the tarsals with open joint spaces
• Sinus tarsi should be visualized
• Open joint spaces of the tarsometatarsal joints</td>
</tr>
<tr>
<td></td>
<td>*Lateral*</td>
<td>Directed perpendicular to the base of the 3rd metatarsal</td>
<td>Lateral projection of the foot and ankle to include the distal tibia/fibula</td>
<td>• Metatarsals should be superimposed
• Distal phalanges, entire foot, and distal tibia/fibula should be included with the tibiotalar joint space open
• Fibula should overlap the posterior aspect of the tibia</td>
</tr>
</table>

		Chart 10–2 ▪ **LOWER EXTREMITY** *Continued*		
	PROJECTION	**CENTRAL RAY**	**STRUCTURES SHOWN**	**EVALUATION CRITERIA**
CALCANEUS (*See Figures 10–6, 10–7*)	*Axial* (plantodorsal)	Directed 40° cephalic to the long axis of the foot entering the level of the base of the 5th metatarsal Watch exit point!	An axial projection of the calcaneus to include the talocalcaneal joint space	• Entire calcaneus to include the talocalcaneal joint • True plantodorsal projection free of rotation • The talocalcaneal joint should be adequately demonstrated without excessive density on the inferior aspect of the calcaneus • Affected foot must be dorsiflexed as much as possible
	Lateral	Directed perpendicular to the midpoint of the calcaneus	True lateral position of the calcaneus and ankle joint	• True lateral projection of the calcaneus and ankle joint • Lateral tuberosity and sinus tarsi should be seen clearly • Proximal tarsals should be included
ANKLE (*See Figures 10–6, 10–7 B & C*)	*AP*	Directed perpendicular to the ankle joint; midmalleoli	AP projection of the ankle joint, including the distal tibia and fibula	• Tibiotalar joint (mortise) visualized with minimal overlap • Superimposition of the fibula over the lateral talus • Medial talomalleolar joint should be open without overlap of the medial malleolus on the talus • Dorsiflex foot as much as possible
	Medial oblique (mortise 15°–20°) (45° oblique)	Perpendicular to the ankle, entering at a point midway between the malleoli	AP oblique projection of the ankle 15° rotation to demonstrate mortise joint and 45° rotation to demonstrate distal tibia/fibula (to include base of 5th metatarsal)	• Distal tibia/fibula demonstrated with adequate density • Talus and distal tibia/fibula should be well visualized • Mortise joint should be completely open • 45° oblique • Distal tibia/fibula may overlap the talus
	Lateral (mediolateral)	Directed perpendicular to the medial malleolus	Lateral projection of the distal tibia/fibula, talus, calcaneus, and proximal tarsals (to include base of 5th metatarsal)	• Fibula superimposed over the posterior aspect of the tibia • Tibiotalar joint well visualized • Include proximal tarsals, calcaneus, talus, distal tibia and fibula, and the base of the 5th metatarsal
TIBIA/FIBULA (*See Figures 10–6, 10–8*)	*AP*	Directed perpendicular to the midpoint of the lower leg	AP projection of the tibial/fibula to include the knee and ankle joint	• AP of the entire lower leg to include the knee and ankle joints • The fibula demonstrates overlap on its proximal and distal articulations with the tibia

Chart continued on following page

	PROJECTION	CENTRAL RAY	STRUCTURES SHOWN	EVALUATION CRITERIA
	Lateral (mediolateral)	Directed perpendicular to the midpoint of the lower leg	Lateral projection of the entire tibia, fibula, to include knee and ankle joints	• Distal fibula is superimposed on the posterior tibia • Ankle and knee joints should be in a true lateral • Midshaft of the tibia/fibula should show some separation
KNEE *(See Figures 10–6, 10–9 B & C)*	*AP*	Directed 5° to 7° cephalic to a point ½″ or 1 cm below the patellar apex; reduces distortion of the joint space due to condylar magnification (superimposition)	AP projection of the knee joint, including the tibiofibular articulation	• Knee joint should be equal and open • Patella completely superimposed over the distal femur • Minimal overlap of the fibula on the tibia
	Medial oblique (internal) (45°)	Directed 5° cephalic to a point just inferior to the patellar apex; reduces distortion of the joint space due to condylar magnification (superimposition)	Oblique projection of the knee joint to include the distal femur and proximal tibia/fibula	• Tibiofibular articulation open • Both tibial plateaus are demonstrated • Femoral condyles are shown in an oblique • Head of the fibula should not overlap the tibia
	Lateral oblique (external) (45°)	Directed 5° cephalic to a point just inferior to the patellar apex; reduces distortion of the joint space due to condylar magnification (superimposition)	Oblique projection of the knee joint to include the distal femur and proximal tibia/fibula	• Tibial plateaus should be demonstrated • Knee joint should be open • Fibula should be superimposed over the lateral tibia
	Lateral (mediolateral)	Directed 5° cephalic to a point ½″ or 1 cm distal to the medial epicondyle; reduces distortion of the joint space due to condylar magnification (superimposition)	Lateral projection of the knee joint to include the distal femur, patella, proximal tibial/fibula	• Femoral condyles should be superimposed • Knee joint should be open and the patella in a true lateral • Knee flexed 15° to 20° • Minimal superimposition of the fibula on the tibia • Patellofemoral joint space should be open
PATELLA *(See Figures 10–6, 10–9 B & C)*	*PA*	Directed perpendicular to the midpopliteal area exiting from the patella	PA projection of the patella providing more detail than an AP projection	• True PA of the patella free of rotation • Patella should be demonstrated with optimal density and minimum magnification • Patella will be located slightly medial on the femur

Chart 10–2 ■ **LOWER EXTREMITY** *Continued*

		PROJECTION	**CENTRAL RAY**	**STRUCTURES SHOWN**	**EVALUATION CRITERIA**

<table>
<tr><td colspan="5">Chart 10–2 ■ LOWER EXTREMITY Continued</td></tr>
<tr><td></td><td>PROJECTION</td><td>CENTRAL RAY</td><td>STRUCTURES SHOWN</td><td>EVALUATION CRITERIA</td></tr>
<tr>
<td></td>
<td>PA axial
(intercondylar fossa)
(tunnel view)</td>
<td>Directed perpendicular to the long axis of the lower leg to the popliteal depression (usually a 40° to 50° caudal angle)</td>
<td>Superoinferior projection of the intercondyloid fossa (used to evaluate the joint space for "joint mice")</td>
<td>• Femoral intercondyloid fossa should be open
• Posteroinferior aspect of the femoral condyles should be demonstrated
• Entire patella should be superimposed over the distal femur
• Femoral tibial joint spaces should be open and without rotation
• Tibial eminence should be well demonstrated</td>
</tr>
<tr>
<td></td>
<td>Tangential
(patellofemoral joint)
(sunrise view)
(skyline)</td>
<td>Directed parallel to pass through the femoropatellar joint space (the degree of angulation will be determined by the degree of lower leg flexion)</td>
<td>Tangential projection of the femoropatellar articulation and evaluation of vertical fractures
Contraindicated for patients with transverse fractures of the patella</td>
<td>• Patella shown in profile
• The femoropatellar joint space should be equal and open
• Patella should demonstrate bony detail
• Projection used for evaluation of vertical fractures</td>
</tr>
<tr>
<td></td>
<td>Lateral
(5° to 10° flexion of knee) mediolateral</td>
<td>Directed perpendicular to the anterior margin of the medial epicondyle</td>
<td>Lateral projection of the anterior knee joint and the entire patella</td>
<td>• True lateral of the entire patella with the patellofemoral joint space open and without rotation
• Anterior femur and lower leg should be included</td>
</tr>
<tr>
<td>FEMUR
(See Figures 10–6, 10–9, 10–10)</td>
<td>AP</td>
<td>Directed perpendicular to the midpoint of the thigh; 15° medial rotation of the leg to achieve a true AP of the femoral neck</td>
<td>AP projection of the femur to include the hip and hip joint and knee joint (this may require more than one film)</td>
<td>• Femoral neck should not be foreshortened
• True AP view of the knee joint
• Greater trochanter should be in profile
• Lesser trochanter should be superimposed on the femoral shaft
• The above criteria depend upon proper rotation of the leg (15° medial rotation of the foot)</td>
</tr>
<tr>
<td></td>
<td>Lateral
(mediolateral)</td>
<td>Directed perpendicular to the midthigh area</td>
<td>Lateral projection of the femur and associated joints; hip and knee (this may require more than one film)</td>
<td>• Unaffected hip should not overlap the affected side
• Greater and lesser trochanter should be well visualized
• Femoral condyles should be superimposed
• Patellofemoral joint space should be demonstrated and open</td>
</tr>
</table>

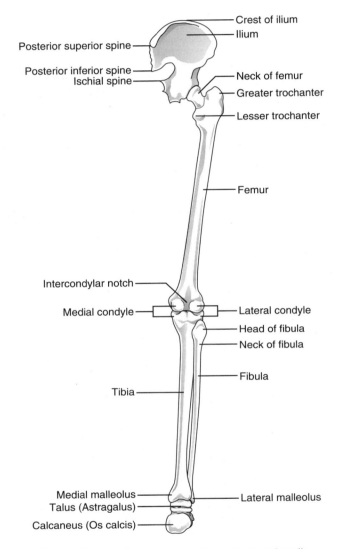

Figure 10-6 ■ Posterior view of the lower extremity.

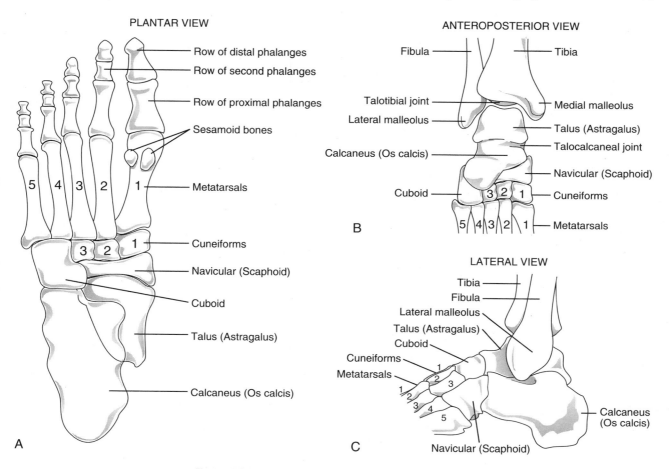

PLANTAR VIEW

Row of distal phalanges
Row of second phalanges
Row of proximal phalanges
Sesamoid bones
Metatarsals
Cuneiforms
Navicular (Scaphoid)
Cuboid
Talus (Astragalus)
Calcaneus (Os calcis)

A

ANTEROPOSTERIOR VIEW

Fibula
Tibia
Talotibial joint
Medial malleolus
Lateral malleolus
Talus (Astragalus)
Calcaneus (Os calcis)
Talocalcaneal joint
Navicular (Scaphoid)
Cuboid
Cuneiforms
Metatarsals

B

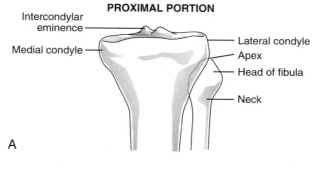

LATERAL VIEW

Tibia
Fibula
Lateral malleolus
Talus (Astragalus)
Cuboid
Cuneiforms
Metatarsals
Calcaneus (Os calcis)
Navicular (Scaphoid)

C

Figure 10-7 ■ Multiple views of the foot and ankle.

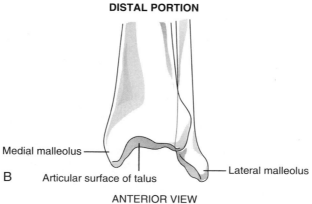

PROXIMAL PORTION

Intercondylar eminence
Medial condyle
Lateral condyle
Apex
Head of fibula
Neck

A

DISTAL PORTION

Medial malleolus
Articular surface of talus
Lateral malleolus

B

ANTERIOR VIEW

Figure 10-8 ■ Proximal and distal views of the tibia/fibula.

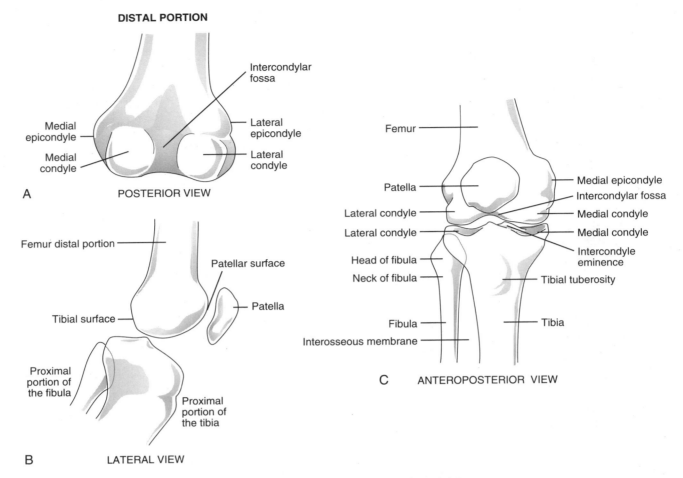

DISTAL PORTION

Intercondylar fossa

Medial epicondyle

Medial condyle

Lateral epicondyle

Lateral condyle

A   POSTERIOR VIEW

Femur distal portion

Patellar surface

Tibial surface

Patella

Proximal portion of the fibula

Proximal portion of the tibia

B   LATERAL VIEW

Femur

Patella

Lateral condyle

Lateral condyle

Head of fibula

Neck of fibula

Fibula

Interosseous membrane

Medial epicondyle

Intercondylar fossa

Medial condyle

Medial condyle

Intercondyle eminence

Tibial tuberosity

Tibia

C   ANTEROPOSTERIOR VIEW

Figure 10-9 ■ Multiple views of the knee joint.

Chart 10-3 ■ **HIPS AND PELVIS**				
	PROJECTION	*CENTRAL RAY*	*STRUCTURES SHOWN*	*EVALUATION CRITERIA*
PELVIS (See Figure 10–11)	*AP* (15° internal rotation of the feet)	Directed perpendicular to the midsagittal plane at a level 2″ above the greater trochanter	AP projection of the pelvis to include L5, the entire sacrum, and the proximal femurs (internal rotation prevents foreshortening of the femoral necks)	• Entire pelvis with the femoral necks in full anteversion to allow visualization of the greater trochanters in profile • Obturator foramen, iliac ala, and ischial spines should be symmetric • Lower lumbar, sacrum, and coccyx should be included
	Lateral	Directed perpendicular to the midcoronal plane at the level of the greater trochanters	Lateral projection of the lower lumbar, proximal femur, and pelvis	• Superimposition of the ischium and ilium • Femoral shafts and heads superimposed • True lateral of the L5, sacrum, and coccyx seen within the pelvis

Chart continued on opposite page

Chart 10–3 ■ **HIPS AND PELVIS** *Continued*				
	PROJECTION	*CENTRAL RAY*	*STRUCTURES SHOWN*	*EVALUATION CRITERIA*
HIP JOINTS (*See Figures 10–10, 10–11*)	*AP* (15° internal rotation to the feet)	Directed perpendicular to a point 2″ medial to the ASIS at the level of the greater trochanter; to pass through the femoral necks	AP projection of the hip joint and the adjacent pelvic girdle and proximal femur	• Femoral head seen within the acetabulum with the greater trochanter in profile • The adjacent ilium and symphysis pubis should be included • Lesser trochanter seen minimally, if at all, medially to the shaft of the femur
	Lateral (frog)	Directed perpendicular to a point midway between the ASIS and the symphysis pubis; to pass through the femoral necks	Lateral projection of the hip joint demonstrating the relationship of the femoral head to the acetabulum	• Hip joint, acetabulum, and proximal femur should be included • Greater trochanter superimposed on the distal femoral neck • Lesser trochanter seen in partial profile
	Lateral (cross-table)	Directed perpendicular to the femoral neck (femoral neck should be parallel to the plane of the film)	Lateral projection of the hip joint to include the relationship of the femoral head to the acetabulum	• Acetabulum with the femoral head should be visualized • Femoral neck seen with minimal overlap of the greater trochanter, distally • Unaffected hip should not overlap the area of interest
SACROILIAC JOINTS (*See Figure 10–10*)	*AP axial*	Directed 30° to 35° cephalic to the midsagittal plane at the level of the greater trochanter	AP projection of the sacrum and sacroiliac joint spaces with minimal overlap	• Sacroiliac joints should be included in their entirety • The junction of L5 and S1 should be included and open • The sacrum and joint spaces should be free of rotation • Technical factors should be selected to demonstrate the joint spaces
	AP oblique (25°–30°) (RPO & LPO) (RAO & LAO if done PA)	Directed perpendicular to a point 1″ medially to the ASIS of the elevated side (part rotation is 25° to 30°)	AP projection of the open sacroiliac joint of the elevated side (side down if done PA)	• Sacroiliac joint should be open without overlap of the adjacent anatomy

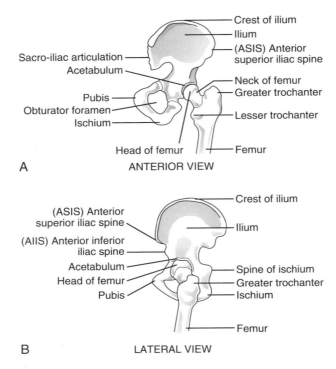

A ANTERIOR VIEW

B LATERAL VIEW

Figure 10-10 ▪ Anterior and lateral views of the hip joint.

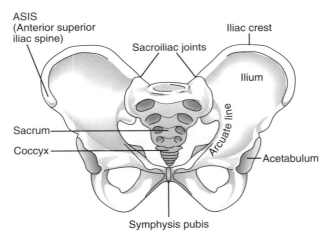

Figure 10-11 ▪ Pelvic girdle.

Chart 10–4 ■ **VERTEBRAL COLUMN**				
	PROJECTION	*CENTRAL RAY*	*STRUCTURES SHOWN*	*EVALUATION CRITERIA*
CERVICAL *(See Figures 10–12, 10–13)*	*AP atlas and axis* (open mouth)	Directed perpendicular to the midpoint of the open mouth	The 1st and 2nd cervical vertebrae projected through the open mouth	• The articulation between the first (atlas) and second (axis) cervical vertebrae • The dens of C2 should be projected through the open mouth without overlap of the base of the skull or the teeth • Lateral masses of C1 should be visualized free of rotation
	AP (axial)	Directed at a cephalic angle of 15° to 20° to the most prominent part of the thyroid cartilage (C5–C6)	AP projection of the lower 5 cervical vertebrae, intervertebral disc spaces	• From C3 to T2 should be visualized • C1 and C2 completely superimposed by the mandible • Intervertebral disc spaces should be visualized open • Spinous processes should be visualized in the midline and en face • May be used to rule out a cervical rib of C7
	AP oblique (RPO & LPO) (45°) (may be done PA oblique RAO & LAO) 72″ SID	Directed 15° to 20° cephalic to the level of the 4th cervical vertebra (may be done PA with a caudal angle)	Oblique projection demonstrating the intervertebral foramina farthest from the film	• Intervertebral foramina farthest from the film (PA oblique will demonstrate foramina closest to the film) • Intervertebral disc spaces should be open • C1 and C2 should not be obscured by the mandible or occipital bone
	Lateral 72″ SID	Directed perpendicular to the midaxillary plane at the level of C4	Lateral projection of the cervical bodies, spinous processes, disc spaces, and articular facets	• Entire cervical column to include the C7–T1 junction • C1 and C2 should not be overlapped by the mandible • Apophyseal articulations should be demonstrated from C2 to C7 • Shoulders should not obscure any part of C7
	Hyperflexion 72″ SID	Directed perpendicular to the midaxillary plane at the level of C4	Lateral projection of the cervical vertebrae demonstrating the range of motion of cervical spine	• Patient's flexion should place the mandible perpendicular to the lower edge of the film • All seven spinous processes should be included and separated from each other
	Hyperextension 72″ SID	Directed perpendicular to the midaxillary plane at the level of C4	Lateral projection of the cervical vertebrae demonstrating the range of motion of cervical spine	• Patient's extension should place the mandible at a 45° angle to the lower edge of the film • All seven spinous processes should be included and demonstrated close together

Chart continued on following page

		Chart 10–4 ■ **VERTEBRAL COLUMN** *Continued*		
	PROJECTION	*CENTRAL RAY*	*STRUCTURES SHOWN*	*EVALUATION CRITERIA*
THORACIC *(See Figures 10–12, 10–14)*	*AP*	Directed perpendicular to the midsagittal plane at a level of the 7th thoracic body	AP projection of the thoracic spine to include C7 and L1	• The entire thoracic spine, along with the junction of the cervical and lumbar spine, should be included • Spinous processes should appear in the midline en face • Density of the upper thoracic spine should not be excessive • Sternoclavicular joints should be symmetric
	AP oblique (RPO and LPO) (70°) (may be done PA RAO & LAO)	Perpendicular to the level of T7	Oblique projection of the entire thoracic spine demonstrating the apophyseal joints farthest from the film	• Apophyseal joints farthest from the film will be demonstrated • Exposure should include from C7 to L1 • Apophyseal joint spaces closest to the film will be demonstrated in PA obliques
	Lateral	Directed perpendicular to the midaxillary plane at the level of T7 CR is angled 5°–10° cephalic, if patient has large shoulders	Lateral projection of the lower 9 thoracic bodies and 1st lumbar body	• T4,5 to the junction of T12 and L1 should be visualized • Posterior ribs should be superimposed to ensure a true lateral position • Intervertebral joint spaces should be open and spinous processes in profile • Breathing technique is helpful to visualize thoracic spine through the blurring of the lung markings and ribs (autotomography)
	Cervicothoracic junction (lateral swimmer's)	Directed 3° to 5° caudally to the cervicothoracic junction; (C7–T1) May be done at 72″ SID	Lateral projection of the lower cervical and upper thoracic spine	• All vertebrae shown should be in a true lateral • An area from C5 to T5 should be included • The shoulders should not be in the same plane

	Chart 10–4 ■ **VERTEBRAL COLUMN** *Continued*			
	PROJECTION	*CENTRAL RAY*	*STRUCTURES SHOWN*	*EVALUATION CRITERIA*
LUMBAR *(See Figures 10–12, 10–15, 10–16)*	*AP*	Directed perpendicular to midsagittal plane at the level of the iliac crest; (L4–L5 interspace)	AP projection of the lumbar spine to include T12, S1, and the sacroiliac joints	• AP projection of the lumbar bodies without rotation, including the junction of the thoracic and sacral spines • Spinous processes should be seen in the midline and en face • The psoas muscles and the sacroiliac joints should be included and symmetric
	AP L5–S1 (may be done PA) (30°–35° caudal)	Directed 30° to 35° cephalic in the midsagittal plane at the level of the ASIS	AP projection of the lumbosacral junction and sacroiliac joints	• Lumbosacral joint (L5–S1) should be visualized and open • Sacroiliac joints should be well visualized and entirely included • The sacrum should appear free of rotation
	AP oblique (RPO & LPO) (45°) (may be done PA RAO & LAO)	Directed perpendicular 2″ laterally from the midsagittal plane toward the elevated side and 1″ above the iliac crest	Oblique projection of the entire lumbar spine demonstrating the apophyseal joints closest to the film (farthest when done PA)	• Apophyseal joints closest to the film should be visualized • Intervertebral joint spaces should remain open • "Scotty dog." EAR: superior articular surface; NOSE: transverse process, NECK: pars interarticularis; BODY: lamina; FRONT LEGS: inferior articular process
	Lateral	Directed perpendicular to the midaxillary plane at the level of the iliac crest (L4–L5 interspace)	Lateral projection of the lumbar bodies, spinous processes, and intervertebral foramina	• True lateral projection free of rotation to include T12 and the junction of the sacrum • Disc spaces should appear open • Intervertebral foramina from T12 to L4 should be well visualized • Spinous processes should be completely viewed in profile
	Lateral L5–S1	Directed perpendicular to a point 1½″ anterior to the spinous process of L5 CR is angled caudad 5°–7° if patient has large hips	Lateral projection of the lumbosacral joint, including the body of L5 and upper sacral spine	• Intervertebral joint space of L5 and S1 well demonstrated and open • Entire visualization of L5 and at least the first sacral segment • Superimposition of the pelvic ilium

Chart continued on following page

	Chart 10–4 ■ **VERTEBRAL COLUMN** *Continued*			
	PROJECTION	*CENTRAL RAY*	*STRUCTURES SHOWN*	*EVALUATION CRITERIA*
SACRUM *(See Figures 10–12, 10–17)*	*AP axial*	Directed 15° cephalic to a point midway between the greater trochanter and the ASIS	AP projection of the sacrum free of superimposition of the anterior pelvis (pubic bones)	• Sacrum projected without foreshortening or rotation • Free of superimposition of the anterior pubic bones • Visualization of the sacral foramina
	Lateral	Directed perpendicular to a point 3″ posterior to the midaxillary plane at the level of the ASIS	Lateral projection of the entire sacrum to include the junction of the lumbar spine and coccyx	• Entire sacrum should be seen in a true lateral projection without rotation • Ischia and ilia should be superimposed • The junction of the lumbar spine and coccyx should be included
COCCYX *(See Figures 10–12, 10–17)*	*AP axial*	Directed 10° caudally to the midsagittal plane at a point 2″ superior to the symphysis pubis	AP projection of the coccyx projected free of superimposition by adjacent anatomy	• All coccygeal segments projected without superimposition • The junction of the sacrum should be included • The symphysis pubis should not superimpose the coccyx • The coccyx should not show rotation • Coccyx segments are projected open unless they are fused
	Lateral	Directed perpendicular to a point 3″ posterior to the midaxillary plane at the level of the greater trochanter	Lateral projection of the entire coccyx to include the junction of the sacrum	• Entire coccyx should be seen in a true lateral projection without rotation • Ischia and ilia should be superimposed • The junction of the sacrum should be included • Coccyx should be projected without excessive density

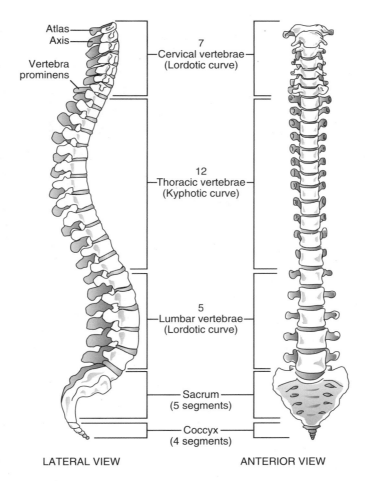

Atlas
Axis
Vertebra
prominens

7
Cervical vertebrae
(Lordotic curve)

12
Thoracic vertebrae
(Kyphotic curve)

5
Lumbar vertebrae
(Lordotic curve)

Sacrum
(5 segments)

Coccyx
(4 segments)

LATERAL VIEW   ANTERIOR VIEW

Figure 10-12 ■ Anterior and lateral views of the vertebral column.

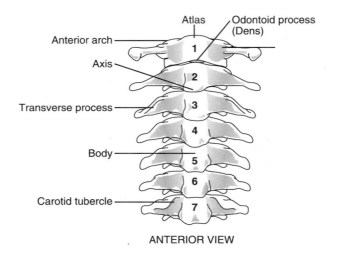

ANTERIOR VIEW

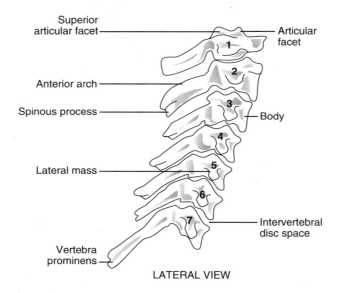

LATERAL VIEW

Figure 10-13 ■ Anterior and lateral views of the cervical spine.

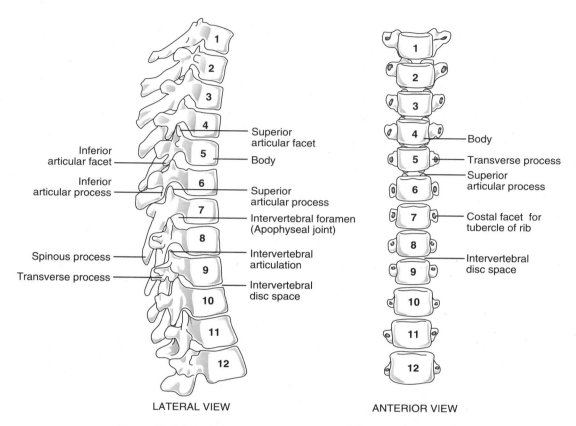

Figure 10-14 ■ Anterior and lateral views of the thoracic spine.

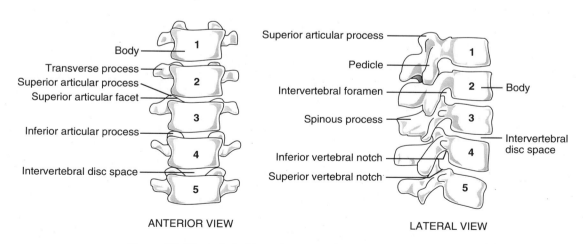

Figure 10-15 ■ Anterior and lateral views of the lumbar spine.

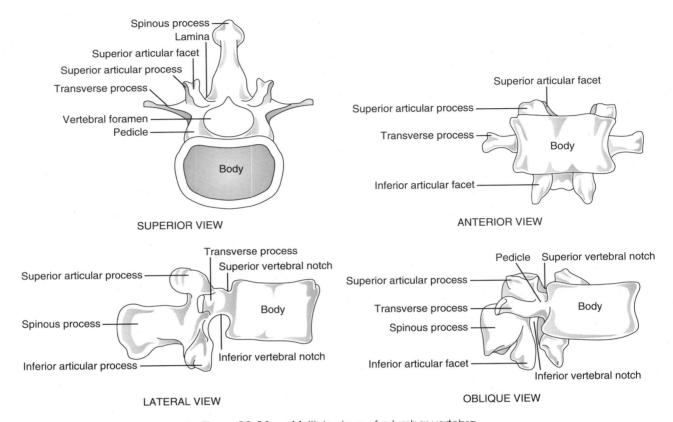

Figure 10-16 ■ Multiple views of a lumbar vertebra.

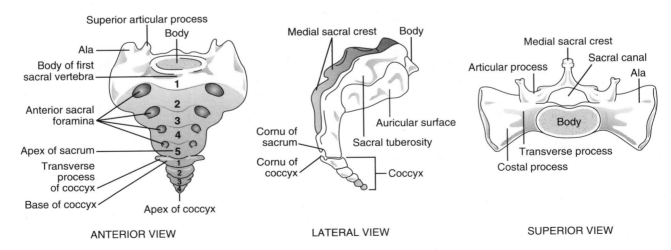

Figure 10-17 ■ Multiple views of the sacrum and coccyx.

Chart 10–5 ■ **CRANIUM**				
	PROJECTION	**CENTRAL RAY**	**STRUCTURES SHOWN**	**EVALUATION CRITERIA**
SKULL *(See Figures 10–18, 10–19, 10–20, 10–21)*	*PA or AP* (Caldwell method)	**PA**—directed 15° caudally to the orbitomeatal line exiting from the nasion **AP**—directed 15° cephalic to the orbitomeatal line entering the nasion	AP or PA projection of the entire cranium and facial bones and sinuses	• Lateral borders of the skull shown without rotation • Orbits demonstrated with the petrous ridges in the lower third • Orbits and petrous ridges should be symmetric • If no angulation is employed, the petrous ridges will fill the orbits • Orbitomeatal line should be perpendicular to the plane of the film
	AP or PA axial (AP Towne) (PA Haas)	**AP**—directed 30° caudally to the orbitomeatal line exiting from the foramen magnum **PA**—directed 25° cephalic to the orbitomeateal line to exit from the nasion	Axial projection of the occipital bone, petrous ridges, and associated anatomy	• Petrous ridges and occipital bone should be symmetric • Visualization of dorsum sellae and posterior clinoid process within the foramen magnum • Exposure should include the entire cranium • Orbitomeatal line should be perpendicular to the plane of the film
	Lateral (right and left)	Directed perpendicular to a point 2″ superior to the EAM	Lateral projection of the entire cranium, facial bones, and sinuses	• Superimposed cranial halves, orbital roofs, mandibular rami, mastoids, EAM and TMJ • Orbital roofs should be superimposed • Sella turcica should be free of rotation • Entire cranium should be included and free of rotations or tilt • Midsagittal plane should be parallel, and interpupillary line should be perpendicular to film plane
FACIAL BONES *(See Figures 10–18, 10–19, 10–21)*	*Parietocanthial* (Waters method) (may be done PA or AP)	Directed perpendicular to exit from (PA) or enter (AP) the acanthion	Axial projection of the facial bones; good visualization of the orbits, maxillae, and zygomatic arches	• Entire cranium should be free of rotation, with petrous ridges projected below the maxillae • The mentomeatal line should be perpendicular to the film plane • Orbits should be projected free of superimposition of the petrous ridges • Maxillary sinuses should be visualized without overlap of the petrous ridges • AP projection will cause considerable magnification of the facial bones

Chart continued on following page

Chart 10–5 ■ CRANIUM Continued

	PROJECTION	CENTRAL RAY	STRUCTURES SHOWN	EVALUATION CRITERIA
	Lateral	Directed perpendicular to the malar surface of the zygomatic arch	Lateral projection of the superimposed facial bones and anterior cranium	• True lateral projection of the facial bones, superimposed • Sella turcica should not be rotated • Superimposition of the mandibular rami and orbital roofs • Exposure should include the mandible and anterior cranium
	PA oblique (53°) (may be done AP)	Directed perpendicular to the infraorbital margin of the orbit closest to the film (rotate part 37° toward the side of interest when done AP)	Oblique projection of the facial bones; both obliques are usually done for comparison	• All facial bones should be demonstrated without overlap of the adjacent side • Both obliques performed for comparative purposes • PA oblique will demonstrate the side closest to the film
ORBITS *(See Figures 10–18, 10–19, 10–21)*	*Parietocanthial* (modified Waters method) (may be done PA or AP)	Directed perpendicular to exit from (PA) or enter (AP) the acanthion	Axial projection of the facial bones; good visualization of the orbits, maxillae, and zygomatic arches	• Entire cranium should be free of rotation, with petrous ridges projected below the maxillae • The mentomeatal line should be placed 55° from the film plane to place orbital floors parallel to plane of film • Orbits should be projected free of superimposition of the petrous ridges • Maxillary sinuses should be visualized without overlap of the petrous ridges • AP projection will cause considerable magnification of the facial bones • Petrous ridges should be in the lower third of the maxillary sinuses when the orbital floors are of interest
	Parieto-orbital PA oblique (Rhese method) (53°)	Directed perpendicular to the affected orbit (orbit closest to the film) (rotate part 37° toward the side of interest when done AP)	Oblique projection of the affected orbit, with the optic foramina located in the lower outer quadrant of the orbit	• Optic foramina seen en face and located in the lower outer quadrant • Entire affected orbit should be included • PA oblique will demonstrate the side closest to the film • Both obliques are performed for comparison • CT and MRI have replaced optic foramina imaging; this is usually performed only status post-trauma for the anterolateral orbital wall
	Lateral (of the affected side)	Directed perpendicular to the outer canthi	Lateral projection of both orbits superimposed	• Entire orbital area should be included • Orbital roofs should be superimposed • Sella turcica should be free of rotation

		Chart 10–5 ■ **CRANIUM** Continued		
	PROJECTION	**CENTRAL RAY**	**STRUCTURES SHOWN**	**EVALUATION CRITERIA**
ZYGOMATIC ARCH (See Figures 10–18, 10–19, 10–21, 10–22)	*Tangential* (basal; SMV) (bilateral examination)	Directed perpendicular to the infraorbitomeatal line in the midsagittal plane and a coronal plane 1″ posterior to the outer canthi	Tangential projection of both zygomatic arches free of superimposition	• Cranium should be free of rotation to project the arches symmetrically • Cranial structures should not superimpose the arches • Both zygomatic arches should be open and well visualized • Zygomatic arches should be demonstrated without excessive density
	Tangential (basal; SMV) (unilateral examination)	Directed perpendicular to the infraorbitomeatal line and centered to the affected zygomatic arch	Tangential projection of the affected zygomatic arch free of superimposition	• Affected zygomatic arch should be open and well visualized • Cranial structures should not obscure the arch • Unaffected zygomatic arch is not visualized • Zygomatic arches should be demonstrated without excessive density
	AP axial (may be done PA)	Directed 30° caudally to the midsagittal plane at a point 1″ superior to the nasion (30° cephalic when done PA)	Axial projection of both zygomatic arches, free of superimposition of the cranial structures	• Zygomatic arches should be projected free of superimposition of the mandible • Arches should be open, well visualized, and symmetric • Cranium should not be rotated • Zygomatic arches should be demonstrated without excessive density
NASAL BONES (See Figures 10–18, 10–19, 10–21)	*Lateral*	Directed perpendicular to the bridge of the nose 3/4″ distal to the nasion	Lateral projection of the nasal bones to include the adjacent soft tissue structures	• True lateral projection of the nasal bones • Exposure must include the anterior nasal spine of the maxilla • Nasofrontal suture should be adequately penetrated • Soft tissue of the nose should be demonstrated
	Parietoacanthial (Waters method) (may be done PA or AP)	Directed perpendicular to exit from (PA), or enter (AP), the acanthion	Axial projection of the nasal septum (coned-down view)	• Nasal septum should be entirely included with adjacent anatomy • Cranium should be free of rotation • Nasal septum should be in the midline • Exposure should be coned down for radiation protection

Chart continued on following page

	Chart 10–5 ■ **CRANIUM** Continued			
	PROJECTION	*CENTRAL RAY*	*STRUCTURES SHOWN*	*EVALUATION CRITERIA*
MANDIBLE *(See Figures 10–18, 10–19, 10–21)*	*PA or PA axial*	**PA**—directed perpendicular to the midsagittal plane at the level of the lips **PA Axial**—directed 30° cephalic to the midsagittal plane at the level of the nasion to exit at the level of the TMJs	PA projection of the body of the mandible or a PA axial projection of the mandibular rami when the central ray is angled	• Mandibular rami should be symmetric • Projection should be free of superimposition and motion • When angulation is employed, TMJs should be visualized inferior to the mastoids • 30° angulation for evaluation of the mandibular rami • AP and AP axial should include the entire mandible
	Axiolateral oblique	Directed 25° cephalic, entering a point just inferior to the mandibular angle farthest from the film Affected area of mandible must be placed parallel to the film	Axiolateral projection of the mandibular body and rami of the side closest to the film	• Mandibular body and rami of the affected side should be free of superimposition of the opposite side • Canine teeth should be included in the exposure • Exposure should be free of motion • Both axiolaterals (right and left) are usually done to include the entire mandible
	Submentovertical (SMV)	Directed perpendicular to the orbitomeatal line in the midsagittal plane at a level midway between the mandibular angles	Basal projection of the mandible to include the mandibular condyle, coronoid, and rami	• Mandible should be projected through the skull, free of rotation, and symmetric • Mandibular condyles should be well visualized • Mandibular symphysis should be in the midsagittal plane
PARANASAL SINUSES *(See Figures 10–18, 10–23)*	*PA axial* *(may be done AP)*	Directed 15° caudally to the midsagittal plane at the level of the nasion (15° cephalic when done AP) (may also be done without an angle)	Axial projection of the frontal and ethmoid air cells (AP projection will cause an increase in magnification)	• Skull and orbits should be projected on a true frontal position • Petrous ridges should be projected in the lower third of the orbits • Frontal and ethmoid air cells should be projected clearly without overlap • Projection should be performed erect and without an angle when air/fluid levels are of interest

	PROJECTION	CENTRAL RAY	STRUCTURES SHOWN	EVALUATION CRITERIA
	Parietoacanthial (Waters and open mouth Waters)	Directed perpendicular to the midsagittal plane exiting from the acanthion (exiting from the open mouth when the sphenoid sinus is of interest)	AP projection of the maxillary and frontal sinuses without overlap of the petrous bones; frontal and ethmoid sinuses are included, sphenoid sinuses are not visualized unless the open mouth projection is performed	• Petrous bones should lie immediately inferior to the apex of the maxillary sinuses • Skull and orbits should be free of rotation • Orbits and maxillary sinuses should be well visualized and free of superimposition of other structures • Sphenoid sinuses are not visualized unless the open mouth projection is employed; if so, the sphenoid sinuses would be projected through the open mouth • Projection should be performed erect and without an angle when air/fluid levels are of interest
	Submentovertical	Directed perpendicular to the infraorbitomeatal line entering the base of the skull, passing through a point 3/4″ anterior to the EAM	Basal projection of the skull, projecting the sphenoid and ethmoid air cells	• Skull should be free of any rotation • The sphenoid and ethmoid air cells should be well visualized and free of superimposition of adjacent structures • Projection should be performed erect and without an angle when air/fluid levels are of interest
	Lateral	Directed perpendicular to the malar surface of the zygomatic arch	Lateral projection of all the sinuses and their relative positions to the adjacent structures	• All sinuses should be included • Sella turcica should be free of rotation • Orbital roofs should be superimposed • Sinuses should be free from overlap of adjacent structures • Projection should be performed erect and without angulation when air/fluid levels are of interest

Chart 10–5 ■ **CRANIUM** *Continued*

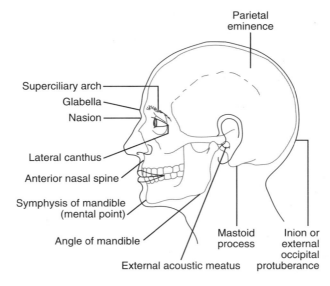

LATERAL VIEW

Figure 10-18 ■ Positioning landmarks of the cranium.

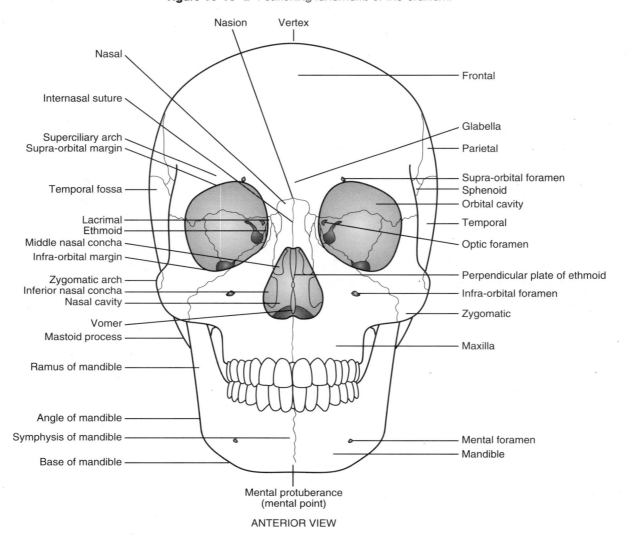

ANTERIOR VIEW

Figure 10-19 ■ Anterior view of the cranium.

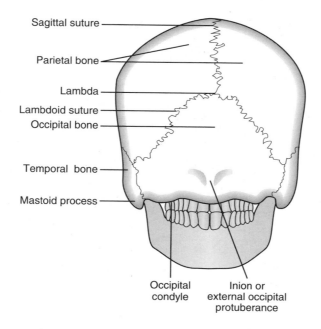

Figure 10-20 ■ Posterior view of the cranium.

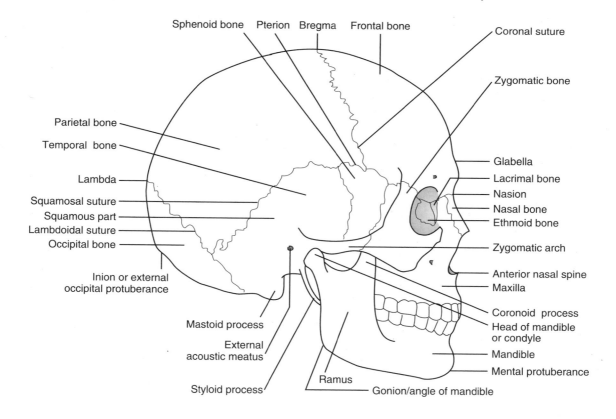

Figure 10-21 ■ Lateral view of the cranium.

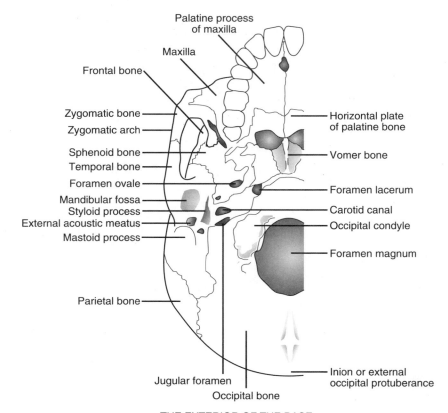

THE EXTERIOR OF THE BASE

Figure 10-22 ■ Basilar view of the cranium.

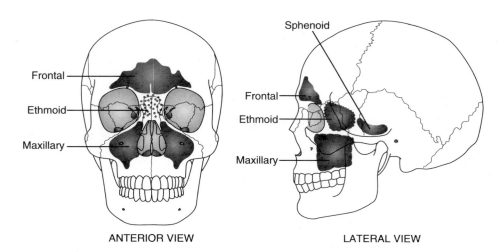

ANTERIOR VIEW   LATERAL VIEW

Figure 10-23 ■ Anterior and lateral views of the paranasal sinuses.

<table>
<tr><td colspan="5" align="center">Chart 10–6 ■ THORAX</td></tr>
<tr><td></td><td>PROJECTION</td><td>CENTRAL RAY</td><td>STRUCTURES SHOWN</td><td>EVALUATION CRITERIA</td></tr>
<tr>
<td>STERNUM
(See Figures
10–25 B & C)</td>
<td>RAO
(may be done
LPO)</td>
<td>Directed perpendicular to the midsternal area (midway between the manubrium and the xiphoid process)</td>
<td>PA projection of the sternum with minimum obliquity (breathing technique will help visualize the sternum by blurring lung markings)</td>
<td>• Sternum should be free of overlap of the vertebral column
• A long exposure time and high mA will increase the visibility of the sternum (breathing technique)
• Entire sternum should be visualized from the manubrium to the xiphoid process</td>
</tr>
<tr>
<td></td>
<td>Lateral</td>
<td>Directed perpendicular to the lateral border of the midsternal area (midway between the manubrium and the xiphoid process)</td>
<td>Lateral projection of the entire sternum
May be done at 72″ SID</td>
<td>• Entire length of the sternum should be visualized, free of motion
• Sternum should not be superimposed by the shoulders, ribs, or arms</td>
</tr>
<tr>
<td>STERNO-
CLAVICULAR
ARTICULATIONS
(See Figures
10–25, 10–26C)</td>
<td>PA
(May be done AP)</td>
<td>Directed perpendicular to the 3rd thoracic vertebra (jugular notch of the sternum)</td>
<td>PA projection of the SC joints, including the medial aspect of the clavicles and the superior sternum (AP will increase magnification)</td>
<td>• SC joints should be visualized through the thoracic spine and without motion
• SC joints should be symmetric
• Exposure should include the superior sternum and medial clavicles</td>
</tr>
<tr>
<td></td>
<td>PA oblique
(RAO and LAO)
(may be done AP;
RPO and LPO)</td>
<td>Directed perpendicular to the SC joint, 3rd thoracic vertebra</td>
<td>Oblique projection of the SC joint closest to the film</td>
<td>• SC joint closest to the film demonstrated with slight rotation
• Medial clavicle and manubrium should be included in the exposure
• SC joint should be projected open and free of the thoracic spine and without motion</td>
</tr>
<tr>
<td>RIBS
(See Figure
10–25 B)</td>
<td>AP
(upper ribs)
(May be done PA and erect to demonstrate the anterior ribs)</td>
<td>Directed perpendicular to the midsagittal plane at the level of the 7th thoracic vertebra</td>
<td>Entire ribs above the diaphragm, 1st through 10th
AP shows posterior ribs
PA shows anterior ribs</td>
<td>• 1st through 8th ribs should be projected above the diaphragm (as many as 10 can be seen)
• Ribs should be projected through the lung fields without motion
• Axillary border to the costovertebral articulations should be included
• Unilateral examination will not include the unaffected side
• Exposure done upon inhalation</td>
</tr>
<tr>
<td></td>
<td>AP
(lower ribs)
(may be done PA and erect to demonstrate the anterior ribs)</td>
<td>Directed perpendicular to the midsagittal plane at the level of the 12th thoracic vertebra</td>
<td>Entire ribs below the diaphragm, 8th through 12th
AP shows posterior ribs
PA shows anterior ribs</td>
<td>• Ribs 8 through 12 should be included in their entirety
• Ribs should be projected through the abdomen to include the costovertebral articulation
• Ribs should be projected without rotation and free of motion
• Unilateral examination will not include the unaffected side
• Exposure done upon exhalation</td>
</tr>
</table>

Chart continued on following page

Chart 10–6 ■ **THORAX** Continued

	PROJECTION	CENTRAL RAY	STRUCTURES SHOWN	EVALUATION CRITERIA
	AP oblique (45°) (axillary ribs) (RPO & LPO) (may be done RAO & LAO) (may be done erect)	Directed perpendicular to a plane midway between the midsagittal plane and the axillary border of the affected ribs Lateral aspect of ribs must be placed parallel to film plane	Oblique projection of the axillary borders of the ribs free from superimposition (anterior obliques will demonstrate side closest and posterior obliques will demonstrate furthest)	• Axillary portions of ribs 1 through 10 should be projected open and free of superimposition • Costovertebral articulation should be included of the affected side • Ribs should be projected clearly through the lung field without motion
CHEST *(See Figures 10–24, 10–25)*	*PA* (may be done AP) (72″ SID)	Directed perpendicular to the 7th thoracic vertebra	PA projection of the thoracic cavity to include the lung fields and adjacent structures (AP projection will result in an increase in magnification of the heart and adjacent structures)	• Apex of the lungs projected above the clavicles and clavicles symmetric from vertebral column • Vertebral borders of the scapulae abducted to avoid superimposition onto lung fields • Lung fields should be symmetric and well inflated (to visualize 10 posterior ribs). Dense heart and mediastinum should be penetrated • Complete lung fields and pulmonary markings • Visualization of the air-filled trachea and bronchi • Right and left diaphragms to include the costophrenic angles • Exposure done on deep inspiration
	PA oblique—LAO 45° (routine) 55°–60° (cardiac studies) (may be done AP RPO) (72″ SID)	Directed perpendicular to the 7th thoracic vertebra at a point midway at the widest part of the body	Oblique projection of the left lung and structures associated with the left lung (for cardiac studies, 55° to 60° LAO will allow better visualization of the heart and great vessels) The right lung to be included	• The off-centered spine allows the left lung to be demonstrated twice as large as the right side • Entire right and left lung fields should be included • Tracheal bifurcation (carina) should be visualized • Right side of the bronchial tree should be demonstrated • Aortic arch and descending aorta projected anterior to the spine • Exposure done on deep inspiration
	PA oblique—RAO 45° (may be done AP LPO) (72″ SID)	Directed perpendicular to the 7th thoracic vertebra at a point midway at the widest part of the body	Oblique projection of the right lung and structures associated with the right lung; to include the left lung	• The off-centered spine allows the right lung to be demonstrated twice as large as the left • Entire right and left lung fields should be included • Air-filled trachea and left main stem bronchi and bronchial tree should be demonstrated • Provides the best projection of the left atrium, left main pulmonary artery, right retrocardial space, and esophagus when filled with contrast

	PROJECTION	CENTRAL RAY	STRUCTURES SHOWN	EVALUATION CRITERIA
	Lateral (72″ SID)	Directed perpendicular 2″ anterior to the midaxillary plane at the level of the 7th thoracic vertebra	Lateral projection of the thoracic cavity used to demonstrate the side closest to the film and interlobular fissures	• Both arms should be raised high enough so they are projected above the lung fields • Long axis of the lung fields should be vertical; lateral view of the sternum; superimposition of the posterior ribs • Entire lung fields visualized to include the apices, costophrenic angles, and hilum • The heart density should be penetrated, with good visualization of both diaphragms
	AP axial (lordotic position)	Directed perpendicular to the midsagittal plane at the level of the body of the sternum	AP projection of the apices of both lungs without superimposition of the clavicles	• Clavicles should be symmetric and projected above the lung fields • SC joints should be symmetric • Used for evaluation of pathology specific to the apices, including interlobular effusions and tuberculosis • Include the superior half of the lung fields
	AP axial Central ray angulation	Directed 15° to 20° cephalic to the manubrium of the sternum	AP projection of the apices of both lungs without superimposition of the clavicles	• Clavicles should be symmetric and projected above the lung fields • SC joints should be symmetric • Used for evaluation of specific pathology to the apices, including interlobular effusions and tuberculosis • Include the superior half of the lung fields
	Lateral decubitus left or right (may be done AP or PA)	Directed perpendicular to the 7th thoracic vertebra	AP or PA projection of the thoracic cavity demonstrating any possible free air or fluid accumulation within the cavity	• True AP or PA projection free of rotation • Left and right lungs should be included in their entirety • Arm shadows should not be overlapping any thoracic anatomy • Technique should reflect the type of pathology suspected: air versus fluid
	Decubitus ventral or dorsal	Directed perpendicular to the midaxillary plane at the level of the 7th thoracic vertebra	Lateral projection used to evaluate fluid levels not visible in other projections	• True lateral view of the entire thoracic cavity; lateral view of the sternum • Arms should not be projected within the thoracic cavity • Technique should be adequate to project the entire lung fields with optimal density

Chart 10–6 ■ **THORAX** *Continued*

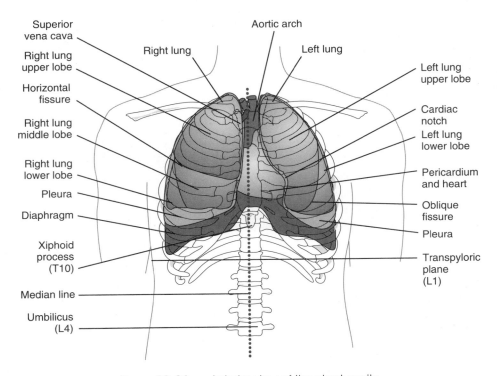

Superior
vena cava

Right lung
upper lobe

Horizontal
fissure

Right lung
middle lobe

Right lung
lower lobe

Pleura

Diaphragm

Xiphoid
process
(T10)

Median line

Umbilicus
(L4)

Right lung

Aortic arch

Left lung

Left lung
upper lobe

Cardiac
notch

Left lung
lower lobe

Pericardium
and heart

Oblique
fissure

Pleura

Transpyloric
plane
(L1)

Figure 10-24 ■ Anterior view of the chest cavity.

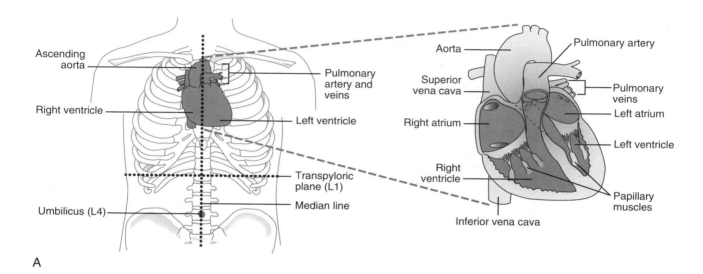

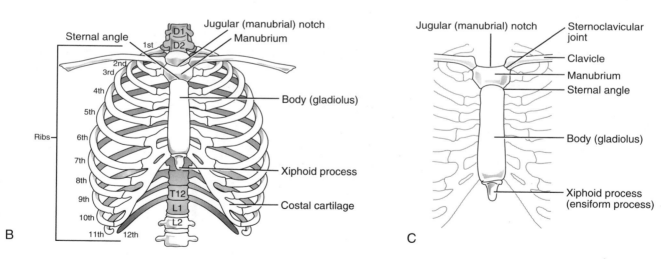

Figure 10-25 ▪ Anterior view of the heart and bony thorax.

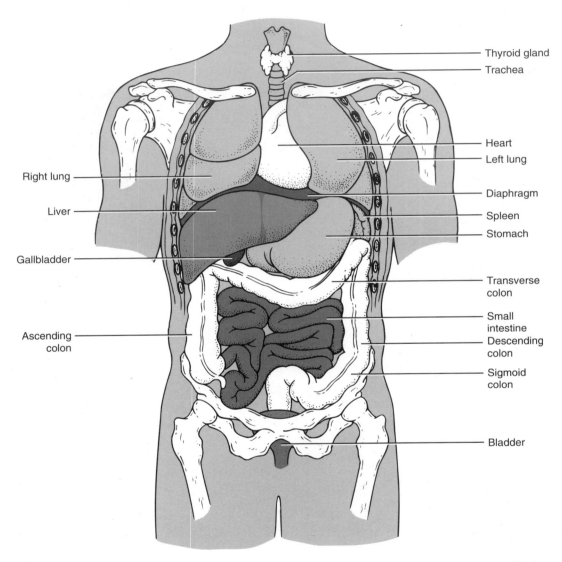

Figure 10–26 ■ Organs of the abdomen and thorax, anterior view. Reprinted with permission from Chabner D-E: The Language of Medicine, 5th ed. Philadelphia, WB Saunders, 1996.

Chart 10–7 ■ ABDOMEN

	PROJECTION	CENTRAL RAY	STRUCTURES SHOWN	EVALUATION CRITERIA
ABDOMEN *(See Figures 10–26, 10–27)*	*AP* (Kidneys, ureters, and bladder, KUB) (may be done PA)	Directed perpendicular to the midsagittal plane at the level of the iliac crests	AP projection of the abdomen demonstrating the intra-abdominal organs to evaluate size and shape	• Symphysis pubis to the diagphragm should be included • Abdomen should be free of rotation, with the spine in the midsagittal plane and symmetric pelvic wings (alae) • Adequate technique should allow visualization of psoas muscles, liver, kidneys, and peritoneal fat • Exposure done on exhalation
	AP erect This can and should be radiographed at 72″ SID to limit magnification	Directed perpendicular to a level 2″ to 3″ above the iliac crests	AP projection of the abdomen demonstrating the intra-abdominal organs to evaluate size and shape (exposure should include both diaphragms in their entirety)	• The diaphragm should be included • Abdomen should be free of rotation, with the spine in the midsagittal plane and symmetric pelvic wings (alae) • Adequate technique should allow visualization of psoas muscles, liver, kidneys, and peritoneal fat • Position used to evaluate free air within the abdominal cavity • Lateral aspects of both diaphragms should be included • Exposure done on exhalation
	Lateral	Directed perpendicular to a point 2″ anterior to the midaxillary plane at the level of the iliac crests	Lateral projection of the abdomen to include the prevertebral space and intra-abdominal organs	• Projected in a true lateral position free of rotation • Diaphragms should be included • Intra-abdominal organs should be visualized • Prevertebral space housing the abdominal aorta should be visualized • Exposure done on exhalation
	Lateral decubitus (right or left)	Directed perpendicular to the midsagittal plane at the level of the iliac crests	AP or PA projection of the abdomen demonstrating the intra-abdominal organs to include the diaphragms The air in the fundus may obscure a free air pattern if a right lateral decubitus is obtained	• Diaphragms included in their entirety and without motion • Both lateral aspects of the abdomen should be included • Most often a left lateral decubitus position is used to evaluate abdominal cavity for fluid and free air (technique should reflect the pathologic condition) • Exposure done on exhalation

Chart continued on following page

	PROJECTION	CENTRAL RAY	STRUCTURES SHOWN	EVALUATION CRITERIA
	Dorsal decubitus	Directed perpendicular to a point 2″ anterior to the midaxillary plane at the level of the iliac crests	Lateral projection of the abdomen to include the prevertebral space	• True lateral position of the abdomen • Abdominal organs should be visualized • Diaphragms should be included without motion • For evaluation of air fluid levels (technique should reflect the pathologic condition • Exposure done on exhalation

Chart 10–7 ▪ **ABDOMEN** *Continued*

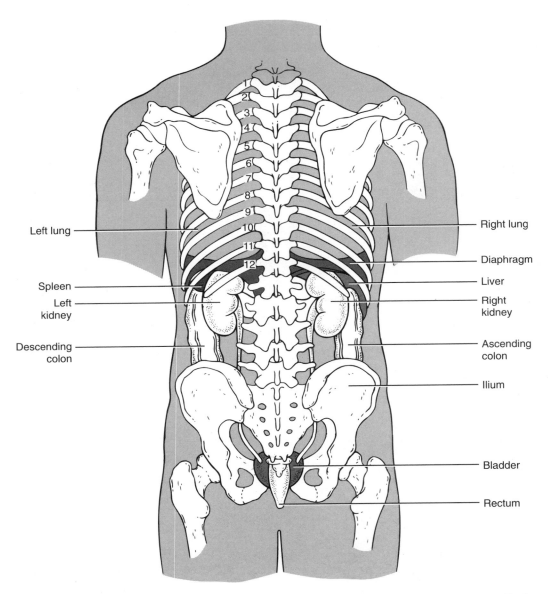

Figure 10-27 ▪ Organs of the abdomen and thorax, posterior view. Reprinted with permission from Chabner D-E: The Language of Medicine, 5th ed. Philadelphia, WB Saunders, 1996.

SKELETAL SURVEYS

Scoliosis Series

This study is performed to evaluate a lateral curvature of the spine. Scoliosis is more common in women than in men. Most often the thoracic spine curves to the right and the lumbar spine curves to the left, but not in all cases. The radiographic evaluation of scoliosis may be done with one AP or PA erect radiograph, but a lateral may also be ordered, especially for an initial screening. A lateral projection will help rule out spondylolisthesis, which is a partial dislocation of one vertebra over the one below it. It is extremely important that the scoliosis examination be performed with the patient erect and feet flat on the floor without shoes. From the radiograph, the angle of the curvature can be measured. If surgical intervention is required, the patient may be sent for magnetic resonance imaging (MRI) to evaluate the integrity of the spinal cord and vertebral foramen.

The radiograph should include all spinal anatomy from C7 to the junction of L5–S1. The iliac crests must also be included for evaluation of fused epiphyses, indicating bone growth cessation. Many facilities will use a special cassette, a 14×36, with a built-in grid, and a graduated screen with increasing speed from top to bottom. This compensates for the increasing tissue thickness. This cassette allows the entire spine to be imaged at one time.

Radiation protection is imperative for this examination. These studies are usually performed on adolescents. Because of their age and the frequency that follow-ups may be needed to show progression, gonadal shielding is required for young men and women. In addition, breast shielding is required for females. The shield may be a shadow shield or a contact shield. Shadow shields may be easier to use because the examination must be performed with the patient erect. Some institutions may perform the examination PA instead of AP because of the decreased dosage the gonads will receive. However, the examination should always be performed at 72 inches SID to minimize the magnification and maximize detail. But other institutions will want the spine as close to the film as possible and do the examination AP.

Long Bone Measurement

This scanogram is used as a method of evaluation of the symmetry of the upper or lower extremity. It is sometimes referred to as orthoroentgenography. The patient is supine on the radiographic table and a radiopaque ruler is placed in the midline, between the extremities being examined. Three exposures are made, each centered over the joint spaces without moving the ruler or patient. For the lower extremity, the ankle, knee, and hip joints are done, and for the upper extremity the wrist, elbow, and shoulder joints are radiographed. The success of this procedure depends greatly on the patient's ability to remain still during and between exposures and the technologist's ability to center accurately over the joint space. The slightest patient movement or improper centering may render this examination useless.

This examination is usually done on pediatric patients as a comparative study for long bone length, but it may also be performed on adults with post-traumatic healing fracture of a long bone to determine limb length. The measurements at each joint will determine whether there is a length difference. These examinations can also be performed with computed tomography (CT), which significantly lowers the patient radiation dosage. The patient is placed on the CT table and a scout film is made. The long bones can be measured with the computer software. Because of the speed of the modern CT machines, the patient does not need to remain still for a lengthy time.

Bone Age

This examination determines whether the skeletal system's developmental age is at a point consistent with the child's chronologic age. A PA projection is taken of the hand and wrist (single exposure). The radiograph is then compared with a skeletal maturation chart to determine whether developmental age is consistent with the child's chronologic age, by evaluating the ossification of the carpal bones.

Bone Survey

This is a general examination of the entire skeletal system. In many cases it is performed on pediatric patients to evaluate for child abuse, but it may also be performed on elderly or mentally challenged people if abuse or nonspecific trauma is suspected. A bone survey may also be clinically indicated for patients with diffuse, progressive bony pathology, such as Paget's disease, metastatic cancer, and osteoporosis. A limited bone survey may also be indicated for children with suspected lead poisoning. Protocols will generally include an AP projection of all long bones, AP abdomen and chest, and an AP and lateral skull. For lead poisoning, the protocol should include an AP film of the knees bilaterally and an AP projection of the abdomen.

CONTRAST

Arthrography

An arthrogram is a contrast-enhanced examination of a joint space and its associated soft tissue anatomy. The contrast is a water-soluble ionic or non-ionic iodinated solution if a positive agent is used, and air if a double-contrast examination is ordered for a negative contrast.

With the patient under local anesthesia and immobilized, the radiologist guides a thin needle into the joint space, usually under fluoroscopy. The radiologist may elect to aspirate some of the synovial fluid from the joint space and have it analyzed by the laboratory. The radiologist will then introduce the contrast into the joint space and the joint is manipulated to distribute contrast throughout. When optimal enhancement is achieved, the radiologist will manipulate the joint under fluoroscopy to evaluate its structure, function, and associated anatomy. Most often the radiologist will make spot radiographs during the procedure under fluoroscopy and require only a limited number of overhead films after the procedure.

Following the inception of MRI, this procedure is now rarely performed. A quality MRI can provide detailed images of the joint and associated anatomy, with much less discomfort to the patient. But the advantage of arthrogram is that it is able to demonstrate the function as well as structure of the joint and its associated anatomy, because the radiologist is able to manipulate the joint under fluoroscopy. Arthrography may also be indicated when the patient's clinical symptoms do not correlate with the imaging results of other tests performed, such as x-ray, CT, or MRI.

Myelography

A myelogram is a contrast-enhanced examination of the spinal canal and associated nerve roots. The contrast used is a non-ionic, water-soluble agent approved for intrathecal injections. The patient may be placed in a number of positions for the injection or puncture. All positions will put the spine in flexion in an effort to open up the posterior spinal components and allow the needle to be passed through. With the patient in this position, a thin, long spinal needle is directed into the subarachnoid space, usually at the level of L2–L3 or L3–L4. Although a lumbar puncture is most common, a cervical puncture (termed a cisternal puncture) may also be performed. The radiologist may elect to aspirate some of the cerebrospinal fluid and have it analyzed by the laboratory. The contrast, which must be checked and confirmed for intrathecal use, is introduced into the same needle and watched under fluoroscopy as it enters the subarachnoid space. The radiologist may request that the patient be rotated or tilted to achieve the maximum contrast enhancement of the area of interest. Spot radiographs will be made during the procedure to document the dynamic flow of the contrast-enhanced cerebrospinal fluid. After spot filming or digital imaging, a translateral view is included.

The myelographic procedure is usually followed up with overhead radiographs, specified by the physician, and a CT of the area of interest. The CT may provide an accurate record of the spinal nerve roots. Throughout the procedure, an effort is made to keep the patient's head elevated to avoid any contrast from entering the ventricles. If contrast does enter a ventricle, it will cause the patient to have severe headaches, which may be accompanied by nausea and vomiting. To avoid these symptoms the patient's head is elevated for up to 24 hours after the procedure.

An MRI examination of the spine and associated anatomy can provide the physician with a high-contrast, high-resolution, multiplanar image. But if the MRI findings do not correlate with the clinical indications, the radiologist may elect to perform a myelogram for better visualization of the nerve roots and the flow dynamic of the cerebrospinal fluid.

Hysterosalpingography

A hysterosalpingogram is a contrast-enhanced examination of the female reproductive organs. It may be performed for many reasons. Hysterosalpingography determines the size, shape, and location of the uterus and fallopian tubes. It is used to help rule out any pathology or anomaly of these organs. Most commonly, it is used to examine for fallopian tube occlusion. When possible, these occlusions are then therapeutically dilated. It may be performed therapeutically if an occluded fallopian tube is suspected. A speculum is placed through the vagina and into the cervix to allow iodinated contrast to be introduced into the uterus. The contrast is allowed to fill the uterus and reflux into the fallopian tubes. When the fallopian tubes are full, the contrast will spill into the pelvic cavity because there is no direct connection between the ovaries and the fallopian tubes. A double-contrast examination may be clinically indicated; air is forced into the uterus and fallopian tubes in an effort to make them patent. Because the contrast may spill into the pelvic cavity, barium sulfate suspensions should never be used. The contrast for hysterosalpingograms is a water-soluble ionic or non-ionic iodinated contrast agent. A hysterosalpingogram is considered a retrograde examination because the contrast is introduced into the uterus and forced to flow backward into the fallopian tubes. Generally, AP and shallow oblique projections are taken after spot or digital images are done.

Venography

A venogram is a contrast-enhanced examination to demonstrate venous flow, usually of an extremity, most often the lower leg. A water-soluble ionic or non-ionic iodinated contrast agent is injected into a vein, distal to the area being examined. The contrast is allowed to flow through the vein, and overhead radiographs are taken. The radiographs will evaluate the integrity of the venous structures. A venogram may be indicated for evaluation of varicose veins, an occlusion, or phlebitis. A vascular examination can also be performed with ultrasound and MRI if a venogram is contraindicated. These examinations may prove safer for a patient who has a history of contrast reactions or renal failure.

Esophagogram

An esophagogram is a contrast (barium, liquid/paste, or oral iodinated medium)–enhanced study of the entire length of the esophagus, from the oropharynx to its termination at the cardiac sphincter.

The patient need not be prepared for this procedure, as long as the esophagus is the only anatomy of interest. If it is combined with an upper gastrointestinal examination, the patient is prepared NPO (nothing by mouth) to insure that the stomach is free of all gastric content.

Esophagograms are requested for the following indications:

1. Impaired swallowing (for example, from foreign body such as a fish bone, epiglottitis, and cancer)
2. Hiatal hernia (the distal esophagus protrudes back up through the diaphragmatic opening into the chest cavity, creating pain and reflux activity)
3. Esophageal varices (varicose veins due to portal hypertension usually, but not

exclusively, associated with chronic alcoholism)
4. Esophageal reflux (gastric contents regurgitate into the esophagus causing "heartburn" and eventual ulceration)
5. Chest pain associated with cardiomegaly (enlarged heart with the increased size affecting the esophagus by applying extrinsic pressure and narrowing the lumen, creating a stricture)

Esophagograms are usually done at 40 inches SID, with the exception of the cardiac esophagogram. This must be done at 72 inches SID to limit magnification, so that the correct heart size can be determined (Fig. 10–28). Most studies are done with the patient erect. Those needed to rule out reflux or herniation may be done with the patient recumbent. The toe-touch maneuver may also be done erect to help rule out reflux. The Trendelenburg position (the patient's head is lower than the feet) is used to demonstrate hiatal hernias, with the force of gravity aiding visual-

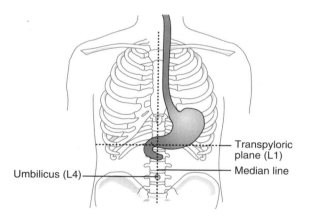
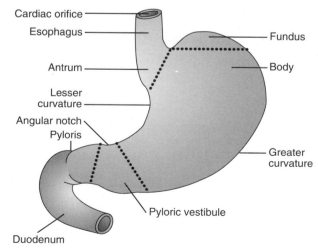

Figure 10-28 ■ Anterior view of the stomach.

ization. The Valsalva maneuver (the patient is instructed to bear down as if to move the bowels) is used to determine the presence of esophageal varices. The increased voluntary pressure causes the varicose veins to dilate with increased blood flow and thus to distend for visualization.

Cine radiography or a video application is frequently utilized when filming these studies, as the actual motion is critical to the diagnosis. The motion may be slowed or sped up as required when viewed afterwards. Digital images as well as traditional spot films are also done. The radiologist instructs the patient to drink or swallow the contrast medium while under fluoroscopy. The patient is asked to rotate into various positions, generally oblique ones, to reduce superimposition of the vertebrae and heart with the esophagus. Overhead radiographs are then taken. The routine positions are AP or PA, left or right lateral, RAO 45°, and LAO 55–60°.

Upper Gastrointestinal Series

This contrast-enhanced study of the stomach and proximal small bowel can be performed as a single- or double-contrast examination to rule out reflux, ulcer, pancreatic disease, and obstructive disease. The patient is instructed to drink a barium sulfate suspension for the single-contrast study or to ingest effervescent crystals to produce air, which distends the stomach lining to aid in visualization of the mucosa while the radiologist watches under fluoroscopy. The patient is rotated into various positions to allow the mucosal lining of the stomach to be coated with the barium for visualization of various structures. Because of the position of the stomach within the body, the barium will fill different structures in different positions, as summarized in Table 10–1.

Small Bowel Series

This contrast-enhanced examination of the small bowel may be performed as a single- or double-

Table 10–1 ■ VISUALIZATION OF BARIUM AND AIR IN GI SERIES

Projection/ Position	Filled with Barium	Empty/Air Filled
AP	Fundus and pylorus	Body
PA	Body	Fundus and pylorus
RAO	Body	Fundus and pylorus
LPO	Fundus and pylorus	Body
Right lateral	Pylorus	Fundus and pylorus

contrast examination. If a double-contrast examination is requested, a gastric tube may be used to introduce the barium as well as the negative air contrast into the small bowel. Enteroclysis is the placement of a French catheter into the small bowel to pass methylcellulose and a barium suspension into it to delineate its contours in specific imaging procedures. This examination is a timed study; films are taken every 15 minutes until the contrast reaches the large colon, the cecum. When the barium is identified in the large bowel, the radiologist will document the ileocecal valve under fluoroscopy with spot films. The patient is usually in a PA position for the entire examination.

Lower Gastrointestinal Series

This is a retrograde contrast-enhanced examination of the large colon, performed as either a single- or double-contrast examination. Air is the negative contrast to delineate the mucosal lining. This approach aids in the visualization of polyps and diverticula. Retrograde means moving backward or against the usual direction of flow and is used here because the introduction of the contrast agent is opposite the normal excretory process of the large intestines. The contrast should be introduced only under fluoroscopy. The contrast used is a barium sulfate suspension plus air if a double-contrast examination is requested. A water-soluble contrast may be used if a perforation is suspected or if surgery is imminent. An enema tip is inserted into the rectum for delivery of the contrast and held in place with a balloon. The patient will be requested to rotate into various positions, which may include being erect, to allow for optimal visualization of the entire colon (Fig. 10–29).

Structures visualized:

AP 30° cephalic angle—sigmoid colon
LAO/RPO—splenic flexure, ileocecal valve
RAO/LPO—hepatic flexure, sigmoid colon
Lateral rectum—rectum

Double contrast:

Right lateral decubitus—lateral aspect of the descending colon
Left lateral decubitus—lateral aspect of the ascending colon
Cross-lateral rectum—better visualization of the rectum

Urologic Studies

These contrast-enhanced studies of the urinary system can be performed many ways. Some uro-

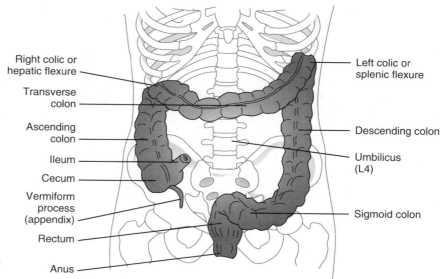

Figure 10-29 ■ Anterior view of the large intestine.

logic studies are retrograde examinations. The contrast agents used for these examinations are water-soluble ionic or non-ionic positive-contrast media (Fig. 10–30).

Cystography. An examination of the urinary bladder. A catheter is placed into the bladder and the contrast is introduced through it into the bladder. The bladder is evaluated for pathology, which may become evident as a filling defect. Because of the way the contrast is introduced

into the bladder, this is a retrograde examination.

Cystourethrography. An examination of the urinary bladder and urethra, very similar to cystography. This test is usually performed as a voiding cystourethrogram. The bladder is filled with contrast, and the patient is instructed to void the contrast while the radiologist observes under fluoroscopy. This may be to evaluate the integrity of the sphincters between the bladder

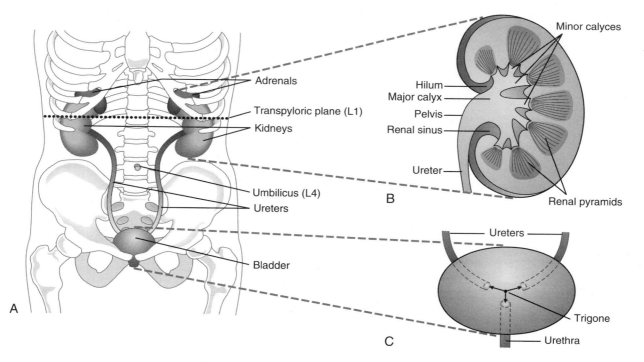

Figure 10–30 ■ Anterior view of the urinary system.

and the urethra as well as the bladder and ureters. This is a retrograde examination.

Intravenous Urography. Also called an IVP (intravenous pyelography). The kidneys are retroperitoneal and are located in the posterior third of the abdominal cavity. A contrast is injected into a vein, either bolus or IV drip, which passes quickly into the urine. This is a timed study in which radiographs are made every 5 to 15 minutes. Tomograms of the kidneys are performed to assess the renal parenchyma or to blur superimposed gas patterns over the kidneys. This examination demonstrates the function of the kidneys and most often will be used to evaluate the collecting system for kidney stones. The most common projections are AP, RPO, LPO, and PA of the full abdomen with collimated projections of the bladder, before and after voiding. Kidney stones may be radiolucent but most often are radiopaque (calcium).

Retrograde Urography. This examination demonstrates the same anatomy as an IVP, but the contrast is introduced into the bladder and ureters. This is a retrograde examination of the urinary system.

Cholecystography

Cholecystography (Fig. 10–31) is a radiographic procedure to evaluate the gallbladder and associated ducts. The contrast used for this examination is a water-soluble iodinated ionic or nonionic positive-contrast agent. This examination may be performed three different ways:

Oral Cholecystography. A contrast-enhanced examination of the gallbladder. The patient is given the contrast in tablet form. The tablets are ingested and absorbed into the portal circulation, collected by the liver, and stored in the gallbladder. This process takes place in 10 to 12 hours; therefore, the patient's intestinal system must be clean, and the patient is on a fat-free diet after the contrast is taken. Extra care must be taken to insure that the patient does not have any adverse reaction to the iodinated contrast medium.

On the morning of the examination, a scout radiograph is made to ensure optimal enhancement of the gallbladder. The radiographic position ante cibum (before the meal) for this procedure may include an erect LAO or a right lateral decubitus. These will allow for the stratification of possible gallstones, which are usually radiolucent due to their bile salt and cholesterol composition. After these radiographs are made, the patient is given a fatty meal that causes the gallbladder to contract and force the contrast out of the gallbladder into the duct system. Radiographs are made in a timed study while this is occurring. The gallbladder will begin to contract about 20 minutes after the fatty meal is eaten. Several positions may be taken post cibum (after

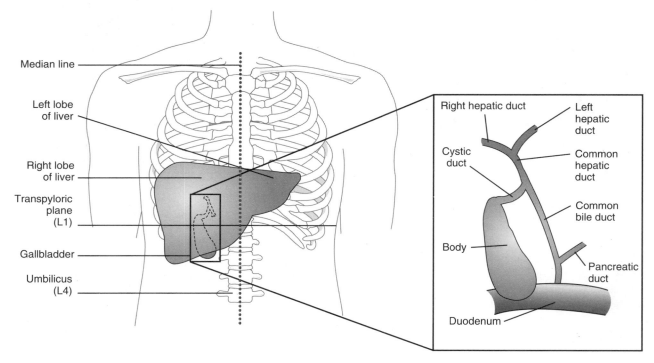

Figure 10-31 ■ Anterior view of the biliary system.

the meal). Fluoroscopy may be included to image the gallbladder and duct system.

Intravenous Cholecystography. This procedure is rarely performed in modern radiology; it has virtually been replaced by ultrasound and endoscopic retrograde cholangiopancreatography (ERCP). The patient's preparation is the same as for oral cholecystography: NPO (nothing by mouth) and a clean colon. An IV iodinated contrast injection is delivered; the contrast is absorbed by the liver and concentrated within the gallbladder. This is also a timed study, with the first radiograph being made 10 minutes after the contrast has been given, with progressive enhancement of the gallbladder until its greatest opacification, occurring at 30 to 40 minutes. A fatty meal is then given, to cause the gallbladder to contract, forcing the contrast into the duct system. The best position for the visualization of the duct system, as it is emptying is an RPO. PIPIDA (*p*-isopropylacetanilido-iminodiacetic acid) scan in nuclear medicine will provide a more sensitive examination of the gallbladder and duct system.

The advantage of oral and IV cholecystograms is that they are examinations of function. They demonstrate the absorption of the contrast, liver function, contraction of the gallbladder, and ejection of the contrast into the duct system.

Percutaneous or T-Tube Cholecystography. This procedure is common practice in the operating room, but within the radiology department it is rarely performed—an ERCP would have much less risk of infection to the patient. It is mainly performed postsurgical (following cholecystectomy). It may be indicated to evaluate the duct system for additional pathology, such as gallstones or pancreatic tumors.

For a percutaneous examination, a long, thin needle is directed through the abdominal cavity and into the gallbladder. Contrast is injected via the needle, filling the gallbladder and duct system. Radiographs are made at optimal visualization of the structures of interest. If a T-tube examination is performed, a T-shaped tube is placed within the duct system of the patient during a surgical procedure in the operating room. It is directed to the abdominal wall, giving access for the injection of contrast. The postsurgical T-tube cholecystogram is normally performed 10 days after surgery. The T-tube may also be used as a drainage system (for bile) after surgical removal of the gallbladder.

Tomography

Tomography is a radiographic procedure that utilizes movement of the radiographic film with an opposing movement of the radiographic tube to create an objective plane of anatomy (everything above and below that level is blurred), decided by a fulcrum selection. The fulcrum selection corresponds to the level of the anatomy of interest. Complex structures such as the inner ear may be evaluated in great detail (although this has been replaced by computed tomography [CT]), while surrounding or overlying structures are blurred or disengage the area of interest. Whatever fulcrum level is selected, in centimeters, in reference to the desired anatomy, becomes the objective plane. It is critical to understand where the anatomy of interest is located in relationship to the tabletop so the fulcrum level can be approximately set. Nephrotomography is a common example and generally misunderstood. The kidneys are retroperitoneal and are located in the posterior third of the abdominal cavity. When you perform nephrotomography, the midline of the kidney corresponds, in fulcrum location, to the pedicle of the lumbar spine. When you visualize in focus the pedicles of the lumbar spine on your preliminary nephrotomogram, you can be certain that you are at kidney mid-cut. However, if the body of the lumbar spine is in focus, appearing as a block, you are too far anterior. If the spinous process is in focus, the fulcrum setting is too posterior.

Measurement of the abdomen is inconsequential in locating the kidneys. Their location rarely deviates above 1 cm or below 8 cm, unless the patient has an inordinate amount of adipose tissue on the back. Many students have been instructed to measure the abdomen carefully with calipers and divide the total measurement by three. The resulting number becomes the correct fulcrum level for kidney location. This "formula," however, is not appropriate. If the patient's abdomen measures 33 cm from posterior to anterior, for example, and is then divided by three, the fulcrum would then be set at 11 cm. It is exceptionally rare, unless the patient demonstrates a large quantity of back fat, that the kidneys would be at this location because it is too far anterior. A patient's abdomen measures 15 cm from posterior to anterior. According to the formula, the kidneys would then be located at 5 cm for fulcrum setting, which is obviously too posterior. Better to use common sense and observe your patient's body type. For most of the general population, the kidney midline fulcrum setting is 7 cm, 8 cm, or 9 cm. It is not dependent upon the measurement of the abdomen, but upon the correlation of the kidney's location in reference to the pedicles of the lumbar spine. Do not forget to compensate for these settings when utilizing a table mat for patient comfort. The mat increases the fulcrum setting to a higher centimeter level because of the addition of height. The objective plane is placed in a more anterior location. Centimeter readings then escalate to an average of 8, 9, or 10 for the mid-cut based upon a standard table mat.

The kidneys are situated at an angle within the body; they are not placed in one plane. The upper poles are posterior, and the lower poles are more anterior. At least three fulcrum settings are required to visualize all the kidney's anatomy and borders. It is therefore essential to locate the midline of the kidneys to determine which additional fulcrum settings are required. Under most circumstances, 1 cm higher and lower then the midline fulcrum setting suffices, as long as the midline fulcrum setting demonstrates the pedicles of the lumbar spine in focus.

The greater the tube amplitude (the distance the tube travels during the exposure) or exposure angle (entire range of movement), the thinner the tomographic cut will be. Also, with thinner cuts and greater tube movement, the amount of heat units produced will increase, as will patient dosage. A hypocycloidal (clover leaf) tube movement makes the thinnest cuts, whereas linear tomography allows for the thickest cuts. With linear tube movements, the long axis of the anatomy of interest must be placed perpendicular to the tube's movement. If the long axis of the anatomy is parallel to the tube movement, the resultant image will demonstrate a streaking or ghosting artifact, obliterating the image.

Zonography is a tomographic procedure that uses a very small exposure angle (5° to 10°) but provides only a thick slice; this is generally acceptable for nephrotomography. This technique depends upon the length of time for tube travel. If the travel time is 1.5 sec then the mA selected must be appropriate for the corresponding mAs. The kVp will be selected based upon the anatomical area being examined or the contrast medium used for anatomical enhancement.

CT and MRI procedures have replaced most of the tomographic procedures with a much higher degree of visibility of structures. The most common tomographic procedure is nephrotomography in conjunction with an IVP examination.

Tomographic Terminology

Amplitude– the amount of speed of the tube movement measured in centimeters per second

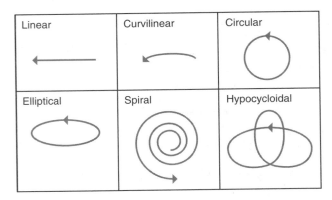

Figure 10-32 ■ Tomographic tube movements.

Blur– the area above and below the focal plane or area of interest

Fulcrum– the distance measured from the tabletop to the area of interest

Objective plane (focal plane)– the plane in which the anatomy is visible, clear, and in focus

Sectional thickness– the slice thickness that is determined by the exposure angle and tube movement

Tube trajectory– the pattern of tube movement: linear, circular, and so on

Tomographic Tube Movements

(Fig. 10–32)

Unidirectional—moves in one direction only:

1. Linear

Multidirectional—moves in more than one direction:

2. Curvilinear
3. Circular
4. Elliptical
5. Spiral
6. Hypocycloidal

Bibliography

Ballinger P: Merrill's Atlas of Radiologic Positions and Radiologic Procedures. 7th ed. St. Louis, Mosby–Year Book, 1991

Bontrager K: Radiographic Anatomy and Positioning. 3rd ed. St. Louis, Mosby–Year Book, 1993

Dorland's Illustrated Medical Dictionary. 28th ed. Philadelphia, WB Saunders, 1994

Gray H: The Classic Collector's Edition of Gray's Anatomy. Avenel, NJ, Crown Publishers, 1977

Section IV **Questions**

1. An AP projection of the first digit should include:

   A. 1st metacarpal
   B. Phalanges
   C. Scaphoid
   D. All of the above

2. A common fracture of the fifth metacarpal is a:

   A. Compound fracture
   B. Boxer fracture
   C. Questionable fracture
   D. Greenstick fracture

3. What radiographic position is demonstrated by radiograph R-1?

   A. AP
   B. Oblique
   C. Lateral
   D. PA

4. The proper obliquity for a posteroanterior projection of the hand is:

   A. 35°
   B. 15°
   C. 45°
   D. 50°

5. Within the wrist, name the proximal row of carpal bones from lateral to medial.

   A. Hamate, capitate, trapezoid, trapezium
   B. Trapezium, trapezoid, capitate, hamate
   C. Scaphoid, lunate, triquetrum, pisiform
   D. Pisiform, triquetrum, lunate, scaphoid

6. Which of the following projections will demonstrate the medial carpal bones with open joint spaces?

   A. PA oblique
   B. Ulnar flexion
   C. PA
   D. Radial flexion

7. Referring to radiograph R-2, what is label *A* pointing to?

   A. Metacarpophalangeal joints
   B. Phalangeal joints
   C. Proximal metacarpals
   D. Sesamoid bones

8. Using radiograph R-2, which carpal is immediately proximal to the base of the first metacarpal?

   A. Trapezium
   B. Hamate
   C. Triquetrum
   D. Scaphoid

9. Using radiograph R-1, which carpal bone(s) are articulating with the radius?

   A. Pisiform
   B. Lunate and scaphoid
   C. Trapezium and scaphoid
   D. Triquetrum

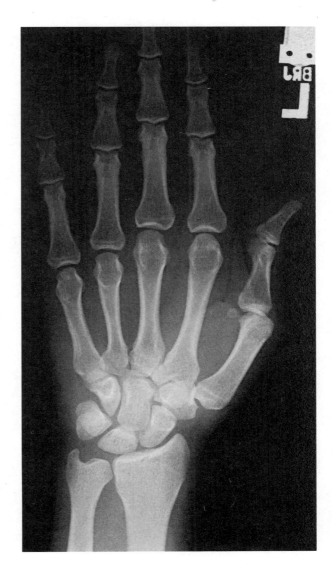

Figure R-1

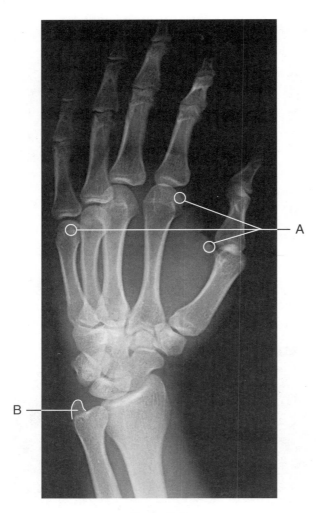

Figure R-2

10. The correct positioning of the hand for an anteroposterior projection of the forearm is:

    A. Supinated
    B. Medial oblique
    C. Pronated
    D. Dorsiflexed

11. A lateral projection of the elbow with less than 90° of flexion will place the olecranon process:

    A. Completely within the olecranon fossa
    B. In profile, posterior to the olecranon fossa
    C. In profile, partially within the olecranon fossa
    D. In profile, anterior to the olecranon fossa

12. Referring to radiograph R-3, which line is pointing to the medial epicondyle?

    A. A
    B. B
    C. C
    D. D

13. Using radiograph R-3, which anatomy is depicted by the letter *C*?

    A. Radial head
    B. Radial neck
    C. Radial tuberosity
    D. Coronoid process

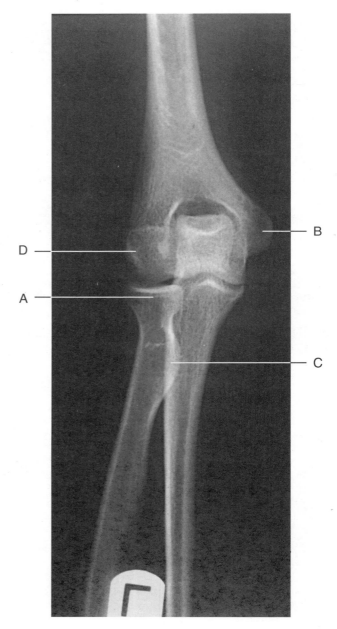

Figure R-3

14. An anteroposterior projection of the shoulder in internal rotation will place the greater tubercle:

    A. In profile laterally
    B. Superimposed over the humeral head
    C. In profile medially
    D. In partial profile inferior to the humeral head

15. The central ray entrance point for an AP projection of the shoulder is:

    A. 2″ below the glenohumeral joint
    B. At the level of the glenohumeral joint space
    C. At the level of the coracoid process
    D. At the level of the coronoid process

16. Name the muscles that make up the rotator cuff.

    A. Supraspinatus, infraspinatus, subscapularis, teres minor
    B. Deltoid, subscapularis, teres major, teres minor
    C. Serratus anterior, supraspinatus, deltoid, teres minor
    D. Pectoralis major, deltoid, teres major, infraspinatus

17. The scapular spine gives rise to which process?

    A. Coronoid process
    B. Lateral process
    C. Acromion process
    D. Coracoid process

18. Using radiograph R-4, Y-view of the scapula, what is the location of the humeral head?

    A. Anterior dislocation
    B. Posterior dislocation
    C. Inferior dislocation
    D. No dislocation

19. Referring to radiograph R-4, the density located within the lung field medial to the scapula can be attributed to:

    A. Normal anatomical variant
    B. A necklace
    C. Pneumonia, in the left upper lobe
    D. Surgical staples

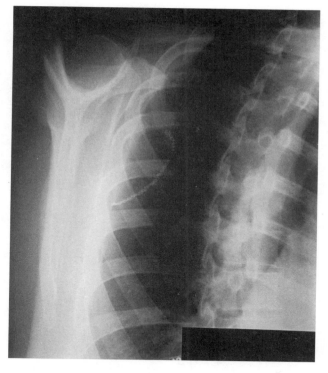

Figure R–4

20. The entrance point for the central ray for an AP projection of the toes is:

    A. 15° caudal to the proximal interphangeal joint
    B. 15° cephalic to the metatarsophalangeal joint
    C. Perpendicular to the proximal metatarsophalangeal joint
    D. 10° cephalic to the metatarsophalangeal joint

21. Referring to radiograph R-5, what are the densities located at the head of the first metatarsal?

    A. Bone cysts
    B. Small benign tumors
    C. Sesamoid bones
    D. Callus

22. What are the names of the tarsals that articulate with the metatarsals?

    A. Navicular, 2nd cuneiform, and cuboid
    B. Calcaneus, navicular, and os calcis
    C. 1st, 2nd, 3rd cuneiform, and navicular
    D. 1st, 2nd, 3rd cuneiform, and cuboid

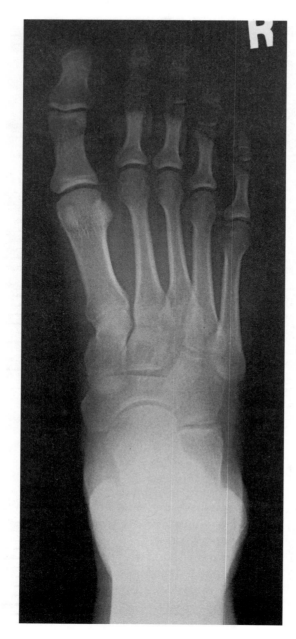

Figure R-5

23. The ankle mortise is the articulation between which three bones?

    A. Calcaneus, fibula, and tibia
    B. Talus, fibula, and tibia
    C. Talus, tibia, and calcaneus
    D. Calcaneus, fibula, and proximal tarsals

24. What is the correct obliquity required to demonstrate the mortise joint of the ankle?

    A. 15°
    B. 30°
    C. 45°
    D. 60°

25. A lateral projection of the tibia/fibula is commonly performed in which position?

    A. Lateromedial
    B. Mediolateral
    C. Anterolateral
    D. Lateroposterior

26. Which of the following projections will demonstrate the tibiofibular articulation open and free of superimposition?

    A. AP projection of the knee
    B. AP tibia/fibula
    C. Medial oblique of the knee
    D. Lateral oblique of the knee

27. Which projection of the patella will aid in the diagnosis of a vertical fracture?

    A. AP projection
    B. Lateral projection
    C. AP axial projection
    D. Tangential projection of the patella

28. Referring to radiograph R-6, what is the name of the pointed processes located on the tibial plateau?

    A. Intercondyloid eminence
    B. Tibial protuberance
    C. Subcondylar eminence
    D. Tibial spine

29. Which of the following will place the greater trochanter in full profile?

    A. Abduction of the affected leg
    B. Adducation of the unaffected leg
    C. Internal rotation of the affected leg
    D. External rotation of the affected leg

30. When the leg is fully extended, the correct anatomical location of the patella is:

    A. Superimposed over the medial aspect of the distal femur
    B. Superimposed over the femorotibial joint space
    C. Superimposed over the tibiofibular joint space
    D. In profile, free of superimposition

31. The lateral projection of the femur will demonstrate the:

    A. Femoral head within the acetabulum
    B. Femoral neck with minimal foreshortening
    C. Femoral condyles superimposed
    D. All of the above

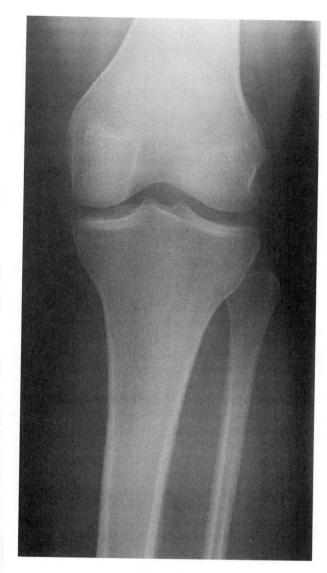

Figure R-6

A. Ilium and ischium
B. Ilium, pubis, and ischium
C. Pubis and ischium
D. Ilium and pubis

35. An AP radiograph of the pelvis reveals that the obturator foramen on the right is considerably smaller than on the left. What is a possible cause of this problem?

    A. Anatomical variation
    B. Patient was rotated toward the right side
    C. Indicates a transverse fracture of the femoral neck
    D. Patient was rotated toward the left side.

36. Which of the following would be required to achieve a true AP projection of the hip joint?

    1. 15° internal rotation of the affected leg
    2. Affected leg fully extended
    3. Central ray entering 2″ superior to the greater trochanter

    A. 1 and 2
    B. 1 only
    C. 1 and 3
    D. 1, 2, and 3

37. In a lateral (frog) hip, the greater trochanter is seen superimposed over the lower third of the femoral neck. Where is the lesser trochanter seen?

    A. In profile, laterally
    B. Superimposed over the distal femur
    C. In profile, medially
    D. Adjacent to the lateral aspect of the femoral head

32. The proper centering point for an anteroposterior projection of the pelvis is:

    A. Anterior superior iliac spine (ASIS)
    B. Symphysis pubis
    C. 2″ below the iliac crest
    D. 2″ above the greater trochanters

33. The most inferior aspect of the pelvic girdle is:

    A. Ischium bones
    B. Pubic bones
    C. Symphysis pubis
    D. Posterior inferior iliac spine (PIIS)

34. Which of the following pelvic bones help form the acetabulum?

38. When evaluating a hip for a fracture, if the patient is unable to abduct the affected side what projection may be substituted for a frog lateral?

    A. Force the leg into the frog position
    B. Cross-table lateral projection
    C. Position for an AP projection and angle the central ray 30° caudal
    D. In cases like this a lateral is not necessary, just do an AP

39. What is the correct central ray angulation for an AP axial projection of the sacroiliac joints?

    A. 15° to 20° cephalic
    B. 20° to 25° caudal
    C. 30° to 35° caudal
    D. 30° to 35° cephalic

40. The sacroiliac joints are the articulations between which of the following bones?

    A. Ischium and sacrum
    B. Ischium, ilium, and sacrum
    C. Sacrum and ilium
    D. Sacrum and pubis

41. Which position will demonstrate the left sacroiliac joint?

    1. Right posterior oblique (RPO)
    2. Left posterior oblique (LPO)
    3. Left anterior oblique (LAO)
    4. Right anterior oblique (RAO)

    A. 1 and 4
    B. 2 and 3
    C. 1 and 3
    D. 2 and 4

42. Which projection of the cervical spine will best demonstrate the odontoid process of C2?

    A. Anteroposterior
    B. AP oblique
    C. Lateral projection
    D. Open mouth projection

43. Referring to radiograph R-7, which letter is pointing to the lateral masses of the first cervical vertebra?

    A. A
    B. B
    C. C
    D. D

44. Referring to radiograph R-7, which letter is pointing to the odontoid process (dens) of the second cervical vertebra?

    A. A
    B. B
    C. C
    D. D

45. Referring to radiograph R-7, what structure is touching the most superior aspect of the odontoid process of the second cervical vertebra?

    A. Maxilla bone
    B. Frontal bone
    C. Occipital bone
    D. First cervical vertebra

46. Referring to radiograph R-8, which of the following structures are visible?

    1. Seven vertebral bodies
    2. Apophyseal joints
    3. Intervertebral foramina

    A. 1, 2, and 3
    B. 1 and 2
    C. 2 and 3
    D. 1 only

47. If the left intervertebral foramina are of interest, which projection would best demonstrate them?

    A. Lateral projection
    B. Left anterior oblique (LAO)
    C. Right anterior oblique (RAO)
    D. AP projection with hyperflexion

48. What is the appropriate location and angulation of the central ray for a PA oblique projection of the cervical spine?

    A. 10° caudal at the level of C6
    B. 15° cephalic at the level of C4
    C. 10° cephalic at the level of C7
    D. 15° caudal at the level of C4

49. What degree of obliquity from the lateral position is necessary to demonstrate accurately the apophyseal articulations of the thoracic spine?

    A. 20°
    B. 70°
    C. 45°
    D. 90°

50. What radiographic position is used to image the cervicothoracic junction in a lateral projection?

    A. Lateral thoracic spine
    B. AP cervical spine
    C. Lateral projection (swimmer's)
    D. More than one, but not all of the above

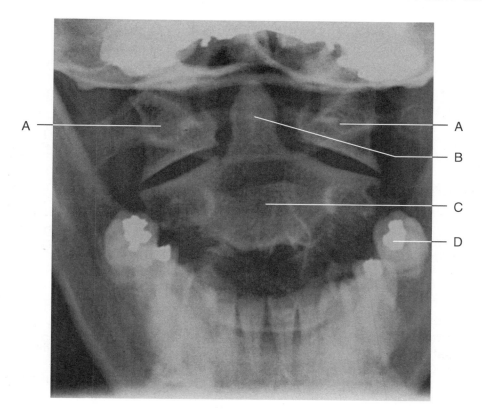

A ——————
A ——————
B ——————
C ——————
D ——————

Figure R–7

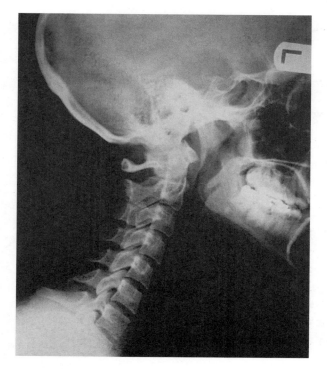

Figure R–8

51. What projection will best demonstrate the intervertebral foramina of the thoracic spine?

    A. AP oblique projection
    B. Lateral projection
    C. PA oblique projection
    D. AP oblique projection with a 30° caudal angle

52. Anteroposterior projection of the lumbar spine should include which of the following:

    1. T12 through L1
    2. Psoas muscles
    3. Sacroiliac joints
    4. Intervertebral foramina

    A. 1, 2, 3, and 4
    B. 1, 3, and 4
    C. 1 and 3 only
    D. 1 and 2 only

53. What is the proper obliquity for an oblique projection of the lumbar spine?

    A. 30°
    B. 70°
    C. 20°
    D. 45°

54. The proper central ray location and angulation for a PA projection of the sacrum is:

    A. 10° cephalic, 2″ below the level of the ASIS
    B. 15° caudal, 2″ above the level of the greater trochanters
    C. 10° caudal, 2″ above the level of the greater trochanters
    D. 15° caudal, 1″ below the iliac crest

55. The evaluation criteria for an AP axial projection of the coccyx includes which of the following?

    1. Free of superimposition of the pelvic bones
    2. Located distal to the sacrum
    3. Joint spaces open without overlap
    4. In the midsagittal plane without rotation

    A. 1 and 4
    B. 2 and 4

C. 1, 2, and 3
D. 1, 2, 3, and 4

56. A true lateral projection of the skull can be identified by which of the following?

    A. Superimposition of the orbital roofs
    B. Sella turcica in full profile
    C. Superimposition of the mandibular rami
    D. All of the above

57. The sella turcica houses which of the following anatomical structures?

    A. Adrenal gland
    B. Thymus gland
    C. Pituitary gland
    D. Thyroid gland

58. Referring to radiograph R-9, what anatomical area is the letter *A* pointing to:

    A. Frontal bone
    B. Ethmoid bone
    C. Sphenoid bone
    D. Occipital bone

59. Referring to radiograph R-9, what anatomical area is the letter *B* pointing to:

    A. Perpendicular plate

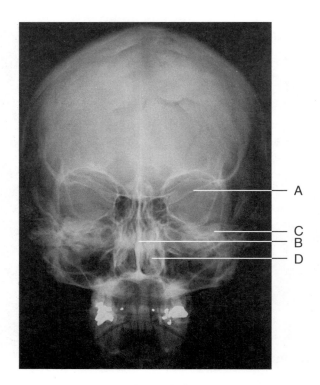

Figure R-9

B. Middle nasal conchae

C. Maxilla

D. Inferior nasal conchae

60. When evaluating the orbits in a PA oblique projection (Rhese method), the proper obliquity of the orbit can be identified by which of the following?

A. The outer rim of the unaffected side

B. The optic foramina in the lower outer quadrant

C. The optic foramina in the lower inner quadrant

D. The foramen of Monro in the lower outer quadrant

61. Which of the following bones contribute to the formation of the orbit?

A. Frontal, sphenoid, zygomatic, maxilla, ethmoid, nasal

B. Frontal, zygomatic, nasal, temporal, ethmoid, maxilla

C. Frontal, sphenoid, zygomatic, lacrimal, maxilla, ethmoid

D. Sphenoid, nasal, lacrimal, ethmoid, sphenoid, maxilla

62. Which of the following projections is best used to evaluate the nasal septum?

A. Lateral projection of the nasal bones

B. Parietocanthal projection

C. AP axial of the skull

D. AP oblique projection

63. Posteroanterior axial projection of the mandible is primarily to evaluate:

A. Mandibular symphysis

B. Mandibular condyles

C. Mandibular rami

D. Mandibular body

64. Why is it preferred to perform a sinus series erect?

A. Erect position will demonstrate air/ fluid levels.

B. Erect position will result in radiographs that have better contrast.

C. This position is more comfortable for the patient.

D. There is no difference between erect and supine sinuses.

65. What position will demonstrate the maxillary sinuses in a frontal projection?

A. Posteroanterior axial projection

B. Parietocanthal projection

C. Submentovertix projection

D. Lateral projection

66. Which of the following radiographic positions will best demonstrate the frontal and ethmoid sinuses in a frontal projection?

A. PA axial projection

B. Parietocanthal projection

C. Submentovertix projection

D. Lateral projection

67. What position will demonstrate all four groups of sinuses?

A. PA axial projection

B. Parietocanthal projection

C. Submentovertix projection

D. Lateral projection

68. Which of the following is the most superior aspect of the sternum?

A. Xiphoid

B. Gladiolus

C. Manubrium

D. Sternal

69. The right PA oblique projection of the sternoclavicular joints will demonstrate the joint space:

A. Closest to the film

B. Farthest from the film

C. Most laterally

D. Most distally

70. A PA projection of the upper ribs will demonstrate which of the following?

A. Posterior ribs above the diaphragm

B. Anterior ribs above the diaphragm

C. Axillary ribs above the diaphragm

D. Posterior ribs below the diaphragm

71. What is the proper obliquity of the patient if the axillary ribs are of interest?

A. 25° to 30°

B. 45°

C. 70° from a lateral position

D. 20° from the supine position

72. A PA chest radiograph should demonstrate a minimum of _____ ribs above the diaphragm.

    A. 8 posterior
    B. 9 anterior
    C. 10 posterior
    D. 11 anterior

73. Which of the following oblique positions would be useful in evaluating the heart and great vessels?

    A. 45° to 55° left anterior oblique (LAO)
    B. 55° to 60° right anterior oblique (RAO)
    C. 55° to 60° left anterior oblique (LAO)
    D. 40° to 50° right anterior oblique (RAO)

74. An AP axial position of the chest would aid the physician in the evaluation of:

    A. Carina and main stem bronchi
    B. Lateral costophrenic angles
    C. Lung apices
    D. None of the above

75. An AP axial of the chest will project the clavicles:

    A. Below the lung fields
    B. Superimposed over the lung fields
    C. Above the lung fields
    D. Laterally to the lung field

76. Which of the following projections would best depict a right-sided hemothorax?

    A. AP projection semierect
    B. Lateral projection erect
    C. Left lateral decubitus
    D. Right lateral decubitus

77. If the patient is unable to be turned from the supine position, what alternative position may be used to evaluate air/fluid levels?

    A. AP axial projection
    B. Ventral or dorsal decubitus
    C. Right or left lateral
    D. AP or PA erect projection

78. The correct centering point for an AP projection of the abdomen (KUB) is:

    A. Perpendicular to the midsagittal plane at a point 1.5″ above the iliac crest
    B. Perpendicular to the midsagittal plane at the level of the iliac crest

C. Perpendicular to the midaxillary plane at the level of the iliac crest
D. Perpendicular to the midsagittal plane at the level of the ASIS

79. The smallest functional unit of the kidney is:

    A. Bowman's capsule
    B. Efferent arteriole
    C. Glomerulus
    D. Nephron

80. Which of the following projections would be useful in the evaluation of free air within the abdominal cavity?

    A. Lateral projection
    B. AP projection erect
    C. Lateral decubitus projection
    D. More than one but not all of the above

81. In what quadrant is the majority of the liver located?

    A. Upper right quadrant
    B. Lower right quadrant
    C. Epigastric region
    D. Upper left quadrant

82. An AP erect projection of the abdomen is performed to rule out free air within the abdominal cavity. If there is free air within the abdominal cavity, where would it be in this projection?

    A. On the left side within the stomach
    B. Just superior to the diaphragm
    C. Within the intestines
    D. Just inferior to the diaphragm

83. Which of the following is the correct anatomical order for urinary excretion?

    A. Kidney, urethra, ureter, bladder
    B. Nephron, pelvis, bladder, ureter
    C. Kidney, ureter, bladder, urethra
    D. Glomerulus, afferent arteriole, nephron

84. Which of the following portions of the aorta is located within the abdominal cavity?

    A. Aortic arch
    B. Aortic root
    C. Descending aorta
    D. Aortic bifurcation

85. With an AP oblique projection of the abdomen, the patient is rotated:

    A. 20°
    B. 55° to 60°
    C. 45°
    D. 30°

86. The abdomen is divided into four quadrants. How many regions is the abdomen divided into?

    A. 4
    B. 6
    C. 5
    D. 9

87. Which of the following is evaluated with a lateral projection of the abdomen?

    A. Kidney function
    B. Flow volumes of the abdominal aorta
    C. The abdominal aorta for possible aneurysm
    D. More than one but not all of the above

88. In the hyposthenic patient, the gallbladder will be placed:

    A. High and lateral
    B. In the midline
    C. Low and in the midline
    D. Low and lateral

89. Which adjuvant imaging modality provides the highest percentage of all gallbladder imaging evaluations?

    A. Magnetic resonance imaging
    B. Computed tomography
    C. Ultrasound
    D. Nuclear medicine

90. Most double-contrast gastrointestinal studies use which of the following contrast medias?

    A. Gadolinium and carbon dioxide
    B. Barium sulfate and air
    C. Methylcellulose and air
    D. Gadolinium and methylcellulose

91. What anatomy does a double-contrast barium enema demonstrate the best?

    A. The mucosal lining
    B. The appendix
    C. The haustra
    D. The rectosigmoidal region

92. Why is an axial projection used during the barium enema procedure?

    A. To elongate the flexures
    B. To open the redundant bowel loops of the sigmoid colon
    C. To increase detail
    D. To eliminate the shadows of the small intestines

93. The position that best demonstrates the retrogastric space during a upper gastrointestinal series is:

    A. LPO
    B. RAO
    C. Left lateral
    D. Right lateral

94. How does the centering differ from a lateral stomach during an upper gastrointestinal series compared with a standard lateral lumbar spine, in relationship to the midaxillary plane?

    A. The centering would be more anterior.
    B. The centering would be more posterior.
    C. The centering would be in the midaxillary plane.
    D. The centering is exactly the same.

95. Which of the following measures the lateral curvature of the spine?

    A. A scanogram
    B. A bone age series
    C. A scoliosis series
    D. A bone survey

96. A radiographic survey of the entire skeletal system is termed a:

    A. Bone scan
    B. Scanogram
    C. Bone survey
    D. Bone age

97. A functional radiographic procedure of the kidneys is called:

    A. A retrograde pyelogram
    B. An intravenous pyelogram
    C. A retrograde urogram
    D. A voiding cystogram

98. The fulcrum setting during tomography determines the:

    A. Exposure factors
    B. Amplitude
    C. Thickness of the tomographic section
    D. Objective plane

99. Which of the following can be considered retrograde examinations?

    A. Voiding cystourethrogram
    B. Barium enema
    C. Hysterosalpingogram
    D. All of the above

100. The thickness of a tomographic cut is determined by which of the following?

    A. The tube angle
    B. The part thickness
    C. The maximum tube limit
    D. The fulcrum setting

Answers appear at the end of the book.

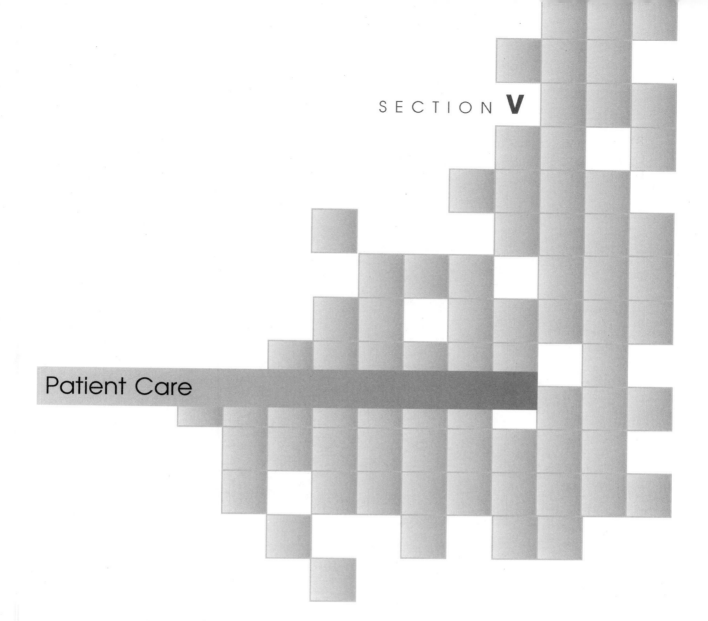

Patient Care

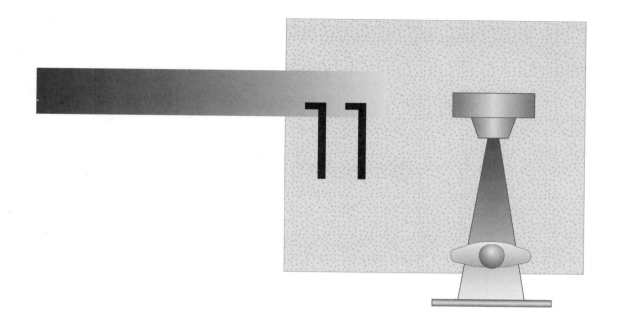

LEGAL AND PROFESSIONAL RESPONSIBILITIES

REQUEST TO PERFORM AN EXAMINATION

How do we begin the process of radiographing a patient? We must receive a formal request or an order from a physician to begin the process legally. The referring physician must place a written prescription, telephone/fax order, or verbal order. That initial order then becomes the starting point for the requisition. This handwritten or computer-generated form contains all the basic information about the patient and the examination: the patient's name, age, date of birth, and medical or radiologic number; patient type (outpatient, house patient, emergency room patient, clinic patient, and so on); date of last menstrual period for age-appropriate females; the name of the ordering physician; and, most importantly, the type of procedure desired.

Sometimes a patient will present an order that requires clarification, as in the case of an order for a "right leg." Is it the femur or tibia-fibula that is required? Or the entire lower limb? Questioning the patient may seem to be the likely choice to gain the answer, but in fact you must contact the doctor directly, because even though the patient may be having pain in the femur, the doctor may be interested in the lower leg as well. The rule is: Don't assume. Always ask.

Just because you now have the requisition in your hand does not mean that you can go ahead and radiograph the patient. The patient must consent to the act.

INFORMED CONSENT

The law recognizes only physicians, of all health care professionals, as legally able to obtain patient consent. It is the doctor who should be providing the patient with enough pertinent information regarding the procedure so that the benefits and risks (however small) may be revealed and the patient can reach an educated decision about care. Most referring physicians may not be familiar with all the inherent risks involved with certain procedures, let alone the procedure itself.

It is imperative that the department delivering the service be forthright with risk information to the patient. Radiology personnel should not rely on the ordering physician to present the entire consent package to the patient. The service area that chooses not to inform the patient may mislead the patient into believing that no risk is involved, thus exacerbating the legal debate should the risk actually manifest itself.

Certain radiographic procedures will require the patient's signature beforehand. Procedures that are invasive, are risky (as in pregnant patients receiving radiation), or employ contrast media generally require written consents. However, prior to the onset of the procedure, you must explain verbally to your patient what he will be experiencing; explain the procedure. If at any time the patient states that he chooses not to have the procedure done, that is a personal choice.

Exceptions

The only exceptions to informed consent are

Emergencies. An unconscious patient is unable to give consent. If the patient's welfare is at stake and the procedure is well recognized as diagnostic to the treatment care plan, the consent will be waived.

Emotional distress/inability to process information. If the physician believes that upon being informed of the procedure/treatment, the patient either will be unable to comprehend the explanation (as in the case of a mentally challenged individual) or that the patient will become emotionally distraught and therefore become unable to consent under self-determination, the consent process may also be waived.

Legal incompetence. The patient is determined to be legally incompetent via judicial pronouncement.

Minor age status. This may vary from state to state. Practitioners must be aware of local laws. Most states recognize emergent situations, and coupled with minor age status and lack of parental consent, one can proceed with medical treatment. If the procedure is routine or elective, it must be postponed until a legal guardian consents to treatment of the minor.

Informed Consent Requirements

- That the ordering physician or point-of-service physician obtain patient consent
- Discussion of benefit vs. risk of the procedure/treatment
- Discussion of alternative treatments/procedures available
- Discussion of possible outcome without consent to procedure/treatment
- Use of layman's terminology, minimal use of medical terminology
- That the area of service fully disclose associated risks to the patient

■ Check your local state policy regarding state-mandated times between the signing of the consent and the actual start of the procedure.

■ That no coercion or scare tactics be employed to gain consent

PATIENTS' RIGHTS

It is possible to think that someone reading this is surprised to learn that the patient has a choice regarding care and treatment. This concept is not new; the American Hospital Association adopted its first Patient Bill of Rights in 1973. The document was brought up to date in 1992 and lists basic rights of hospital patients.[2]

Most states have tailored the basic bill for their own use. It is beyond the scope of this book to list every states' bill of patients' rights, but please familiarize yourself with your local policy.

Patients are generally intimidated while hospitalized. They do what is asked of them, sometimes without question. Some patients believe that doctors are omnipotent. The patient bill of rights is changing that belief system. It allows patients the ability to be self-directed in their health care journey. Beyond the issue of informed consent, other areas are addressed. Advance directives, living wills, appointed surrogates, confidentiality, privacy, access to their own medical records, and access to health care itself are just some of the "rights" appointed.

ETHICS

In addition to relying on the Patient Bill of Rights, our professional society, The American Society of Radiologic Technologists, developed a code of ethics that helps define our role in the health care delivery system. In this review, the ASRT code of ethics is not listed in its entirety, but certain aspects of it are emphasized.

Code of Ethics (condensed)

The ten principles of the ASRT Code of Ethics are

1. Act as a professional.
2. Respect the dignity of all mankind.
3. Deliver care without discrimination.
4. Practice competent technology.
5. Practice responsible decision making, act on behalf of your patient.
6. Recognize that diagnosis and interpretation are beyond the scope of this profession.
7. Practice *current* technology and *current* radiation safety policy.

8. Provide the patient with quality care and ethical behavior.
9. Respect the patient's privacy and maintain confidentiality.
10. Participate proactively in continuing education.

Two of these essential points require further comment.

Confidentiality. Often students and radiographers get into trouble by not maintaining this principle. Keep what you know about the patient to yourself. Do not offer information to others outside the clinical arena. An exception to this principle is legally required reporting, which occurs in suspected abuse or communicable disease cases.

Diagnosis/Interpretation. We are radiographers employing a technology. We are not diagnosticians. Although some radiographers have become quite good at film interpretation, we may only *aid* in the diagnosis through observation of the patient and our clinical notes directed to the radiologist. We cannot formulate diagnostic conclusions.

Obviously the code has been tightly condensed but delivers the essential points of what our profession is all about. By respecting the Patient Bill of Rights and practicing the ASRT Code of Ethics, you will be providing your patients with the best radiologic experience possible.

LIABILITY

We need to present this topic as two separate categories:

■ Civil liability
■ Professional liability

Civil Liability

Civil liability is in itself defined by torts. We are not referring here to some amazing three-tiered sponge cake (torte!) with hazelnut mocha ganache, however pleasing that may sound. We are referring to a legal term defined as "A civil wrong, other than a breach of contract, for which the court will provide a remedy in the form of an action for damages."[3] In other words, if you are unreasonable in your code of conduct either intentionally or out of negligence, you may be held responsible for financial recompense to the injured party (your patient). Torts are also divided by category:

Intentional Torts

These are acts committed on purpose. They are committed with the *intent* to interfere with a person's bodily freedom. People are granted the inalienable right to freedom from interference with their person. Intentional torts are assault, battery, false imprisonment, intentional infliction of emotional distress, and defamation.

Let's look at each of these individually.

Assault. Assault may be explained as the apprehension involved with the *threat* of a physical attack. No *actual* physical act of violence needs to take place, just the *threat* that one may occur. An example of assault, in relationship to health care, would be holding a fist up to an uncooperative patient while telling him that he had better behave. Another scenario would be attempting to force-feed barium to a patient who has emphatically stated her refusal to drink it. Although a charge of assault will stand alone, it is usually coupled with battery.

Battery. This is the most common tort resulting in a liability charge and recovery against radiographers.[4] Battery may be defined as an "offensive contact, made without regard for reasonable dignity of the person's body; unwanted contact."[5] A radiographer's palpating for the symphysis pubis without asking the patient's permission could be construed as an act of battery. The contact does not have to be made by bodily touch alone. The application of adhesive tape to an elderly patient that results in adhesive burns and skin desquamation could lead to charges of battery. Striking out at a wheelchair or crutches resulting in patient injury is another example. *Civil* assault and battery requires only unconsensual touch. No physical injury has to take place for a damage award. *Criminal* assault and battery requires actual injury to substantiate financial or punitive damages.

False Imprisonment. This tort consists of confining patients against their will, without privilege, violating the patients' right to freedom. Like assault, the patient's *perception* of the confinement is enough to levy a tort of false imprisonment. Let's use the example of the patient who is receiving a magnetic resonance imaging (MRI) procedure. The patient becomes claustrophobic during the examination. The patient requests to leave, but the MRI technologist refuses. The patient becomes more agitated and once again is denied termination of the examination. Depending on the mood and legal expertise of the patient involved, a tort could be realized.

Restraints placed on the patient can also be interpreted as false imprisonment. The fine line here, however, is whether they've been placed for the patient's protection. In most radiology departments, restraints are placed for such a brief period of time, and for the safety of the patient and the technical necessity of obtaining radiographs without motion, that there needs to be little concern. Nurses must be wary of restraining their patients for *brief or extended* periods without a written order from the physician. The restraint order must be explicit as to the type: two-point, four-point, Posey, and so on, and as to the length of time. The stereotypical image of the elderly stroke victim restrained by Posey to a chair all day long so that the bed linens stay clean is why orders must be documented and why a tort like this exists. Unjustified or threatened restraint of a patient may also be interpreted as assault.

Damages may be recovered for the patient when a jury declares that the radiographer's actions were unreasonable, unjustified, and unprivileged.[6] Financial claims are awarded for bodily injury, physical discomfort, inconvenience, loss of time and wages, emotional distress, harm to one's reputation, and loss of time with family.[7]

Intentional Infliction of Emotional Distress. This tort has limited application to radiography. Intentional outrageous or extreme conduct by the defendant must be evidenced as inflicting severe emotional distress in the plaintiff up to and including resultant bodily harm for liability. If a radiographer willfully decided to threaten and badger a patient, for whatever reason, this tort may apply. Generally the behavior has to be so outrageous or heinous that it would be a rare occurrence. An example of this tort, outside of radiology's scope, is a parent who chains a child inside a closet, without food or clothing, beating and sexually abusing the child until near death.

Defamation. Simplistically, this tort requires that someone place another person in a false light or actually lie about the person or their behavior. Allegations do not have to be proved, they may be assumed. Both methods of defamation *require a third person* to read or overhear the information. Two types of defamation (damaging the reputation) are:

Libel—defamation by unprivileged publication. A letter containing degrading remarks or commentary may be considered "published" even if dictated to a secretary (she becomes *the third person*).

Slander—defamation by unprivileged speech. If two radiographers are discussing a patient in a way that could be considered damaging, it would result only in slander if made in the presence of *a third party* and overheard.

Professional Liability

Negligence

There are four elements of negligence:

1. Duty
2. Breach of duty
3. Causation
4. Damages

Your *duty* must be defined, as a radiographer, through a specific standard of care. That standard must be *carried out while the patient is your responsibility.* Should your standard *lapse,* resulting in *patient injury or harm,* you may then be considered negligent. Policy and procedure become one of the fundamental guidelines for practice here. Generally policy and procedure will be scrutinized during an investigation. Was the radiographer abiding by directed policy for the procedure? If the policy is there and is clearly written, an obvious *breach* may be construed as negligent behavior. An example might be determining your own protocol for a radiographic procedure. You decide that lateral chest films aren't necessary for the patients. Should a radiologist miss a diagnosis of a neoplasm due to your newly defined protocol, the act would be considered negligent after the investigation demonstrated your alteration of the accepted and written code of practice.

A person may or may not be considered negligent if no harm was involved. Let's use the previous example. You are now in the radiologist's office being advised that lateral chest films ARE a necessity. The radiologist found three examinations demonstrating your "new" protocol. All three patients are recalled, and laterals are now included. All three patients exhibit normal findings. If one of those patients realizes that you made an error, he could try to claim that you were negligent. Damage outcomes are highly subjective and depend primarily upon the jury's interpretation in response to your actions.

Medical Negligence

The basic points of negligence also apply to medical negligence, which is termed malpractice. The burden of proof is usually with the person initiating the charges. The person must address all four elements of negligence: duty, breach of duty, causation, and damage. Malpractice is negligence in the professional arena.

A Latin term closely associated with medical negligence is *res ipsa loquitur,* translated as *the thing speaks for itself.* This means that the situation is so obvious that there is no other explana-

tion than negligence. A good example of this in radiology would be the incorrect insertion of a barium enema tip into a woman's vagina rather than her rectum. Once the barium starts to flow and the initial spot film is exposed, there is little doubt of the error taking place. The damage may be unwanted assault or resultant problems with conception. The documentation is strong and obviously indicates negligence.

Another doctrine of negligence is termed *respondeat superior,* translated as *let the master answer.* What this means is that the health care facility is held accountable in an act of negligence committed by the radiographer. The injured party has only to prove that the radiographer was negligent and the facility may share in the liability as the ultimate overseer of its personnel. The radiographer can be sued as well as the facility.

Malpractice is also closely aligned with scope of practice. Scope of practice defines what particular responsibilities a health care professional has toward the patient. This is generally mandated by the professional accrediting agency licensing and providing professional certification. Obvious examples of a radiographer performing outside the recognized scope of practice are a radiographer performing neurosurgery, writing or filling narcotic prescriptions, or providing psychiatric counseling. Less obvious examples may be radiographic interpretation, cast application, intravenous injection (if not condoned by the state's licensing agency), or performing adjuvant procedures, such as radiation therapy, ultrasound, or nuclear medicine if the radiographer is not licensed in those specialty areas.

Risk Management

This is so intertwined with negligence that it must be included here. Risk management is a holistic approach to total liability. Every aspect of liability is defined and researched to determine how it can be reduced or eliminated. Health care is a field inundated with liability. This can cost the facility millions of dollars annually, depending upon its size and scope of practice. With budgetary restraints being what they are these days and insurance providers using liability percentages as determinants to providership, this has become one of the most critical nonpatient care departments.

Incident reporting is also crucial to track risk. Any occurrence that is considered out of the ordinary should be reported via incident report. Departments that demonstrate zero incidents for the year are probably not initiating reports when necessary. Contrary to popular belief, an incident report is not an admission of fault or liability. The ramifications of the absence *of one* will always return when you least expect them to. Incident documentation is one of the most powerful tools to define, measure, and reduce liability. Use it.

Total Quality Improvement and Total Quality Management

Other considerations closely aligned with risk management include total quality improvement (TQI) and total quality management (TQM).

TQI includes a menu of quality indicators that help define sensitive areas for quality control and improvement within each department. These indicators allow us to *measure,* through various means, our continued improvement, if necessary, in the specific area studied. The newest terminology for this is now *performance improvement.*

TQM is the holistic approach to quality improvement. It defines high-risk problems and studies them through teams made up of associated personnel. The reports that are generated from their study help identify problems and provide improved solutions. TQM continues after the solution has been reached and put into process, by evaluating outcomes in the future to insure continued commitment to quality. Many existing styles of TQM are published for use, so it is up to the facility's discretion which program they choose to initiate. The basic concept is universal—only the program design differs. TQM originated the concept of plotting quality and productivity for customer satisfaction. It works, especially in the production of goods, but inherent trade-offs exist in service industries such as health care. Without proper tracking and measurement of actual improvement following a proposed and activated solution, there is no guarantee of its benefit.[8]

It is important for everyone to remember that we do not produce widgets in the health care profession. We *serve* humanity. What may be good corporate medicine for IBM or Toyota may not help cure what is ailing the American health care system. Only time and our own demand for quality medical practice will help steer our customer service business in the best direction. Strong vocal protest over the 24-hour length of stay for C-section births, by patients and health care professionals alike, altered an insurance dictate and increased patient stay to a longer, more realistic one. The system will be molded by just such events. Exactly what the end result will be is yet to be determined.

References

1. Rozovsky FA: Consent to Treatment: A Practical Guide. 2nd ed. New York, Little, Brown; 1994
2. The Patient's Bill of Rights. American Hospital Association, 1992
3. Prosser, Keaton: The Law of Torts. 5th ed. St. Paul, MN, West Publishing Company, 1985
4. Obergfell AM: Law and Ethics in Diagnostic Imaging and Therapeutic Radiology. Philadelphia, WB Saunders, 1995, p 44
5. Ibid, p 44
6. Ibid, p 46
7. Goldstein LS, Zaremski MJ: Medical and Hospital Negligence. Deerfield, IL, Callaghan, 1990, p 35
8. Huff L, Fornell C, Anderson E: Quality and Productivity: Contradictory and Complementary. Quality Management J 96:4, 1996

Bibliography

Campion FX, The Risk Management Foundation of the Harvard Medical Institutions Inc, The American Medical Association: Grand Rounds on Medical Malpractice. Milwaukee, WI, American Medical Association Publications, 1990

Creighton H: Law Every Nurse Should Know. 5th ed. Philadelphia, WB Saunders, 1986

Huff L, Fornell C, Anderson E: Quality and productivity: Contradictory and Complementary. Quality Management J 96:4, 1996

Obergfell AM: Law and Ethics in Diagnostic Imaging and Therapeutic Radiology. Philadelphia, WB Saunders, 1995

Rozovsky FA: Consent to Treatment: A Practical Guide. Supplement. New York, Little, Brown, 1994

Chapter 11 **Questions**

1. The only person/people that is/are legally recognized to order radiographic procedures is/are:

    1. The physician
    2. The registered nurse
    3. The unit clerk
    4. The patient care associate

    A. 1, 2, and 4
    B. 2 and 4
    C. 1 only
    D. 1 and 4

2. An order arrives stating: "spine x-rays, please." This indicates to you that:

    A. Thoracic lumbar–spine radiographs are required.
    B. Cervical spine radiographs are required.
    C. All areas of the spine must be radiographed.
    D. Clarification is necessary from the physician.

3. Invasive and high-risk procedures require:

    A. Written patient consent
    B. Oral patient consent
    C. Physician's order only
    D. The radiologist's consent

4. An unconscious female patient who is 3 months pregnant arrives in the emergency department after a motor vehicle accident. This situation would be an exception to the legal requirement of:

    A. Negligence
    B. Informed consent
    C. Res ipsa loquitur
    D. False imprisonment

5. A child requires suturing and the family cannot be reached. The medical staff must:

    A. Proceed with the procedure; minors do not require informed consent.
    B. Postpone the procedure until a family member will consent.
    C. Be familiar with their state's legal guidelines for minor consent and proceed accordingly.
    D. Ask the child if it is all right to suture.

6. The Patient Bill of Rights was instituted by:

    A. A grass roots patient advocacy group
    B. The American Medical Association
    C. The American Hospital Association
    D. The Better Business Bureau

7. The Patient Bill of Rights insures that:

    A. The patient is in charge of his or her own health care plan.
    B. The patient's bill will not be sent out until the patient is satisfied.
    C. Patients cannot request physician-assisted suicide.
    D. A patient cannot leave the hospital without medical advice.

8. Advance directives, living wills, surrogate appointments, and medical records access are all associated with:

    A. The Patient Bill of Rights
    B. The hospital-patient contract
    C. The Patient Advocacy Bill
    D. The physician-patient contract

9. The ten principles developed by the American Society of Radiologic Technologists focus on:

    A. Patient rights
    B. Technical issues
    C. Ethical issues
    D. Society entrance requirements

10. Which of the following embody the ASRT's Code of Ethics?

    1. The radiographer will interpret basic trauma and pathology.
    2. The radiographer will wear his/her film badge.
    3. The radiographer will maintain confidentiality.
    4. The radiographer will maintain a professional dress code.

    A. All of the above
    B. 1 and 3
    C. 2 and 3
    D. 2, 3, and 4

11. A tort helps define:

    A. Criminal behavior
    B. Malpractice
    C. Civil liability
    D. More than one, but not all of the above

12. Intentional torts include:

    A. Assault and battery
    B. False imprisonment
    C. Malpractice
    D. More than one, but not all of the above

13. Assault may be defined as:

    A. Physical molestation
    B. Restraint without order
    C. Apprehension from the threat of physical molestation
    D. More than one, but not all of the above

14. Threatening to tape an elderly patient's mouth shut and then proceeding to do it, with resultant injury to the patient, would be:

    A. Assault
    B. Assault and battery
    C. False imprisonment
    D. Disregard for informed consent

15. Confining and physically restraining a 5 year old for a small bowel series that takes several hours may be considered:

    A. Assault
    B. Negligence
    C. Disregard for informed consent
    D. False imprisonment

16. Negligence claims are based upon:

    A. Duty and breach of duty
    B. Causation
    C. Damage
    D. All of the above

17. One of the most critical areas to be investigated during negligence claims is:

    A. Time and attendance
    B. Policy and procedure
    C. The employee handbook
    D. Personnel records

18. Which *one* factor will *most* influence the resultant outcome incurred for a negligence claim?

    A. Breach of duty
    B. Erroneous standard of care practice
    C. Harm to the patient
    D. The subjective nature of the jury

19. A patient required an appendectomy 6 months ago, and the resultant radiograph today demonstrates surgical gauze pads remaining in the abdominal cavity. This illustrates which legal term?

    A. Respondeat superior
    B. Bis dat qui cito dat
    C. Res ipsa loquitur
    D. Rem acu tetigisti

20. A legal term that relates to shared negligence between the individual health care employee and the facility is:

    A. Res ipsa loquitur
    B. Carpe diem
    C. Respondeat superior
    D. E pluribus unum

21. The basic reporting mechanism that is *essential* to risk management to measure and help reduce liability is the:

    A. Incident report
    B. Pareto chart
    C. Quality indicator
    D. Excel computer program

22. An example of a radiographer performing outside of her or his scope of practice would be the following:

    A. Assisting in catheter placement
    B. Operating a C-arm during surgery
    C. Suturing the incision after the removal of a foreign body
    D. Assisting the orthopedic physician with a cast application

23. TQI refers to:

    A. Quality control of the processor
    B. A comprehensive quality or performance improvement program
    C. Indicators for film critique
    D. Total quality management

24. TQM refers to:
    A. A management style encompassing quality built by teams
    B. Quality control
    C. Quality indicators
    D. Total quality management by department directors

25. The success of TQI/TQM is dependent upon:
    A. The darkroom technician
    B. The densitometer being used
    C. H&D curve
    D. Monitoring outcomes after solution implementation

Answers appear at the end of the book.

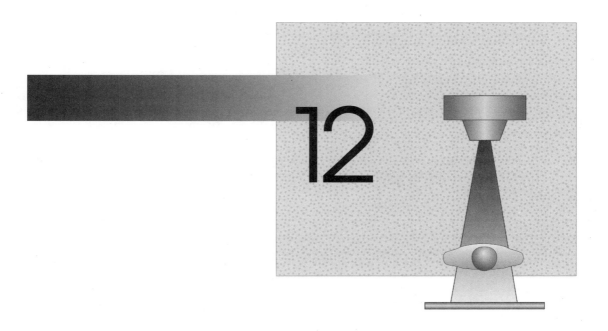

PATIENT EDUCATION, SAFETY, AND COMFORT

COMMUNICATION WITH PATIENTS

Review of Patient History

It is important to obtain a clear and concise patient history, whether your patient is an inpatient or an outpatient. This information is essential to the radiologist for image interpretation. Without it, the radiologist has to guess why the patient presented and why the procedure was requested.

Outpatient History

The following information should be collected at time of service and is generally obtained through verbal communication with either the patient or the physician requesting the examination:

- If the patient is female and within childbearing age, a status of pregnancy should be established. Example: *Ten-day rule or pregnancy test.*
- Assess patient's compliance with preparation for procedure.
- Chief complaint. What is the patient's problem, why is the patient here, and what are the associated symptoms? Example: *"CC: Patient states involved in MVA, lower back pain."**
- Duration of condition or date of trauma. Example: *"Patient complains of (c/o) dysuria for 5 days"* or *"MVA, 3/3/99."*
- Explain visible signs of injury or associated discomfort. Example: For an ankle injury: *"Lateral malleolus appears swollen and tender."* For sinus study: *"Patient c/o frontal headache and associated bloody mucosal discharge."*
- Medication history review. Example: *Contrast media reactions or present medications that would affect the procedure.*

Inpatient History

The following information is obtained by reviewing the patient's medical chart or electronic record and through verbal communication with the patient, physician, and/or nursing personnel. Accurate and complete clinical histories must be obtained for inpatients as well.

- Consent for treatment or procedure
- Date of previous procedure, to be used for comparison
- Laboratory test results that may have an impact on the present procedure. Example:

BUN and creatinine results prior to an IVP study.
- Standing medication orders that contraindicate the present procedure. Example: *Glucophage order not discontinued before the study and held for at least 48 hours afterwards, contraindicating intravascular iodinated contrast medium injection.*
- Patient condition that may warrant canceling or delaying the procedure. Example: *Pacemaker insertion will cancel a scheduled MRI procedure. Substitution of a procedure may occur: An ultrasound, doppler, or MRA (magnetic resonance angiography) when an angiogram is contraindicated; an MRI with contrast for a CT with contrast when the patient has renal insufficiency.*
- Patient information that will alter the patient's course of treatment. Example: *A documented notation of DNR (do not resuscitate) will determine whether a resuscitation code should be initiated if the occasion requires it.*

Explanation of Current Procedure

You must educate your patients and their families or significant others regarding the procedure you are about to do.

- Ask if they are familiar with the procedure.
- Find out if someone else explained it to them.
- Explain it to them in layman's terms.
- Stress important instructions, such as holding the breath during exposure.
- Have them explain it back to you. They should demonstrate instructions back to you, when necessary.
- Keep the discussion open-ended; allow questions throughout the procedure, if possible.

In the same vein, you must be educated in relation to procedures of other modalities, so that you can intelligently explain them to your patient, should they ask. Keep explanations brief.

Magnetic Resonance Imaging

MRI utilizes a magnetic field and a radiofrequency signal interfaced with a computer software package to image the body. No ionizing radiation is involved. Soft tissue studies are especially well defined, due to the subtle contrast variations visualized. Coils are also used to increase visualization and are adapted for specific body areas.

---

*CC, Chief complaint; MVA, motor vehicle accident.

Gadolinium is used as the contrast medium for MRI scans. Adverse reactions to this material are rare, unlike iodinated products used in radiography. There are other concerns, however: magnetic fields create inherent problems with metallic objects inside and outside the body. Scissors can fly across the room, magnetic strips can be erased, and patients with metallic clips or devices can be placed in mortal jeopardy if an MRI procedure is initiated. Another issue is the tight imaging space of the gantry. Claustrophobia is not an unusual side effect of these procedures. Premedication and conscious sedation are often a necessity to provide the patient enough tranquility to maintain composure throughout the entire procedure for imaging success. MRI has virtually replaced arthrography for soft tissue joint visualization.

Computed Tomography

Computed tomography, CT, as this modality is commonly referred to, is also a computer-assisted technology. It utilizes highly collimated, pencil-point beams of radiation, as well as slip ring technology (in helical delivery), to deliver the radiation dose required for computer-calculated imaging in mere seconds. Three-dimensional imaging is also available through the use of this modality. This becomes important in the treatment of cancer, as the entire lesion can be measured from all angles and treated accordingly through the use of sophisticated stereotactic treatment planning.

Axial images are obtained, and image reconstruction can then be applied to reveal images in other planes as well. Iodinated contrast medium is used to enhance tissue differentiation. Motion is a factor, even in helical acquisition, so patient cooperation is essential. Premedication and conscious sedation, again, become important in aiding the successful outcome of the scan.

Ultrasound

Medical sonography uses high-frequency soundwaves and the capture of their return echo to image the body. After the echoes return through the transducer, they are assigned values by a computer software interface. Most applications are for soft tissue visualization, but bone can also be detected. Once a noninvasive technology, ultrasound has expanded its role into invasive procedures, such as biopsy retrieval, intravaginal imaging, and transesophageal echocardiography.

Contrast medium is on the horizon for ultrasound examinations, but currently water is ingested for certain studies, to allow the full bladder to function as a window for increased visualization. Ultrasound is the desired modality for fetal imaging. Pelvimetry, a method of radiographically measuring the maternal pelvis, provided limited information regarding gestational status and is no longer performed.

Nuclear Medicine

Radiation is once again introduced in this modality, but instead of the equipment producing the radiation, the patient is injected with radioisotopes and emits radiation (gamma) particles to a scintillation camera for image construction, via software. The radioisotopes act as nuclear tracers, metabolizing into organs. Healthy metabolism will reveal a negative examination. Dysfunctional organs or areas of disease will demonstrate differently, either by no or limited visualization or "hot spots," demonstrating an area of increased metabolic rate.

The Nuclear Regulatory Commission (NRC) regulates this modality, and stringent records and procedures must be adhered to in order to maintain a license to operate. Radioactive waste is also regulated, and proper disposal methods must be followed.

Nuclear medicine technologists inject the radioisotopes, and that function is exclusive to their professional scope of practice. Recently, radiographers' scope of practice has been expanded to include venipuncture and injection as well. This regulation varies per state. All these digital modalities (CT, MRI, ultrasound, and nuclear medicine) lend themselves to picture archiving and communications system (PACS) application.

Mammography

Mammography has become so regulated and its programs so sophisticated that it has its own registry and is actually treated as a separate section or modality. The federal government regulates mammography with the MQSA (Mammography Quality Standards Act) of 1994, and the American College of Radiology (ACR) also applies its own mandatory regulations. Additional continuing education is required for mammographers and radiologists interpreting the images.

Special equipment that delivers a low dose to the patient has been implemented, and immaculate record keeping is essential for a successful program. Biopsy retrieval is part of this modality, through stereotactic means or needle localization and surgery. Ultrasound localization is often an adjuvant to imaging the breast. Nuclear medicine's mammoscintigraphy and lymphoscintigraphy also help to determine false-positive findings and reduce unnecessary invasive biopsies. Additionally, MRI, utilizing dedicated breast coils, can aid in imaging women who have had breast implants or can help clarify questionable breast lesions or lesions located in close proximity to the chest wall. Holistic breast centers or women's centers are emerging to provide the patient with all imaging modalities in one location, for customer convenience as well as increased patient care outcomes.

Patient confidentiality and comfort are paramount requirements in this modality. The anxiety level of the patient is high, and any way to provide a soothing and private environment must be maximized.

Generally two projections per breast are utilized per examination. One is craniocaudad; the second is mediolateral. Compression is also used to maximize detail by maintaining uniformity of tissue thickness. This is one modality that does not yet apply to electronic imaging via PACS. Too much detail is compromised, and traditional film-screen combinations still afford the best imaging detail for interpretation. Magnification projections using a fractionated focal spot to enhance detail are also done to clarify questionable areas of the breast image.

Sequencing of Multiple Procedures

Because of the use of contrast media and their natural retention in the body cavity, sequencing patterns have been formatted to aid in the scheduling process for successful examination outcomes. In order, they are as follows:

1. Intravenous pyelogram (IVP)
2. Gallbladder (GB) study (if applicable; most gallbladders are visualized using ultrasound)
3. Barium enema (BE)
4. Upper gastrointestinal study (UGI)

IVPs and BEs may be ordered in combination on day 1. GBs and UGIs may be ordered in combination on day 2.

Computed tomography studies also have to be considered, as oral contrast medium in the bowel will limit visibility of other studies scheduled afterward.

PATIENT ASSESSMENT

It is obvious that not all conditions or injuries are alike; neither are the patients. You must assess each patient individually for his or her specific needs. The Joint Commission on Accreditation of Healthcare Organizations (JCAHO) has recently addressed patient needs assessment, and most facilities now have specific chart documentation for this. Basically, it will advise you as to the patient's condition upon admission, the religious and cultural disposition, any impairments to learning such as hearing loss or language barriers, the level of the ability to learn, and actual physical limitations, such as right-sided paralysis, requires support to stand, colostomy bag present, and so on. Allergy status will also be noted. Although this information is handy for inpatients, you must still assess the patient yourself, including all outpatients. Through the assessment process you will learn how to make the radiographic procedure as easy and as successful as possible for that particular individual. Please refer to Chapter 9 for application of specific criteria for special patient requirements.

BODY MECHANICS

Back injuries are the most common injuries of health care professionals. Proper use of body mechanics will not eliminate all back injuries but will certainly reduce them. It also will benefit the safe transfer of the patient from one area to another and help reduce any unintentional injury. Some basic guidelines for body mechanics are

- Assess the load. Ask yourself the following questions before lifting:
- Can I lift this alone?
- Will I need mechanical help?
- Is it too awkward for one person? Shall I ask for help?

If the load is manageable, then proceed with these guidelines:

- Provide a wide base of support; stand with your feet slightly apart.
- Tuck your pelvis in and straighten your back. Avoid twisting.
- Bend your knees. This keeps your center of balance and allows your strong thigh muscles, rather than your back, to help in the lift.
- Keep the load as close to your body as possible. It becomes part of the center of gravity.
- Maintain a sure footing and a clear path for movement.
- Follow these same guidelines when placing the load down.

It requires the same amount of time to lift

safely as it does not to, so use these guidelines for a safe lift every time.

Patient Transfer

In radiology, there are basically two types of transfer options:

- Wheelchair to table/standing and vice versa
- Stretcher to table and vice versa

Before attempting any transfer, make certain that you have the correct patient by checking the ID band or questioning the patient. Assess your patient to see how much help the person is capable of during the move. This will alert you to the option of getting additional help. Make sure that all wheelchair or stretcher locks are locked before attempting to move the patient. Always check all patient lines (intravenous, Foley catheter, oxygen tube) to be sure that they do not become caught or pulled out. Last but not least, explain to the patient precisely what you are intending to do and what his or her role in this will be. Provide your patient with clear instructions.

It is beyond the scope of this review book to provide graphic demonstration of these procedures. Should you require a review of these transfers, several references are available to you (see Bibliography).

PATIENT PRIVACY, SAFETY, AND COMFORT

Privacy

All patients require and deserve privacy. It is important to remember these points:

- Provide a private area for a dressing room.
- Provide a dressing gown that has a closure.
- Provide two gowns if the patient is very large.
- Use a sheet to cover the patient's exposed legs and feet.
- Offer disposable slippers if the patient will be walking in the department.
- Only expose that portion of the body area that is absolutely necessary for the procedure. Keep the rest of the body draped or covered.
- Have only the necessary personnel in the room. Do not encourage people to use your procedure room as a short-cut. Do not engage in private conversation with a coworker in front of your patient.
- If you must assist the patient during an excretion process, provide as much privacy to the person as possible.

- Restrict the patient's chart only to personnel requiring it for the procedure.
- Respect the patient's confidentiality. Do not discuss the patient with others.
- Treat your patients as you yourself would like to be treated.

Safety

The following list provides important safety concerns:

- Identify the patient properly.
- Assess your patient. Be aware of skin fragility, allergies, stomas, and so on.
- Use proper body mechanics and transfer procedures.
- Use side rails on all stretcher patients. Do not allow them to ambulate.
- Use the safety strap on the table or provide personnel to stay with the patient. Do not leave patients unattended.
- Use immobilization devices, when necessary, for pediatric patients.
- Use restraints, if necessary. You must have a written order by the physician, unless you are restraining the patient for radiographic positioning only.
- Be aware of moving tabletops and Bucky trays and the location of the patient's hands.
- Always place the patient's personal items in the proper receptacle and label it with the patient's name. Make certain that it is secure.
- Document any injury/property loss, no matter how trivial, via incident report.

Comfort

Radiographic procedures are, by their very nature, uncomfortable. It is up to us, as professionals in our field of service, to attempt to comfort our patients as much as feasible. Radiolucent table mats and positioning sponges can help provide comfortable positions for the patient before, during, and after the procedure, or during waiting time. Any patient with decubitus ulcers must have additional comfort aids placed under these stressed areas. Sometimes an oblique position is more comfortable than the patient being supine. Offer an angle sponge to a patient while they are waiting—it sometimes helps. Every patient and every situation is different.

Use pillows when you can to elevate the patient's head. This is necessary when the patient's breathing is compromised or the person is experiencing nausea or vomiting. If the patient is being positioned for skull radiographs, consider how you push in the Bucky tray. It can be very loud and uncomfortable for a patient already experiencing a headache from a skull injury or sinus infection.

Comfort extends into other areas besides the obvious. Remind your patient to void prior to an IVP study. If the patient begins this procedure with a full bladder, he or she will be uncomfortable in a short time and probably will have to void prior to the study's end. A full bladder also may obscure pathology on the preliminary radiograph.

After a UGI series, offer your patient a wet cloth and clean the barium from the lips. Apply a lip balm to soothe parched lips. Offer tissues to someone coughing or sneezing and blankets to someone shivering. Provide a cool, wet cloth for a febrile patient. Offer water to the emetic patient for the purpose of rinsing the mouth. The options are endless. When your patient is struggling to try to tuck in the chin for a PA axial of the skull, observe the rest of the body. A sponge placed under the chest will assist in accomplishing that body position. Again: treat your patients as you yourself would like to be treated.

Bibliography

Ballinger PW: Merrill's Atlas of Radiographic Positions and Radiologic Procedures. 7th ed. St. Louis, Mosby–Year Book, 1991

Brust DJ, Foster JA: From Nursing Assistant to Patient Care Technician; New Roles, New Knowledge, New Skills. Philadelphia, WB Saunders, 1997

Ehrlich RA, McCloskey ED: Patient Care in Radiography, 3rd ed. St. Louis, Mosby–Year Book, 1989

Perry AG, Potter PA: Clinical Nursing Skills and Techniques. 3rd Ed. St. Louis, Mosby–Year Book, 1994

Chapter 12 **Questions**

1. A clinical history for radiology should include all but the following:

   A. The patient's chief complaint
   B. Duration of condition or date of trauma
   C. Contact person to reach in the event of an emergency
   D. Explanation of visible signs of injury or associated discomfort

2. A child fell and injured his mandible; a deep gash is evident at the mental point. He says that his lower teeth hurt and are loose. He is an emergency department patient and was transported by ambulance from his school. His mother informs you that a week ago he had the flu and a high fever. Your best clinical history would include:

   A. Pt. c/o pain and fever.
   B. Pt. fell today, lacerating mental protuberance, c/o pain lower alveolar process, states teeth are loose.
   C. Patient cut his mandible, his teeth are loose. He had the flu 1 week ago.
   D. Pt. fell today, lacerating mental point, c/o pain in his lower teeth, they are loose, notice high concentration of plaque formation on lower incisors.

3. A female patient presents for an abdominal radiograph. She complains of RLQ pain. Just as you are about to take the exposure, she tells you that, yes, she might be pregnant. You would:

   A. Shield her ovaries and take the exposure.
   B. Cancel the examination.
   C. Establish her pregnancy status prior to the examination.
   D. Send her to ultrasound.

4. Educating your patient requires the following:

   1. A technical explanation of the procedure
   2. Have patient give a return explanation and demonstration of instructions
   3. Time for questions

   A. 1 only
   B. 1, 2, and 3
   C. 1 and 3 only
   D. 2 and 3 only

Questions 5 through 10. Match the following:

5. Slip ring technology is used in which modality?
   _____

   a. Ultrasound
   b. MRI
   c. CT
   d. Nuclear medicine

6. Radio frequency signal applies to:
   _____

7. Radio isotopes are used in which modality? _____

8. Gadolinium applies to: _____

9. A transducer applies to:
   _____

10. Claustrophobia may affect patients in:

    _____

11. Breast imaging is available in all but the following modalities:

    A. Computed axial tomography
    B. Ultrasound
    C. Magnetic resonance imaging
    D. Nuclear medicine

12. The MQSA and ACR regulate which modality?

    A. Mammography
    B. Ultrasound
    C. MRI
    D. Nuclear medicine

13. Craniocaudad projections are used routinely in:

    A. Mammography
    B. Ultrasound
    C. MRI
    D. Nuclear medicine

14. A breast coil would be used in which modality?

    A. Mammography

B. Ultrasound
C. MRI
D. Nuclear medicine

15. Select the correct order of procedural sequencing:

    A. IVP, BE, UGI
    B. UGI, IVP, BE
    C. IVP and UGI on day 1, BE on day 2
    D. BE on day 1, IVP and UGI on day 2

16. Assessing patients addresses their:

    A. Insurance provisions
    B. Medical and personal needs
    C. Previous medical bills
    D. Ability to pay for medical coverage

17. Which combination applies to good body mechanics?

    A. Wide support base, bend knees, carry load close to the body
    B. Straight back, bend knees, use arms as a lift, extended from the body
    C. Narrow support, bend knees, twist back slightly from side to side, keep load close to body
    D. Straighten pelvis and knees, wide support base, carry load close to body

18. You are about to begin an IVP. While you are setting up for the preliminary film, your friend comes in to ask you to go to lunch with her. You would:

    A. Let her know that you'll be free at noon to have lunch with her.
    B. Ignore her and keep talking to your patient.
    C. Tell her you are busy and cannot discuss this now and apologize to your patient.
    D. Report her to your supervisor.

19. A grandmother is accompanying her grandson to Radiology for some femur radiographs. While she is in the room, you notice she is looking in his chart. You would:

    A. Tell your supervisor.
    B. Tell her that she isn't allowed to look in the chart and ask her to leave the room.
    C. Ask her to close the chart and explain to her that she will have to request information about her grandson's condition from the nurse or doctor. Remove the chart from the area.
    D. Let her take a quick peek; she is family.

20. The patient you are radiographing hits her head on the x-ray tube while getting onto the table. She assures you that she is fine. You would:

    A. Continue with the procedure.
    B. Cancel the examination.
    C. Complete the examination, have the injury assessed, and fill out an incident report.
    D. Not be required to fill out an incident report because she said she was fine.

21. A patient requiring skull radiographs is wearing glasses and earrings and has dentures. You would:

    A. Remove them and place them on her stretcher until the end of the case.
    B. Remove them and place the dentures in a cup, and the glasses and earrings in another receptacle, well marked with her name.
    C. Have her remove them and hold them.
    D. Not remove them.

22. The same patient returns later for cervical spine radiographs and states that she is missing her earrings. You know that you returned them to her. You would:

    A. Tell her that she forgot and she must have misplaced them.
    B. Tell her you will look for them and then just forget about it.
    C. Tell her that you will have to fill out an incident report.
    D. Tell the nurses to look for them.

23. Another patient needs to urinate. The person is on a stretcher in the hallway. You would:

    A. Get the patient up and escort him or her to the bathroom.
    B. Provide the patient with a urinal or bedpan.
    C. Move the stretcher into an empty room and provide the patient with a urinal or bedpan.
    D. Tell the patient you'll be back in a

few minutes and hope someone else helps.

24. If breathing is compromised and the patient cannot sit up, to aid in breathing you would:

    A. Place pillows under the head.
    B. Administer oxygen.
    C. Provide an inhaler.

D. Place the patient in the Trendelenburg position.

25. Patient comfort, safety, and privacy will be:
    A. Exactly the same for each patient
    B. Varied for each individual circumstance and patient
    C. Sacrificed if the department is busy
    D. Documented on every requisition

Answers appear at the end of the book.

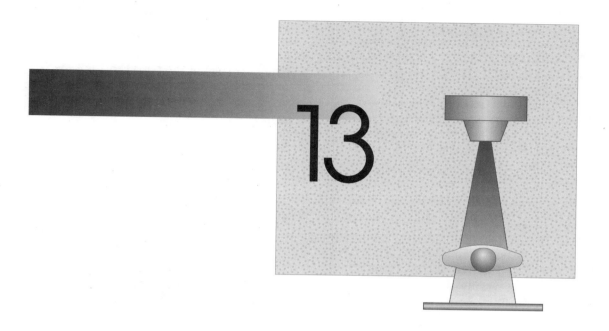

PREVENTION AND CONTROL OF INFECTION

TRANSMISSION OF INFECTION

We do not live in a sterile world. Microbes, bacteria, viruses, and other assorted pathogens are part of everyday life and are located everywhere. There is no escaping them. Usually they do not pose a threat of constant disease, and for the most part we mutually inhabit the earth without serious conflict. Unfortunately, we are not all healthy with perfect immunity, and at times, if our immune system is compromised or we break our most protective shielding, our skin, we set up an invitation for invasion, creating illness or infection. A cycle of infection actually exists to allow for infection to occur, and it is described here.

Cycle of Infection

1. The pathogen must exist.
2. A source or origin for its growth and reproduction must exist.
3. An exit must be present from the growth source.
4. A transportation mode for transmission must exist.
   a. Direct—Pathogen delivered straight to host by infected carrier.
   b. Indirect
      1. Fomite—An object that is contaminated with pathogens delivers pathogen when touched by a host. Example: hands
      2. Vector—An organism in which the pathogen multiplies or develops (not necessarily affecting it) before infecting the new host. Example: mosquitoes/malaria
      3. Airborne—Droplet/dust/spore contamination. Example: cough
5. A host entryway must be present.
6. The host must be susceptible.

All these must be present for the infection to take place. If one element of the cycle is absent, the infection cannot take hold and its cycle is broken. This is the basis of *infection control*. As health care workers we have to be especially vigilant to minimize *nosocomial infection* (resultant infection from hospital health care delivery). Nosocomial infection tends to inhabit the following body sites: urinary tract, blood stream, respiratory tract, and wound locations. We attempt to break at least one link of its cyclical chain to *prevent* the infection. We may use one of two types of infection control practice: *medical* and *surgical asepsis*.

MEDICAL AND SURGICAL ASEPSIS
Medical Asepsis (Table 13–1)

This is referred to as *clean technique* or *aseptic technique* and refers to all procedures that cannot be accomplished in a sterile environment for whatever reason. The idea here is to reduce as many microorganisms as possible and limit the spread of the ones that "got away." Let's examine each criterion for infection and see what mechanism of aseptic technique could be employed.

The most critical mechanism that can be used to ward off infection is *hand washing. It is, by far, the most effective.* Just simple rinsing will not reduce the bacterial count.

An established procedure must be followed for proper hand washing. This will vary according to each facility's policy and procedure for infection control, but the basic gist is that warm water and antiseptic cleaner must be used, jewelry should be removed, fingernails should be specifically cleaned as they harbor the highest content of microbes, and the washing action must continue for a specified time: minimally, at *least* 10 to 15 seconds. Cross-contamination by touching the faucets should be avoided. Always use paper toweling to turn off the faucet, and then dispose of it.

Hand washing should be performed by healthcare workers for these situations:

▪ Before and after each patient contact or associated patient care procedures.
▪ After contact with organic material or containers holding these materials.
▪ After handling contaminated equipment.
▪ After removal of sterile and nonsterile gloves.

The following pointers will assist in reducing nosocomial infection:

▪ Wash hands!
▪ Assess your patient's susceptibility to infection. Identify high-risk patients.
▪ Be dogmatic in your approach to aseptic practice. Do not relax standards.
▪ Stay home if you are ill. Bringing a known infection into the workplace is unacceptable.
▪ Identify body sites that tend to develop nosocomial infection so that you can intensify infection control when necessary.

Isolation precautions will be covered independently and are an integral piece in the control of all infectious disease processes.

Surgical Asepsis (see Table 13–1)

Surgical asepsis is more stringent in practice than medical aseptic technique. In this practice,

Table 13-1 ■ **MEDICAL/SURGICAL ASEPSIS**

Infection Criterion	Infection Control Practice Mechanism
Existence of the Pathogen	Cleanliness (keep objects and areas as clean as possible) Antiseptic use (**inhibits** microbial growth) Germicide use (disinfects—**destroys pathogenic** microbes) Sterilizing (when possible: **destroys all** microbes; heat, gas, or chemical solutions)
Source or Growth Origin	Change, capture, and dispose of soiled dressings, linens, and clothing Contain soiled tissues and dispose of promptly Dispose of needles and syringes into moisture-/puncture-proof containers Check the integrity of all bodily fluid drainage systems Dispose drainage systems as biohazardous/medical waste Keep bottled solutions closed tightly as much as possible Maintain a clean and dry environment Patient must be kept clean and dry
Exit at the Growth Source *(Exit for escape of pathogens)*	Cover nose and mouth during sneezes or coughs Limit talking/sneezing/coughing over open wounds or sterile fields Use a mask or place a mask for URI (upper respiratory infection) Wear gloves if handling blood/bodily fluids Use gowns/eye shields if bodily fluids may spray/splash Approach all handling of bodily fluids/specimens as if infectious
Spread or Transmission Mode	Wash hands! Avoid shared use of personal care items Confine contaminants: do not shake linens, clothing, or dustcloths Avoid cross-contamination of soiled articles with clean ones Discard/disinfect or resterilize any item that falls onto a septic area Adhere to isolation guidelines
Host Entry	Maintain skin integrity. Keep clean and lubricated If skin is broken, clean thoroughly and apply dressing, if applicable Limit exchange of bodily fluids Dispose of sharps in the proper containers. Don't assume that others will; keep an eye out for misplaced or ill-disposed sharps in bed linens and gowns, and so on
Susceptible Host	Maintain good nutrition, sufficient rest, vitamin and mineral therapy, exercise, and wear season-appropriate apparel Keep stress to a minimum or learn stress management techniques Attend to health requirements promptly

also referred to as *sterile technique,* microorganisms are all eliminated from an object, and the surgical area is protected from outside contamination through the use of sterile draping. If an infraction occurs during this technique, it greatly increases the patient's odds of becoming infected. This process is strictly utilized under the following conditions:

- Any time the patient's skin is broken for an intentional procedure. Example: sutures
- Any time the skin is damaged during trauma, surgery, or burns
- Any time a procedure requires insertion of a device or instrument into a body cavity

All instrumentation must be autoclaved or sterilized via a sterilizing gas or chemical solution. Sterile paper, cloth or plastic gowns, masks, booties and caps, as well as paper drapes assist in protecting sterility. Sterile gloves must be worn, and specific instructions must be adhered to for setting up a sterile field. Patients who are anesthetized for a procedure cannot contaminate

the field, but patients who are under a local anesthetic and receiving treatment outside the operating room must be educated in their role, so they don't contaminate the field without thinking.

Surgical asepsis is a mind set. The more frequently it is practiced, the more it becomes ingrained in the health care worker's behavior.

Principles of Surgical Asepsis

- The most important concept is: *a sterile object remains sterile only by coming in contact with another sterile object.*
- Sterile in contact with clean is contaminated.
- Sterile in contact with contaminated is contaminated.
- Sterile in contact with questionable is contaminated.
- Only sterile items may be placed in a sterile field.
- Sterilized packaging must be checked for its

integrity. If there is any question regarding it, the object is rendered unsterile.

■ Sterile objects held below waist level or out of the field of vision are considered unsterile. Sterility is assured only when the objects have remained in full view.

■ Heavy air movement or prolonged exposure to air also provides contamination.

■ Personnel not considered essential should be kept away from the sterile preparation.

■ Avoid extending your reach over the sterile field. This may cause contamination.

■ A sterile object is never returned to its original packaging.

■ Saliva droplets also carry microbes. Talking, singing, laughing, and sneezing/coughing should be minimized over and around the sterile field.

■ Moisture will wick its way to the sterile object and create contamination. Any solution that is spilled, unless on a moisture-proof surface, will cause contamination. Radiographers must be diligent in observing for moisture contamination, either in packaging or created during the procedure.

■ After hand washing, it is critical to keep the hands at a level above the elbows. This prevents contamination of the scrubbed hands from water that may run downward from the *un*scrubbed arm.

■ Sterile field borders (1″) from the edge are considered contaminated. They act as a buffer between the unsterile and sterile; it is added protection. It is important that sterile protective wear or sterile objects do not touch this unsafe space.

■ Edges of sterile containers are also considered contaminated. During uncapping of a sterile syringe, if it touches the outside edge of the paper package, it is no longer sterile. Another one must be used. Xylocaine gel derived from a multiuse tube must be extruded and discarded and a second amount extruded again for the procedure.

■ Solutions must also be poured for discard and then poured again from the same area of the bottle lip for the procedure.

It is always helpful to have someone else help you set up the sterile area, as two sets of eyes are better than one in evaluating possible contamination. Sterile trays or drapes are always opened with the top flap folded back, away from you first, then the side flaps are opened, and finally the one on the bottom and closest to you is then opened toward you. This helps reduce how many times you must reach over the tray or drape, thus reducing the chance of contamination.

UNIVERSAL PRECAUTIONS/STANDARD PRECAUTIONS

Years ago, isolation was assigned for patients exhibiting specific diseases. There were varying degrees of isolation, becoming more elaborate as the severity of the illness increased. Years ago, HIV (human immunodeficiency virus) and AIDS (acquired immunodeficiency syndrome) were not epidemic. Tuberculosis (TB) was epidemic and mandated by the government to be reported to public health officials. It was followed on a per case basis. There are TB survivors from an outbreak in the 1950s residing in northern California who are still being followed today. There are also arguments, pro and con, about the constitutionality of such a protocol. In 1991, when the Occupational Health Administration (OSHA) and the Centers for Disease Control (CDC) and Prevention mandated that *health care workers approach every patient and body specimen as if infected,* and that is when *universal precautions* for isolation techniques were born. Universal precautions were renamed *standard precautions* in 1995. Both names are used within this text, as the terminology is still considered relatively new.

Fact List for Universal Precautions/ Standard Precautions

Universal precautions/standard precautions apply to all patients with:

■ Any dressing, tissue or body fluid visibly contaminated with blood

Precautions must be taken for contact with all of the following:

■ Peritoneal, amniotic, vaginal, and seminal fluid; synovial fluid and saliva (dental)
■ Cerebrospinal fluid
■ Pleural and pericardial fluids

Personal protective equipment (PPE), hand washing, and other preventative measures include the following:

■ Gloves must be worn when encountering any of the aforementioned patients or specimens.
■ Gloves must be worn for phlebotomy.
■ Gloves must be changed between each patient and removed while performing other

tasks that do not require them to prevent cross-contamination.

- Hands and other skin surfaces must be washed immediately if contaminated.
- Masks and protective eye shields must be worn when splashing/spraying of bodily fluid is predicted. TB filtration (respirator) masks must be worn if TB is suspect.
- Protective gowns and related items must be worn if splashing/spraying of bodily fluid is predicted.
- Used needles are not to be recapped or removed from the used syringe. Dispose of sharps in a protective container designed for that purpose. Use self-sheathing sharps when available.
- Resuscitation masks or other protective barriers should be available for use.
- Specimens must be transported in a leakproof, sturdy container. Care must be instituted to prevent outside contamination of the container or paperwork.
- Personnel must report exposure to blood/bodily fluids or incidents regarding sharps to their supervisors, with anticipated follow-up with infection control and employee health services.
- Any health care worker with weeping skin lesions/dermatitis should be relieved from direct patient contact care and from handling equipment.

Universal/standard precautions, however standard they may appear, are still not standard enough. Other patient conditions warrant additional isolation and protective measures. Additional isolation measures are required for specific disease transmission (see Isolation Guidelines Flow Chart).

Isolation Guidelines Flow Chart

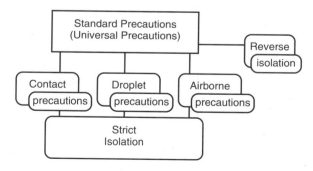

Contact Isolation Precautions

Address MRSA (methicillin-resistant *Staphylococcus aureus*)–infected patients and those afflicted with *Salmonella* or *Escherichia coli* who suffer from infectious diarrhea. Included in the contact category would also be patients with hepatitis A, severe herpes simplex, as well as those with lice and scabies. Gloves must be worn upon service with the patient or upon entering the patient's room. Gloves must be changed after contact with infectious material. Gowns are worn during patient care or when touching infectious environmental surfaces.

Droplet Isolation Precautions

Address disease processes that are spread by droplets. These would include meningitis (*Haemophilus influenzae*/*Neisseria meningitidis*), *Mycoplasma* pneumonia, rubella, and group A strep. Patients must be sequestered in private rooms. Masks must be worn by health care providers. Gloves must be worn for contact with every patient.

Airborne Isolation Precautions

Address tuberculosis, measles, and varicella. Employ contact precautions. These infections require strict isolation, as they are transmitted by *droplet nuclei particles*. These nuclei particles are so microscopic that they must be filtered from the air by special equipment. Negative pressure (6 or more air exchanges per hour) rooms are designed to have all the air in the room filtered and vented to the outside so that the pathogens do not float in the air, out into the hallways, afflicting others. Respiratory (N95) masks must be worn by all who enter into service with these so infected individuals.

Reverse Isolation

This precaution is designed to *protect the patient* from the health care worker or visitor. It is termed *reverse isolation*. Positive pressure rooms are designed to prevent the air from the adjacent hallway to enter the room and possibly compromise the patient's health. This room is used for the severely immunosuppressed individual (leukemic/bone marrow patient) or the organ transplant recipient. When strict isolation is enforced, few, if any visitors are allowed. This has an impact on the mental and emotional status of the patient and, at times, will prolong the disease process because of a stress reaction and depression. Most facilities have an infection control policy; become familiar with it.

ISOLATION/INFECTION CONTROL PRACTICE DURING RADIOGRAPHIC PROCEDURES

Some guidelines must be adhered to when radiographing a patient:

- Always wash your hands before seeing every patient; allow them to see you do this; and wash hands after the procedure has ended.
- Always change the pillowcase between patients, and clean the table surface. It is reassuring to the patient to witness the pillowcase change.
- If the patient must place the face or open mouth against the table or upright Bucky for a projection, demonstrate, in front of the patient, the actual cleaning process.
- A sheet placed on the tabletop aids in keeping the surface clean.
- Provide the patient with a cup for dentures or container specifically designed for that purpose. Do not add jewelry or hairpins to this container.
- Always place the cassette in a pillowcase or behind the sheet rather than directly against the patient's skin. This will keep the cassette cleaner and be more comfortable to the patient.
- Clean cassette or table surfaces promptly, should they become contaminated.
- Reverse isolation precautions require equipment cleaning prior to the procedure.
- Full protective barrier dress may be required for strict or reverse procedures.
- Remember to discard all protective gear properly by removing it so that the "clean" side winds up on the outside. Consolidate it, if possible, and remove promptly.

Follow all isolation precautions to a "T." Stop at the nurses' station to check the chart or ask specific questions regarding the patient's condition. Most health care personnel will help one another by alerting you to the status of the patient, even if it is questionable, so that you may take the necessary precautions. But there is always the patient who surprises everyone after the battery of tests is completed and the results are in.

The best advice is to use common sense. If you are radiographing an emergency room patient who is coughing and spitting up mucus, who really knows what he or she has? Maybe it will turn out to be TB, or maybe just the flu. Do you want to take the risk of contracting either? Even prior to the diagnosis being formally made, it is completely acceptable to wear a mask for yourself or ask the patient to please wear one during the procedure. An old but true adage still applies: An ounce of prevention is worth a pound of cure.

BIOHAZARDOUS MATERIALS

It used to be that garbage was garbage. No matter what it was, you threw what you didn't want into the trash and it magically disappeared. Or so we thought. We are now running out of dumping ground for garbage, and nobody wants it. More importantly, receivers want only specific garbage. Organic garbage is still okay. Recyclables are still in demand. But biohazardous or medical waste is in a different league. No one wants it, and, in fact, it costs medical facilities millions of dollars every year to find someone to dispose of it, and only if it is disposed of properly. Should a hospital be identified as a facility that has mixed the biohazardous waste with the regular trash, watch out! Heavy monetary fines are now levied, and in fact that facility will likely have all the contaminated garbage delivered back to its own doorstep! Not a pretty picture on the front page of the local newspaper. Or worse: on the national news.

It is imperative that all medical waste be disposed of in the proper receptacle appointed for that particular function at your facility. Most medical waste is mandated as such if it is saturated with or contains blood or other bodily fluid. Some facilities have big red garbage containers, imprinted with the universal biohazard insignia, for just that purpose. Sharps, however, do not go into that container. They must be disposed of into the sharps box, designated for that particular purpose. The sharps boxes have reduced needlesticks dramatically. Many facilities subcontract outside companies to pick up and replace these containers.

Some sophisticated equipment exists for garbage identification prior to release to the carter company. Conveyor belts will send the garbage through an inspection line of workers looking for biohazards that don't belong. Radioactivity can also be detected by scanners that will alert, via alarm, any level of radiation required. This material is then allowed to decay and be disposed of safely at a later date. These systems are generally set up through the facility's safety and/or radiation safety committee. The Environmental Protection Agency (EPA), OSHA, and Nuclear Regulatory Commission (NRC) are responsible for most of these garbage initiatives. It is important for you to think, before you throw anything away, about where it will finally end up.

Bibliography

Ballinger PW: Merrill's Atlas of Radiographic Positions and Radiologic Procedures. 7th ed. St. Louis, Mosby–Year Book, 1991

Ehrlich RA, McCloskey ED: Patient Care in Radiography. 3rd ed. St. Louis, Mosby–Year Book, 1989

Garner JS: Guidelines for isolation precautions in hospitals. Infect Control Hosp Epidemiol 1996;17(1):53–80. *Erratum* Infect Control Hosp Epidemiol 1996;17(4):214.

Gurley LT, Callaway WJ: Introduction to Radiologic Technology. 3rd ed. St. Louis, Mosby–Year Book, 1992

Perry AG, Potter PA: Clinical Nursing Skills and Techniques. 3rd ed. St. Louis, Mosby–Year Book, 1994

1. The best "defense against infection" organ that humans possess is:

   A. The liver
   B. The skin
   C. The heart
   D. The spleen

2. Which of these do not belong in the cycle of infection?

   A. A susceptible host
   B. An existing pathogen
   C. Medical asepsis must exist
   D. A source for growth and reproduction must exist for the pathogen.

3. Infection control hopes to:

   A. Eliminate all microbes from the work environment
   B. Control only existing infections
   C. Break one of the links in the infection cycle
   D. Control infection by using only standard precautions

4. Infection specifically related to health care delivery is termed:

   A. Sepsis
   B. Enteric infection
   C. AIDS
   D. Nosocomial

5. Medical asepsis is also referred to as:

   A. Aseptic or clean technique
   B. Sterile technique
   C. Surgical asepsis
   D. Universal precautions

6. Aseptic technique is meant to:

   A. Eliminate all pathogens
   B. Be used during surgical procedures
   C. Be used only for syringe preparation
   D. Minimize as many microbes as possible and limit infection spread

7. If you wish to inhibit microbial growth, which control will be used?

   A. An antiseptic
   B. A germicide
   C. An autoclave
   D. An ultraviolet light

8. Disinfectants are used to:

   A. Destroy all microbes
   B. Inhibit microbial growth
   C. Destroy all pathogenic microbes
   D. Balance the pathogenic microbes for immediate control

9. Sterilization is the only process that:

   A. Destroys all microbes
   B. Balances microbial population
   C. Is used for medical asepsis
   D. Allows good bacteria to survive

10. What helps minimize the growth of pathogenic bacteria in a patient environment?

    A. A good diet
    B. Use of gloves
    C. Maintaining a clean and dry environment
    D. Maintaining at least 80% humidity in the patient environment

11. The most effective method to control the spread of infection is:

    A. Use of antiseptics
    B. Hand washing
    C. Face masks
    D. Proper sharps disposal

12. Most antiseptic wash solutions take at least _____ to begin their effectiveness.

    A. 3 to 5 sec
    B. 10 to 15 sec
    C. 30 to 60 sec
    D. 5 min

13. To limit cross-contamination at the sink:

    A. Use paper towels when touching the faucet
    B. Use a new bottle of antiseptic scrub at every wash
    C. Always prepare to wash with gloves on
    D. Use only hot water

14. You must wash your hands for which of the following conditions?

A. Before and after patient contact
B. After touching each cassette
C. After removal of sterile or nonsterile gloves
D. More than one, but not all of the above

15. Coming into the health care workplace with an active cold will:

    A. Help you gain *employee of the month* status for not using your sick time
    B. Probably help promote nosocomial infection
    C. Only make you uncomfortable while working
    D. Allow you to be sent home early by your supervisor

16. Surgical asepsis is the same as:

    A. Aseptic technique
    B. Clean technique
    C. Sterile technique
    D. Standard precautions

17. Sterile technique is required for which of the following situations?

    1. Insertion of an IV
    2. Foley catheter placement
    3. Assessing the patient's temperature

    A. 1 only
    B. 3 only
    C. 1 and 2
    D. 1 and 3

18. A discoloration appears on the outside of the sterile instrument you are about to open. In which category would you place this instrument?

    A. Sterile
    B. Questionable, therefore contaminated
    C. Questionable, but sterile
    D. Fine

19. A piece of tape on the sterile packaging has lost its adhesiveness and fallen off. All other tape is intact. In which category would you place this instrument?

    A. Sterile
    B. Questionable therefore contaminated
    C. Questionable but still sterile
    D. Contaminated

20. Universal/standard precautions are employed for:

    A. Patients who are HIV positive
    B. Patients who have TB
    C. Patients who are immunosuppressed
    D. Every patient

21. If a patient has TB, they may be placed in:

    1. A negative-pressure room
    2. A positive-pressure room
    3. Strict isolation

    A. 1 only
    B. 2 only
    C. 1 and 2
    D. 1 and 3

22. Contact precautions are initiated when the patient has:

    A. *E. coli*
    B. Lice
    C. MRSA
    D. All of the above

23. A liver transplant recipient would most likely be placed in:

    1. A positive-pressure room
    2. Reverse isolation
    3. A negative-pressure room

    A. 1 only
    B. 2 only
    C. 1 and 2
    D. 1 and 3

24. Band-aids should be discarded in the:

    A. Regular trash
    B. Biohazard container
    C. Sharps container
    D. Toilet

25. Biohazard disposal laws were initiated by:

    A. The garbage companies
    B. OSHA, NRC, and the EPA
    C. The FDA
    D. The FBI

26. A contaminated cassette is an example of which indirect infection transmission?

    A. Vector
    B. Fomite
    C. Air-spore
    D. It is an example of direct transmission.

27. Which of the following diseases is spread by vector transmission?

A. Malaria
B. Genital herpes
C. Pneumonia
D. Whooping cough

28. Fomites, vectors, and airborne transmission are all examples of:

A. Methods of direct contact infection
B. Methods of indirect contact infection
C. They can be direct or indirect methods of contact infection.
D. They are the only methods applied to viral contact infection.

Answers appear at the end of the book.

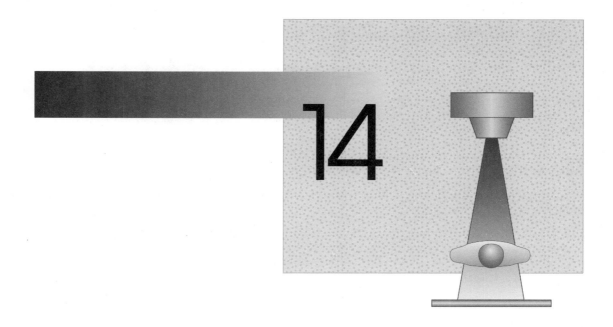

PATIENT MONITORING

ROUTINE MONITORING

As health care responds to the new demands placed upon it by government and insurance providers, through managed care, so must radiographers respond to their new, amplified role. Medical professionals are being asked to expand their traditional responsibilities into other arenas. Cross-training and multiskill performance are now being implemented everywhere. Technologists are being asked to provide more clinical nursing duties than in the past. This chapter addresses those duties.

Vital Signs

Vital signs are primary indicators of the patient's health status. They include

- Temperature
- Respiration
- Pulse
- Blood pressure

These must be measured and documented under the following conditions:

1. On the patient's admission to the health care facility
2. In hospital, on routine schedule according to the physician's order or hospital policy
3. During the patient's visit to the clinician's or physician's office
4. Before and after any surgical procedure
5. Before and after any invasive diagnostic procedure
6. Before and after any administration of medications affecting cardiovascular, respiratory, or temperature control function
7. When the patient's general physical condition changes. E.g., pain increase, loss of consciousness, reaction to medication
8. Before and after clinical intervention influencing the vital signs
9. Whenever a patient reports a change or a clinician observes a change, of nonspecific nature, creating distress. E.g., odd sensations, or feeling "funny"[1]

Vital signs are measured and have specific numerical ranges that are considered normal. To measure some of them, special equipment is re-

Table 14–1 ■ **BASICS OF VITAL SIGNS**

Vital Sign	How to Measure	Normal Range
Temperature	Thermometer	Oral: 98°–99°F/37°C Rectal: 99°–100°F/38°C Axillary: 97°–98°F/36°C Tympanic: 98°–99°F/37°C
Respiration	Wristwatch Visual observation Count respirations for 30 sec; multiply by 2 for exact count	Neonate: 30–60/breaths/min Children: 20–26/breaths/min Adolescent: 16–18/breaths/min Adult: 12–20/breaths/min
Pulse	Wristwatch Visual observation Point of contact: 　Radial artery (use fingers, not thumb) 　Carotid artery (use fingers, not thumb) 　Count pulse for 30 seconds, multiply by 2 for exact count	Normal falls between 60–100/beats/min 　Tachycardia—over 100/beats/min 　Bradycardia—under 60/beats/min
Blood Pressure	Stethoscope Sphygmomanometer (blood pressure cuff) 　Position cuff above antecubital space 　Position stethoscope at brachial artery 　Inflate cuff to 180 mm Hg 　Pulse first heard = systolic (top number) 　Pulse disappears = diastolic (bottom number)	**Diastolic** ≤85　Normal BP 85–89　High normal BP 90–104　Mild hypertension 105–114　Moderate hypertension >115　Severe hypertension **Systolic, If Diastolic BP Is <90** ≤140　Normal BP 140–159　Borderline, isolated systolic hypertension >160　Isolated systolic hypertension
Oxygen Saturation (medical order required)*	Pulse oximeter measures arterial O_2 saturation	Normal SaO_2 >90% If SaO_2 is <85%, medical intervention is required

*This measurement is generally ordered for critical care patients and monitored by a registered nurse. It is included here because it is used frequently within a radiology department. It is *not* considered a standard vital sign.

Data from Perry AG, Potter PA: Clinical Nursing Skills and Techniques. 4th ed. St. Louis, CV Mosby, 1998.

quired. You should be aware of the equipment's location and accuracy.

Table 14–1 provides the basics of vital signs. Remember to document your outcomes!

Patient Assessment

Now that we have a baseline for normal measurement in patient assessment, let's discuss abnormal conditions and how to identify them (signs and symptoms):

Temperature. Elevated temperature, fever/febrile:

Skin

- may be flushed
- may be warm/hot
- may be dry/diaphoretic
- may demonstrate "goosebumps" (piloerection)

Other

- patient will shiver, have chills
- tachycardia
- malaise/restless

Response. Remove as much exterior clothing/coverings as possible. Keep room cool.

Decreased Body Temperature, Hypothermia:

Skin

- pale
- cool and dry

Other

- patient will shiver, have chills
- shallow respiration rate
- compromised mental response

Response. Cover with additional sheets/blankets. Try to keep room warm.

Respiration. Any of these signs and symptoms may alert you to a respiratory problem.

- cyanosis (hypoxia, blue cast to skin)
- restless, irritable, confused, compromised level of consciousness
- difficult/painful breathing (dyspnea)
- excessive sputum production during cough
- inability to breathe (apnea)
- trouble breathing unless upright (orthopnea)
- apnea and hyperventilation pattern in alternate periods (Cheyne-Stokes breathing)
- hypoventilation (respiratory rate too low)
- hyperventilation (respiratory rate elevated)

Response. When possible, elevate patient's head. If oxygen administration is required because of hypoxia, remember that it is considered a medication and must be ordered by a physician.

Patients suffering from COPD (chronic obstructive pulmonary disease), which includes emphysema, cannot tolerate high-oxygen therapy. In an emergency, high-dose oxygen therapy is initiated despite preexisting conditions. If complications develop, the patient can be intubated and ventilated mechanically.[2]

The usual dose of oxygen therapy is between 2 and 4 liters/min. This can be delivered by nasal cannula, face mask, or tent. All this information will be documented in the patient's chart. It is important to check this information in the radiology department, because many times a patient will present with a portable tank that is almost empty. Generally, you will have access to wall oxygen, but if the patient is delayed for the procedure or delayed in transport back to the room, you must calculate whether there is adequate oxygen reserve in the tank.

Use these formulas:

$$\text{Pressure of the cylinder tank} = \text{PSI (pounds/square inch)}$$

For E cylinder tanks (hold 625 liters of oxygen): cylinder factor = 0.3

For H cylinder tanks (hold 6600 liters of oxygen): cylinder factor = 3.1

$$\frac{(\text{PSI}) \times \text{cylinder factor}}{\text{liters/minute}} = \frac{\text{remaining minutes}}{\text{of available oxygen}}$$

Example:
An **E cylinder** contains 1800 psi
The flow rate for the patient is 4 liters/min
$1800 \times 0.3 = 5400 \div 4 = 135$ min.

Pulse

Peripheral pulse is an indication of the level of function of the cardiovascular system. It is actually a wave formation originating from the blood volume released from the ventricle against the aortic wall. As the blood surges against the aorta, it extends and creates the pulse wave that will instantly travel to the distal arteries. The following symptoms and signs may indicate a change in status of the cardiovascular system:

- dyspnea
- fatigue
- chest pain
- heart palpitations
- jugular distention
- edema
- cyanosis or pallor

Response. Compare pulse rate to previously recorded rate. If it is significantly altered, seek assistance from nursing. Always document your findings.

Blood Pressure. Blood pressure is the measurement of the force of blood against the vessels' walls. The sphygmomanometer contains mercury in a sealed tube. The blood pressure actually causes that mercury to move upward, resulting in a measurement standard. The systolic pressure originates when the left ventricle releases the blood into the aorta. This is considered the maximum pressure of the cardiac pumping cycle. The diastole is the relaxing stage, or minimum pressure of that cycle. This occurs as the ventricles relax.

Signs and symptoms of blood pressure complications are

Hypertension (high blood pressure)

▪ not unusual for patient to be asymptomatic
▪ headache
▪ flushed face
▪ epistaxis (nosebleed)
▪ fatigue

Hypotension (low blood pressure)

▪ lightheaded/dizzy
▪ restless
▪ pale
▪ cool, especially extremities (they may appear mottled)
▪ change in mental status

Response. Other than the obvious comfort response, if the patient complains of any of these changes or an obvious change in status occurs during the procedure, check the blood pressure. Compare it with what is documented in the chart, if that is available. If an appreciable difference is detected, seek medical assistance. Always document your findings in the medical record and contact the patient's unit nurse/attending physician.

SUPPORT EQUIPMENT

When certain functions of the body are compromised because of illness, specific equipment can be implemented to assist the patient in recovery. Let's review them.

Intravenous Devices

Patients require IV fluid administration to maintain body fluid, electrolytes, nutritional requirements, and access for medications; generally these are injected through a heparin lock. When medication access is required, it is referred to as PIV (peripheral *intravenous*) therapy. Most patients arriving in the radiology department have IV pumps (electronic infusion devices, or EID) if they are on IV therapy. These are awkward and troublesome but highly reliable. Every pump is designed differently, so instruction must be provided for each one to determine its use. It is critical to check the medication order for volume and flow rate prior to restarting the unit. This will insure that the patient is receiving the proper prescription. It is also imperative that when a solution bag empties and must be replaced, it is noted in the patient's chart. Observe the IV site when the patient arrives and once again at the end of the procedure. Check for redness or swelling from infiltration. Make sure the line is open and not occluded with blood. Always ask for nursing assistance if you are unsure or require help.

Vascular Access Devices (VADs)

Patients who are critically or chronically ill require these devices. They are catheters that are placed in a central venous line so that the patient no longer requires venipuncture. Many drugs or prolonged use of specific venous sites deteriorate the veins so badly that they can no longer be accessed successfully. There are three main types of VADs (although there are numerous brand names, such as Hickman, Port-A-Cath, Swan-Ganz).

Central Venous Catheters. These are inserted into a large vein, commonly the superior vena cava that leads to the right atrium of the heart. Because the lumen of the vessel is large, it minimizes irritation, inflammation, and sclerosis. It is used to administer medications, parenteral nutrition, and blood products. It is also accessed for blood samples. These catheters can also be tunneled or surgically implanted. The chance of infection is now reduced.

Percutaneous Central Venous Catheter. This is placed through the skin directly into the subclavian vein. It can also be threaded into the antecubital fossa and go directly into the right atrium. They are generally called PICC (peripherally inserted central catheter) lines. These are initially placed under fluoroscopic conditions in the interventional radiologic suite.

Implanted Infusion Port. This is the third type of VAD. It is inserted during a surgical procedure and is located in the infraclavicular fossa but threaded via a large vein into the right atrium. Special needles (Huber) must be used to gain access to this port. They are needles that do not core the rubber stoppers of medication, inadvertently introducing foreign particulate matter.

All of these special access devices require care to prevent infection and clotting. Heparin is used to maintain patency. The access port must be kept clean. Care should be taken with patients who have these devices. Move patients gently on the radiographic table; do not disturb these sites.

Nasogastric Tube

This tube is threaded into the nasopharynx and on into the stomach. It allows fluid in and out (with suction) of the stomach. It is very uncomfortable for the patient, and care must be taken not to displace or remove the tube. The NG tube is also called a Levin tube. Nasoenteric tubes are also utilized. They are destined for the small intestine and may be placed under fluoroscopy. Their tip is radiopaque for ease in visualization. Barium must never be used in these tubes. Oral iodinated contrast medium that is water soluble is the medium of choice.

Urinary Bladder Catheter (Foley Catheter)

This is a catheter attached to a bag. The catheter tip is inserted into the urinary bladder, and the urine is then able to drain into the bag. This is especially helpful to incontinent patients as well as postsurgical patients who do not have voluntary control of their bladder because of anesthesia. It is critical to note whether this device is being used by your patient. It must be clamped off if the patient is having an IVP and unclamped for the postvoid film. It is also critical not to tug or pull on this tube or have the bag drop when close to full. The weight may sometimes dislodge the catheter.

Closed-Chest Drainage Systems

When air or fluid leaks into the intrapleural space, either because of trauma, surgery, or disease, a chest drainage system is required to restore the closed environment. If such a system is not inserted, the patient will experience a collapsed lung, infection, or other problems. There are various systems. Some have a water suction, and others are waterless. A tube is placed into the pleural space, which attaches to a drainage receptacle that measures output. Care must be taken not to disturb this assembly. Serious injury will occur to the patient if either attachment becomes dislodged. Be certain to maintain the level of the fluid container lower than the patient's lungs to avoid backflow into the lungs.

Make a mental note of the fluid level at the onset of the procedure. If excessive fluid, especially if it is bloody, drains during the procedure, contact the patient's physician immediately.

Ostomy Construction

An ostomy is a surgically created opening to allow the passage of feces, urine, or air. Although this is not a device, it is a means of aiding the patient's health status, as the patient, for whatever reason, cannot manage the natural function. Typical created ostomies are:

Colostomy/Enterostomy. This opening is surgically created through the abdominal wall into the colon. It can be made into any portion of the colon: ileostomy, transverse colostomy, and sigmoid colostomy. An external bag must be worn as an attachment to collect the feces and be emptied as needed and replaced. Sigmoid colostomies don't always require a bag. Because of the location and formation of the stool, the colon can be irrigated daily to remove the feces on a schedule.

Ureterostomy. This is generally performed only on infants. It is a surgical procedure that brings the ureter up to the abdominal surface, and the urine is collected in the diaper. No bag is required. As the child approaches school age, another procedure takes place: a urinary diversion called the ileal loop.

Ileal Loop/Incontinent Urinary Diversion. The ileum of the small bowel is resected and a small section removed and positioned as a graft to the abdominal wall. Both ureters are repositioned surgically to drain into it and allow the urine to drain out of the abdominal wall. An ileal stoma is generally located in the right lower quadrant of the abdomen; a colon loop is generally located in the left lower quadrant. This necessitates a bag termed an Indiana pouch for collection of constant urine output.

Continent Urinary Diversion. An internal pouch is surgically placed to function as a reservoir for urine that must be drained periodically via catheter. The stoma is placed in the lower right quadrant and is flush with the skin.

Radiographers must be especially diligent not to dislodge any of the pouches or tubes during procedures. Patients have a difficult time adapting to these ostomies and may feel very self-conscious about them. These devices must be kept clean. Remember, water-soluble contrast media are preferable to barium for lower bowel imaging.

Tracheostomy

A surgical opening is made into the trachea so that an artificial airway is created (tracheotomy).

If a tube is placed in the opening so that the airway is more permanent, it is termed a tracheostomy. Tape anchors the tubing. Patients may require suction and/or oxygen maintenance, so have it available (set up) for any procedure that a tracheostomy patient may require.

A tracheostomy is vulnerable due to its location and lack of secure attachment. Extreme care must be taken by the technologist performing a procedure. Watch cassette placement for chest radiography and general patient movement in regard to the equipment.

COMMON MEDICAL EMERGENCIES AND THEIR MANAGEMENT

Let's look at the worst-case scenarios first. Trauma patients and critically ill patients are generally accompanied to the radiology department by at least a nurse. Generally the radiographer spends much of the time trying to perform her or his duty while other health professionals crowd around. In this type of situation, if the patient's status deteriorates, many people are available and able to help. Under these circumstances, the technologist will not have to respond initially because there will be many qualified professionals immediately available.

The most serious radiographer response situations occur with the patient whose trauma is not considered major. Many times the impact of that trauma has not been fully evaluated, and you now have the patient in the x-ray room alone. These are the patients that must be assessed continuously by you. The patient may still be in shock but able to stand or sit for the radiographs, when all of a sudden he or she may collapse or begin to vomit blood or have a seizure. This is the time when you, the radiographer, must know what to do.

Head Injuries

Patients that present with any type of head trauma, however minimal, should not be left unattended. If you must leave the area to develop the radiographs, ask for someone to stay with your patient in your absence. Many times these patients will need to vomit. When they do, it is generally projectile in nature. Generally an emesis basin will not be adequate to contain the vomitus. If a large basin or bedpan is available, use that instead. If the patient is supine, turn him or her onto the left side to vomit. Due to the configuration of the bronchi, turning the patient onto the right side actually increases the chance

of aspiration. Shock (neurogenic) may also be secondary to head trauma.

Shock

Shock is hypotension. It may originate from several situations:

Low blood volume/hypovolemic shock

- vomiting
- diarrhea
- hemorrhage

General collapse of the circulatory system/septic shock

- overwhelming infection

Failure of arterial resistance/neurogenic shock

- head/spinal trauma
- neurotransmitter failure

Failure of the heart to pump/cardiogenic shock

- pulmonary emboli
- myocardial infarct
- pericardial edema

Allergic response reaction/anaphylactic shock

- bee stings
- medications
- contrast media
- peanuts
- any foreign substance introduced into the body that the body has not yet been particularly histamine sensitized

Emotional/psychologic response reaction/syncope

- fear
- pain
- unpleasant events

Management of Shock

The signs and symptoms of shock are identical, regardless of which type of shock the patient is experiencing. They include:

- Hypotension (low blood pressure, under 90 mm Hg/systolic)
- Tachycardia (pulse rate over 100/minute)
- Cool, moist, pale skin
- Increased respiration
- Decreased mental status
- Anxiety
- Thirst

Recognition by the radiographer of these signs and symptoms is critical to the welfare of the patient. If you see that the patient is deteriorating, **by all means stop the procedure and *get help***. If the patient is standing or sitting, lower him directly onto the floor and elevate the feet into the Fowler position. Take the blood pressure and continue to assess for changes. It is much better to call a code and have it be a false alarm than for the patient to experience the alternative consequences. Knowledge of the correct method of calling in a code, the code cart's location, and your role during the code is essential. Review your facility's code policy. Allergic response reactions are discussed in Chapter 15.

Other Emergency Situations
Epistaxis/Nosebleed

- Have the patient sit up, if possible, or elevate the head.
- Provide gauze—tissue will adhere to the blood and stick.
- Instruct the patient to apply pressure against the nasal septum.
- If ice is available, place an ice pack on the nose; this will constrict blood vessels.
- Provide an emesis basin for the patient to spit blood into.
- Provide the patient with water to rinse the mouth.
- Get help if the bleeding doesn't stop after 10 minutes or worsens.

Seizures

- Have the patient lie down.
- Cushion the head.
- Turn patient onto the left side to avoid aspiration.

- Do not attempt to restrain the patient.
- Have suction ready and available.
- Use oxygen therapy if necessary.
- Time the seizure, if possible.
- After the seizure, check vital signs.

Hypoglycemia/Low Blood Sugar

- Determine diabetic status.
- Be alert for symptoms such as sudden onset of weakness, tremors, sweating, hunger, and syncope.
- Administer orange juice or provide a piece of hard candy.
- Use glucose gel on the inner cheek, if available.
- Check vital signs.

It is important to note that if the patient is injured when collapsing, an incident report must be documented. Any unusual occurrence in the radiology department must be reported to the patient's unit and documented in the chart.

CPR/American Heart Association Abdominal Thrusts

Cardiopulmonary resuscitation (CPR) has dedicated classes provided by the American Heart Association. In order for you to be ready and able to intervene and help during a cardiopulmonary arrest, you must be certified. It is beyond the scope of this book to provide you with all the CPR essentials. Table 14–2 provides vital CPR *review* information only.

The American Heart Association has also endorsed the use of their abdominal thrusts for dislodging foreign matter from the choking victim's airway. It is beyond the scope of this text to teach this maneuver, as it requires hands-on

Table 14–2 ■ **AMERICAN HEART ASSOCIATION'S ABCS OF CARDIOPULMONARY RESUSCITATION**

	Adult	*Child*	*Infant*
Airway	Head tilt–lift chin (no cervical trauma) Jaw thrust (cervical trauma)	Place hand under neck, elevate chin slightly	Place hand under neck
Breathing	Pinch nose, cover mouth with yours Two full initial breaths 0.5–2 sec Then: 10–12 breaths/min	Place your mouth over patient's nose and mouth Two full initial breaths 1–1.5 sec duration Then: 20 breaths/min	
Circulation	Place hands: 1–2 cm above xiphoid process Compress:* 1.5–2″ Rate: 80–100/min	Use heel of 1 hand: 1–2 cm above xiphoid ¾–1.5″ 100/min	Use index and middle finger: 1 cm below nipple line 0.5–1″ 100–200/min

*Maintain proper rate of compression!
Compression to breath ratio/2 rescuers = 5:1.
Compression to breath ratio/1 rescuer = 15:2.
Data from The American Heart Association: Textbook of Basic Life Support for Healthcare Providers. Dallas, The American Heart Association, 1994.

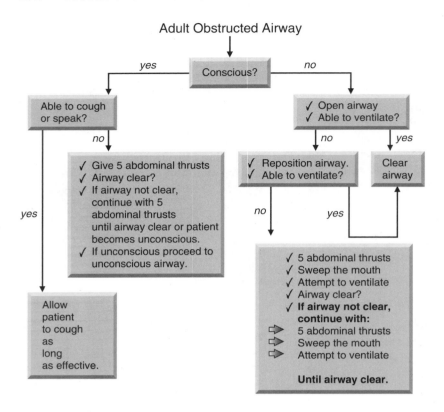

Adult Obstructed Airway

Figure 14-1 ■ Adult obstructed airway action chart. (From Brust DJ, Foster JA: From Nursing Assistant to Patient Care Technician. Philadelphia, WB Saunders, 1997.)

instruction. The flow chart in Figure 14–1 reviews the process.

ELECTROCARDIOGRAMS

This section provides an overview of the electrocardiogram (ECG). It is not meant to serve as a teaching exercise, only as a review of the basic elements: An electrocardiogram is a graphic representation of the heart's electrical energy that is produced during the cardiac cycle. A cardiac cycle is defined as diastole (resting or filling stage) and systole (contracting or emptying stage). During diastole, blood enters the right atrium from the superior and inferior vena cava. This blood fills and distends the right atrium, surging blood through the tricuspid valve into the right ventricle. Concurrently, blood is filling the left atrium from the pulmonary veins. As blood distends the left atrium, it is forced through the bicuspid valve into the left ventricle. The ventricles then contract (systole) causing the blood to surge out into the pulmonary and systemic circulation.

This cycle relies on electrical impulses to regulate the heart muscle continuously to rest and contract (Fig. 14–2). When this function becomes abnormal, a pacemaker is inserted to regulate the cardiac cycle artificially. The contraction phase originates in the sinoatrial node (SA node) located in the right atrium near the superior vena cava. The electrical impulse then travels to the atrioventricular node (AV node). The impulse continues through the bundle of His and on through the Purkinje network. The impulse spreads throughout the heart, and the heart muscle contracts shortly thereafter. The voltage produced can be detected on the skin by the electrode/sensor leads and then displayed on the monitor or paper.

The trick is to interpret these wave forms on the paper and correlate them with the actual event (see Fig. 14–2). Variations in these normal waves (Fig. 14–3) indicate specific problems, depending upon their rhythm and rate. It is the physician's role to interpret the abnormal findings.

Basic Procedure for the 12-Lead ECG

The patient must be made comfortable and provided with as much privacy as possible. The examination is done with the patient supine and covered with a sheet when not placing/accessing the electrodes. Because skin is a poor conductor, gel is applied to the skin before the electrode

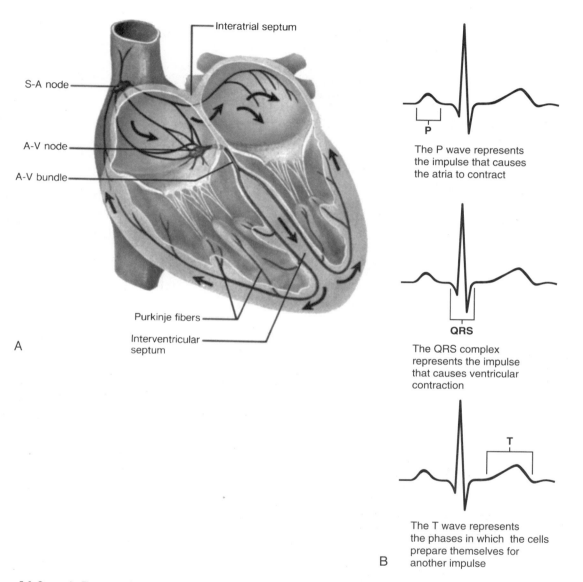

Interatrial septum

S-A node

A-V node

A-V bundle

Purkinje fibers

Interventricular septum

A

The P wave represents the impulse that causes the atria to contract

QRS

The QRS complex represents the impulse that causes ventricular contraction

T

The T wave represents the phases in which the cells prepare themselves for another impulse

B

Figure 14-2 ■ *A,* The conduction system of the heart. (From Creager JG: Human Anatomy and Physiology, 2nd ed. Dubuque, Wm C Brown Publishers, 1992.) *B,* Relationship between rhythm strips and electrical activity. (From Brust DJ, Foster JA: From Nursing Assistant to Patient Care Technician. Philadelphia, WB Saunders, 1997.)

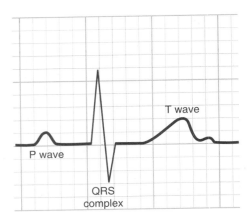

Figure 14-3 ■ Normal ECG waves. (From Brust DJ, Foster JA: From Nursing Assistant to Patient Care Technician. Philadelphia, WB Saunders, 1997.)

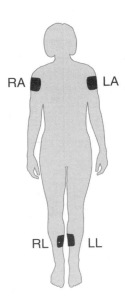

Figure 14-4 ■ Electrode placement for limb leads. (From Brust DJ, Foster JA: From Nursing Assistant to Patient Care Technician. Philadelphia, WB Saunders, 1997.)

application to increase conductivity. Skin areas where the electrodes are to be placed should be swabbed with alcohol and allowed to dry before placing the gel and sensor. Skin areas with hair must be shaved. Ten color-coded leads are placed at various locations. Limb leads are placed on the right and left upper arms and right and left lower legs (Fig. 14–4). They should be placed on the fleshiest area, never on the wrists, ankles, or shins; this helps minimize artifact production. The remaining leads, called chest leads, are placed at strategic locations on the chest (Fig. 14–5). Even though there are only 10 actual electrodes, they provide 12 separate "leads," or graphic indicators of the heart's electrical activity. The four limb leads provide six graphic indi-

cators, and the additional six chest leads total twelve.

Improper electrode placement will produce less than desirable results. Artifacts are also an inherent problem. A skilled ECG operator will know how to recognize these erroneous tracings, correct the problem, and repeat the procedure. When cardiac monitoring must be done for an extended time period, Holter monitors are used. These can provide a continuous, 24-hour ECG, recorded on magnetic tape.

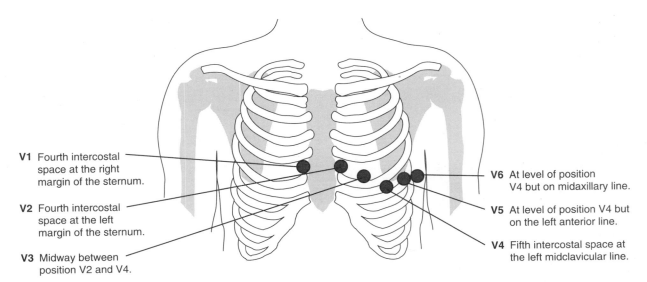

V1 Fourth intercostal space at the right margin of the sternum.

V2 Fourth intercostal space at the left margin of the sternum.

V3 Midway between position V2 and V4.

V6 At level of position V4 but on midaxillary line.

V5 At level of position V4 but on the left anterior line.

V4 Fifth intercostal space at the left midclavicular line.

Figure 14-5 ■ Placement of chest electrodes. (From Brust DJ, Foster JA: From Nursing Assistant to Patient Care Technician. Philadelphia, WB Saunders, 1997.)

References

1. Perry AG, Potter PA: Clinical Nursing Skills and Technique. 3rd ed. St. Louis, CV Mosby, 1994
2. Cohan RH, Leder RA, Ellis JH: Treatment of adverse reactions to radiographic contrast media in adults. Radiol Clin North Am 34:(5), 1055–1076, 1996

Bibliography

American Heart Association: Textbook of Basic Life Support for Healthcare Providers. Dallas, The American Heart Association, 1994

Ballinger PW: Merrill's Atlas of Radiographic Positions and Radiologic Procedures. 7th ed. St. Louis, Mosby–Year Book, 1991

Brust DJ, Foster JA: From Nursing Assistant to Patient Care Technician: New Roles, New Knowledge, New Skills. Philadelphia, WB Saunders, 1997

Ehrlich RA, McCloskey ED: Patient Care in Radiography. 3rd ed. St. Louis, Mosby–Year Book, 1989

Perry AG, Potter PA: Clinical Nursing Skills and Techniques. 3rd ed. St. Louis, Mosby–Year Book, 1994

Persing G: Respiratory Care Review, Study Guide, and Workbook. Philadelphia, WB Saunders, 1992

1. Patient Jones is in need of a vital signs assessment; you will perform the following:

   A. Clinical history, temperature, pulse, and weight
   B. Weight, height, temperature, and pulse
   C. Pulse, respiration, temperature, and blood pressure
   D. Pulse, respiration, blood pressure, and an ECG

2. "Normal" rectal temperature is:

   A. Lower than oral
   B. Higher than oral
   C. Lower than axillary
   D. Lower than tympanic

3. You are counting respirations of your adult patient. You have counted 12 in 30 seconds. This indicates that:

   A. The respiration rate is 12, and it is within normal limits.
   B. The respiration rate is 24 and is normal.
   C. The respiration rate is 12 and is abnormally low.
   D. The respiration rate is 24 and is abnormally high.

4. The newborn patient has a respiratory rate of 50. This indicates that:

   A. The rate is within normal limits, for the younger the patient, the higher the respiratory rate.
   B. The rate is too low; the normal range is between 60 and 100.
   C. The rate is too high; the patient must be febrile.
   D. The rate is out of normal limits; the younger patient always has a lower rate.

5. Your adult patient has a carotid pulse of 120. This indicates:

   A. A normal count for the carotid pulse
   B. An abnormal count, indicating tachycardia
   C. An abnormal count, indicating bradycardia
   D. An abnormal count; try the radial pulse

6. A sphygmomanometer is an instrument used to:

   A. Measure intraspinal pressure
   B. Measure oxygen saturation
   C. Measure blood pressure
   D. Time respiration during a stress test

7. The blood pressure reading is 130/70. This indicates that:

   A. The diastole is greater than the systole—abnormal results, indicative of hypertension.
   B. The systole is greater than the diastole—normal blood pressure results.
   C. The diastole is greater than the systole—normal blood pressure results.
   D. The systole is greater than the diastole—abnormal results, indicative of hypotension.

8. The systolic number can be much higher and still remain normal, if:

   A. The patient is taking blood pressure medication.
   B. The patient is an athlete.
   C. The diastolic number is below 50.
   D. The diastolic number is below 90.

9. A pulse oximeter measures the:

   A. Pulse electronically
   B. Blood pressure
   C. Arterial oxygen saturation
   D. All blood gases

10. If your patient is febrile, you should:

    A. Summon help STAT.
    B. Provide the patient with additional blankets.
    C. Administer oxygen.
    D. Remove outer coverings, blankets, sheets, and so on.

11. Cheyne-Stokes breathing is defined as:

    A. Hypoventilation
    B. Hyperventilation
    C. Hyperventilation alternating with periods of apnea
    D. Apnea

12. Your patient refuses to remain supine. He insists that he can breathe only when he is standing up. His condition is termed:

A. Orthopnea
B. Hypothermia
C. Gastritis
D. Hypoxia

13. If your patient is complaining of dyspnea, it is sometimes helpful to:

A. Provide spirits of ammonia.
B. Elevate the patient's head.
C. Take the patient's blood pressure.
D. Have the patient void.

14. Your patient has COPD. Her oxygen consumption:

A. Must be low-dose therapy
B. Must be a very-high-dose therapy
C. COPD patients should never receive oxygen therapy
D. Must alternate between high-dose and low-dose therapy

15. If the patient, on 4 liters of oxygen therapy per minute, is required to wait for 30 minutes in the radiology department for a delayed small bowel radiograph and the E tank has 550 liters of oxygen remaining, how many minutes are in reserve?

A. 4.1 min
B. 5.5 min
C. 8 min
D. 10 min

16. Systolic pressure corresponds to:

1. The relaxing phase of the cardiac cycle
2. The top number charted for blood pressure
3. The bottom number charted for blood pressure

4. The ventricle releasing blood into the aorta

A. 1 and 3
B. 1 and 2
C. 2 and 4
D. 3 and 4

17. When a patient presents in the radiology department for a procedure with an EID, it is essential to:

A. Confirm pregnancy status.
B. Check the site for swelling and/or redness pre- and postexamination.
C. Set the drips to a maximum.
D. Replace the solution prior to returning the patient to her unit.

18. A VAD is:

A. A PICC line
B. A Hickman catheter
C. A Port-A-Cath
D. All of the above

19. The following special care is required for central venous lines, regardless of type:

A. Special needles must be used to access the port.
B. The line must be irrigated daily with saline.
C. The line must be kept patent and clean.
D. The line must be changed daily.

20. Which catheter must be clamped during an IVP?

A. Levin tube
B. PICC
C. Bardex
D. Foley

Answers appear at the end of the book.

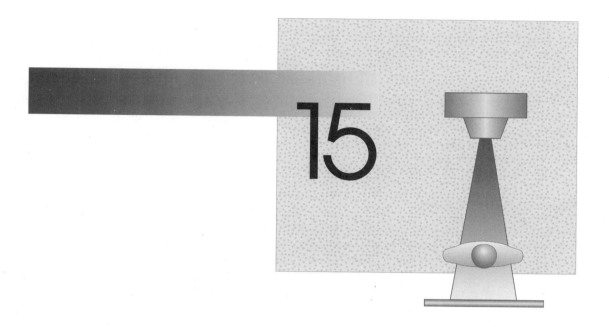

CONTRAST MEDIA

TYPES AND PROPERTIES OF CONTRAST MEDIA

Contrast media are used in radiography to enhance visualization of an organ or tissue, by increasing or decreasing the attenuation (kilovoltage dependent) of radiation for that particular area of the body via the photoelectric effect. The area or organ of interest will now be delineated and become highly visible due to increased contrast for radiographic interpretation. There are probably hundreds of contrast media available for use. This chapter reviews the most common varieties and concentrates on what is commonly used by today's standards.

Basic Principles

Let's review some basic principles that apply to contrast medium use and its importance.

- The *atomic number* and periodic chart location of the primary element being used is of great import. Remember that the atomic number refers to the amount of protons in the nucleus. The higher the atomic number, the greater the binding energy of the K shell electron, due to the increased nuclear forces.
- *Photoelectric effect* determines the attenuation of the incident radiation, thus the resultant scale of contrast. The characteristic photon emitted, after interaction has occurred, is unique to each individual element, due to the inherent binding energy of the K shell electron.
- *kVp selection* is critical for obtaining optimal contrast and limiting ionization damage to the patient. The kVp must be of an energy equal to or more than the binding energy of the element's K shell, in order to dislodge the electron. Care must be taken to provide at least that much energy: increasing kVp slightly allows for adequate penetration; increasing it too much will produce unnecessary scatter.

Contrast Medium Selection

In selecting an iodinated product, we can refer to the periodic table and note that iodine is number 53. The minimum kV that can be used to displace the K shell electron is 65 kV. This will afford the best attenuation, resulting in a high level of contrast and/or short-scale contrast. You may, however, require additional penetration due to patient size. As you increase your kV, attenuation will still occur, but additionally the byproduct will be unwanted scatter.

A selection of 70 kV will be radiographically adequate, but 90 kVp would render the resultant radiograph useless due to scatter and radiographic fog.

Similarly, should you select barium, with a higher atomic number, the kV range will increase accordingly in order to obtain the same optimal contrast for the resultant radiograph. More energy is required to displace the K shell electron.

This is why when you perform an upper gastrointestinal (GI) series using barium sulfate, your kV range is above 100. When the same procedure is done using an oral iodinated contrast medium, the kV range reduces to 65 to 75. Gases, with low atomic numbers, require far less kV to obtain the optimal contrast, as their K shell electrons are loosely bound, requiring less energy for displacement and minimal attenuation, rendering it a radiolucent medium.

It is hoped that this clarifies the importance of the matched union between contrast media and kV selection.

Here are the different types of contrast media and their uses:

1. *Barium sulfate products.* These are available in powder, premixed liquids, and pastes. The powders may be mixed to any desired density. Premixes are also available in thick and thin varieties. They can be administered orally or rectally. The paste form is thick and comes in a tube. It is used for oral procedures, generally to depict the esophagus. Some barium products are flavored. They are not water soluble or easily eliminated. They are in suspension. Reactions do occur but are extremely rare.
2. *Oral ionic iodinated products.* These products are available in powder and liquid forms. They are iodine based, water-soluble products that may be used orally (they taste bitter) or rectally, or they may be injected via catheter or syringe into fistulas, sinus tracts, or stomas (because of their water-soluble properties). They are absorbed and eliminated readily from the body. Their high-osmolar ionic iodinated base may cause reactions, but the percentage of occurrence is less than with iodinated intravenous products. These can never be injected intravenously.
3. *Iodinated products.* These products vary greatly because of their chemical composition. They can be ionic or non-ionic, monomers or dimers. This depends on the

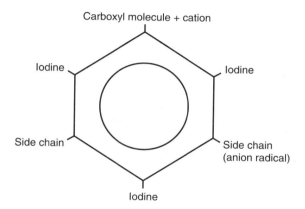

Figure 15–1 ■ Chemical configuration of an ionic monomer contrast medium. From Tortorici M: Administration of Imaging Pharmaceuticals. Philadelphia, WB Saunders, 1996.

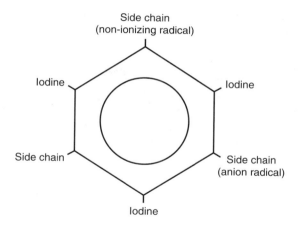

Figure 15–3 ■ Chemical configuration of nonionic monomer contrast medium. From Tortorici M: Administration of Imaging Pharmaceuticals. Philadelphia, WB Saunders, 1996.

actual *chemical configuration* of the iodine atoms and to what else they are attached. Pure iodine cannot be injected into the body. It must be configured with other molecular substances. These configurations may be either an *ionic* monomer or dimer molecular configuration (Figs. 15–1, 15–2) or a *non-ionic* monomer or dimer molecular configuration (Figs. 15–3, 15–4). It is the other "stuff" (ions and free radicals) that create the reaction probability. The best design is one that increases the iodine atoms over foreign particles or ions.

The higher the number of iodine atoms to particles, the better and less reactive the contrast medium. This is expressed as a ratio. The higher the ratio, the better. For example, a ratio of 6:1 means that there are six iodine atoms to one particle; 3:2 indicates that there are three iodine atoms to two particles. Obviously, the 6:1 would be a less reactive contrast medium (see Fig. 15–2).

This also dovetails with the *osmolality* issue. The more particulates that occur in solution, the greater the osmolality. Again, the desired effect is to have the maximum number of iodine atoms

and the least amount of particles. Human plasma is about 300 milliosmoles (mOsm) per kilogram (kg). Ionic contrast media have a minimum osmolality of 1000 mOsm/kg. Non-ionic contrast media have a minimum osmolality of 600 mOsm/kg. High osmolality indicates that contrast medium penetrates the blood cell wall, creating discomfort and possible reactivity. Rigidity of red blood cells is a toxic response. A pharmaceutical company has recently released a contrast medium with the same osmolality as human plasma. It is a new product and will have to be evaluated as to its speculated improvement.

Another variation among products is *iodine concentration*. The higher the iodine concentration, the better the visualization due to greater attenuation, but the greater the reaction occurrence. The product will also have a higher viscosity. Concentration levels of iodine vary among products. Check with your own facility's representative for specific mg/ml product information. All iodinated media are radiopaque because of their inherent high atomic number, the binding energy of the K shell, and the attenuation properties during photoelectric effect.

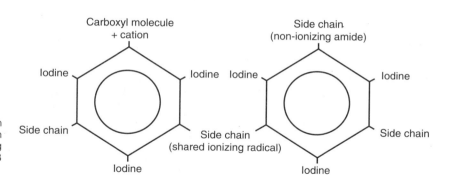

Figure 15–2 ■ Chemical configuration of an ionic dimer contrast medium. From Tortorici M: Administration of Imaging Pharmaceuticals. Philadelphia, WB Saunders, 1996.

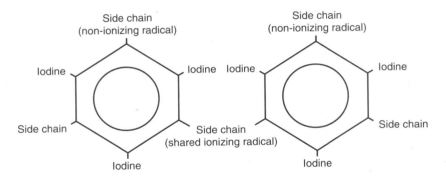

Figure 15-4 ■ Chemical configuration of a nonionic dimer contrast medium. From Tortorici M: Administration of Imaging Pharmaceuticals. Philadelphia, WB Saunders, 1996.

These products are used for many procedures. All can be used for intravenous (IV) studies. Intra-arterial examinations also utilize these products, as do biliary, urinary, athrography, bronchography, and hysterosalpingographic studies. Intrathecal studies are limited to non-ionic, iodinated, low-osmolality media. Ionic iodinated products CANNOT be injected intrathecally. This error might prove fatal to the patient. Most of these products are water soluble and are easily absorbed and eliminated from the body. There is, of course, always one exception: ethiodol, an oil-based iodinated medium, is used exclusively for infrequently performed lymphangiograms because of its oily, retentive qualities.

Gases

Air and carbon dioxide are also used as contrast media. These are radiolucent rather than radiopaque. They are easily penetrated because of their inherent low atomic numbers and corresponding low attenuation factors and will appear as black, rather than white, on the resultant radiograph. Air will inflate the area of interest and allow maximum visualization of the mucosal lining, especially the GI organs, when used in conjunction with barium as a double-contrast study. Bromo-Seltzer–type crystals can be used for upper GI series; also, a straw with a needle hole is effective for adding air for a double-contrast study. Air insufflator bags are used to insert air for double-contrast enemas.

Carbon dioxide is being used for digital subtraction angiography (DSA). This is a new method of performing the procedure; outcome results need to be evaluated. Both this and air are readily absorbed and in moderation have little toxicity.

Gadolinium

Gadolinium, as a pure element, is highly toxic to humans. It has been paired with another chemi-

cal set, called diethylenetriamine pentaacetic acid (DTPA), which minimizes the toxicity. It is a paramagnetic contrast medium, used exclusively for magnetic resonance imaging (MRI). It decreases the relaxation time of the T_1- and T_2-weighted images, affecting and increasing the visualization. Reactions are rare.

APPROPRIATENESS CRITERIA OF CONTRAST MEDIA TO PROCEDURE AND PATIENT CONDITION

Barium Procedures/Oral Iodine Procedures

Barium can be used for most adult GI examinations without concern. Barium sulfate and water provide a suspension of an inert, nontoxic element. The exceptions to its use are

- Suspicion of existing perforation. (Barium is not absorbed or soluble.)
- Fistula, stoma, and sinus tract studies. (Barium will sometimes be used.)
- Severe fecal impaction of the bowel. (Will exacerbate condition.)
- Some pediatric cases. (Depends on clinical history or child's compliance.)
- Patients who may require abdominal operative procedures.

Pediatric doses are calculated per kilogram of body weight; follow product insert recommendations.

Intravenous and Other Iodinated Contrast Medium Procedures

It is important to check all existing history of the patient. Many contraindications exist for these procedures (refer to Relative Risk Factors). Patients tolerate the low-osmolar, non-ionic contrast medium much better than ionic products. Reactions are not as frequent or severe. The cost of this product is much higher than that of the ionic version. Many facilities are premedicating their patients prior to the procedure and using ionic material. Premedication protocol may include:

- Mild sedatives (to alleviate anxiety)
- Diphenhydramine HCl (antihistamine)
- Corticosteroid (to reduce inflammation and suppress immune response)

The medications must be prescribed according to the patient's history, weight, age, physical condition, allergy status, and medication use. The actual schedule will vary, but these are generally given 1 to 24 hours prior to the procedure. The iodinated contrast media, ionic or non-ionic, are all administered according to the patient's weight. Refer to the package insert for recommended guidelines for administration.

It is important to remember the proper sequential ordering protocol for contrast medium procedures. They are listed here from "schedule first" to "schedule last."

- Iodine uptake studies
- Urinary tract procedures
- Biliary tract procedures
- Computed tomographic (CT) procedures requiring contrast media
- Lower GI procedures
- Upper GI procedures

CONTRAINDICATIONS

The contraindications for barium studies are discussed in the previous section. There were few associated risks. Patients requiring iodine-based contrast media must be screened for risk.

Relative Risk Factors

The following patient conditions/medical histories preclude the use of iodinated contrast media. They are contraindications to its use.

- Experience of a previous contrast medium reaction (histamine trigger)
- Asthma (bronchial compromise)
- Multiple food and medication allergies (sensitivity, especially to iodine in any form)
- Azotemia (renal impairment)
- Cardiac patients (especially congestive heart failure [CHF])

The following diseases or conditions will heighten reaction and/or may be exacerbated by the iodinated contrast medium:

- Pheochromocytoma (risk of hypertensive crisis)
- Multiple myeloma (risk of renal failure)

- Sickle cell anemia (sickle cell crisis)
- Active hyperthyroidism (thyroid storm—T_3 and T_4 increase uncontrolled)
- Azotemia (contrast-induced renal failure)
- Myasthenia gravis (symptoms exacerbated)
- Beta-blocker–medicated patients (incidence of bronchospasm will increase)
- Diabetic patients on metformin/Glucophage (lactic acidosis/fatal)
- Cancer patients receiving interleukin-2 (delayed anaphylactoid response)

The following laboratory values are also helpful in assessing iodinated contrast medium use:

Blood urea nitrogen (BUN)—normal values: 6 to 20 mg/dl. This lab test checks the metabolic function of the liver and excretory function of the kidneys. *Abnormal values* may indicate CHF, renal disease, renal failure, myocardial infarction, dehydration.

Serum creatinine—normal values: 0.5 to 1.1 mg/dl. This lab test checks renal excretory function. *Abnormal values* indicate dysfunction of the kidneys and/or dehydration.

Generally, dialysis patients can tolerate contrast media despite abnormal BUN and creatinine levels because of the dialysis exchange postprocedure. These issues must be discussed with the physician prior to injecting. After a thorough review of the patient's clinical history, the physician and patient ultimately decide whether the benefit is worth the risk.

PATIENT EDUCATION
Preprocedure

Patient preparation is critical to most radiographic procedures. If the patient is noncompliant in regard to the preparation, the procedure will be either canceled or of suboptimal quality for diagnosis. Most contrast medium procedures require the following preparation.

Dietary Restrictions

- A clear liquid diet or strict NPO instructions
- No cigarette smoking or gum chewing

These restrictions keep the digestive organs empty, limit gas production, and minimize peristalsis, gastric enzyme production, and vomiting.

Laxatives/Cathartics

- Castor oil, citrate of magnesia, Dulcolax: one of these will be prescribed.

■ Suppositories of various types may also be prescribed in addition to the oral laxative.

They empty the colon of all contents, eliminating feces/gas from obstructing information.

Enemas

■ A soapsuds, tap water, or Fleet enema may be prescribed.

This will be the final cleansing of the colon, preparing the abdomen for optimal visualization.

Explanation of Procedure

This information is reviewed in Chapter 12. It is essential to provide the patient with as much information about the procedure as possible. It is just as essential to provide yourself and the radiologist with as much information *about the patient* as possible. This level of preparation helps minimize failure of the examination and maximize optimal results and accurate diagnosis. This is especially true when you are about to perform a contrast media procedure, which is not easily repeated. Preprocedural preparation, once accomplished, cannot be easily repeated once the contrast medium has been introduced. You and your patient's mutual goal is to get it right the first time.

Postprocedure

For most barium studies, you must instruct the patient to increase fluids (if that is permissible). This helps hydrate the patient, as barium tends to absorb water. Sometimes another laxative is prescribed to hasten the barium's removal.

Iodinated contrast medium tends to dehydrate patients. Increased fluid intake instruction is also required for the postexamination patient. Patients who required air insufflation during an examination could be prescribed Mylicon drops or another product with simethicone to break down the gas and limit flatulence and cramping.

Certain therapies must be closely monitored. Glucophage (metformin), used in the treatment of Stage II diabetes, must be withheld for at least 48 hours postprocedure when an iodinated contrast medium is used intravascularly. Renal function must be assessed and deemed normal before resuming the drug order. If Glucophage is continued after the procedure, lactic acidosis may develop because of renal insufficiency. If the lactic acidosis reaches a toxic level, 50% of these patients do not survive. Every facility should address this issue in policy and procedure.

ADMINISTRATION OF CONTRAST MEDIA

Primary Drug Routes

There are four *primary* routes of drug administration.

1. Enteral

   ■ Oral (PO)
   ■ Sublingual (under the tongue)
   ■ Buccal (drug placed between gum and cheek)
   ■ Rectal

2. Parenteral (injection)

   ■ Intravenous (IV)
   ■ Intra-arterial
   ■ Intramuscular (IM)
   ■ Intradermal
   ■ Intrathecal
   ■ Subcutaneous (SQ)

3. Pulmonary

   ■ Inhalation

4. Topical

   ■ Application to the skin, eyes, ears

The IV and intra-arterial routes are the fastest absorption methods; usually the medication is absorbed within 1 minute. There are two natural barriers to drug absorption:

1. The blood-brain barrier (only fat-soluble drugs enter; it may be bypassed by intrathecal injection)
2. The placental barrier (only some drugs are excluded; alcohol will pass)

Supplies

For enteral administration, the following supplies may be used:

Cup
Straw
NG tube
Tapered adapter
Syringe/spoon
Enema bag
Catheter/syringe

For parenteral administration, the following supplies may be used:

Syringe
Needle
Angiocath
Tourniquet

Alcohol wipe
Band-Aid/tape

Syringes come in all sizes (tuberculin to 50 ml), and the selection is based on need. Needles also come in varying sizes. The size indicates the lumen of the needle, or gauge. The higher the gauge number, the smaller the lumen opening. A 23-gauge needle is a finer needle than an 18-gauge. Needles can be attached to minicatheters, such as a butterfly infusion set or Angiocath. The latter can be taped to the patient's skin and left in for the duration of the test, so that if additional medication must be given, there is an access port.

For pulmonary medication administration, the following supplies may be used:

Inhaler
Tent or face mask

For topical medication administration, the following supplies may be used:

Dropper
Applicator
A spray bottle or atomizer
Premedicated wipes
Transdermal patch

It is critical that during any medication administration, you comply with **The Five Rights**:

1. The right patient
2. The right drug
3. The right dose
4. The right route
5. The right time

You must always TRIPLE-CHECK when administering or preparing medication!

1. Check the drug order.
2. Confirm the medication.
3. Re-confirm the drug at time of administration.

You must check the label and

- Verify the drug—keep the container until the drug is given.
- Check concentration/strength vs. dose.
- Check expiration date. (The expiration date on the container applies *only* to an unopened, untampered with medication.)
- Single or multidose vial? Verify sterility. Is it dated? (Medication dating will vary by institution. Unit dose dispensing is considered the best technique for patient and medication safety.)
- Date any multidose vial when opened; refrigerate if necessary.

- Verify route ordered with the appropriate drug. Is it safe?
- Check control or lot number—use when reporting adverse drug reactions (ADRs) or product-related problems.

It is critical to keep in mind when NOT to give a drug. Such situations are

- Label illegibility (if you can't clearly read the label, don't give the drug).
- If someone other than you prepared the drug, don't administer it.
- Do not chart a drug as part of the medical record until given.
- Do not leave the patient with the drug to take alone; insure compliance.

Venipuncture

The actual clinical technique of venipuncture is beyond the scope of this book. Refer to the Bibliography if you require more information. Some basics are provided here.

Preparation of Medication/Contrast Medium

- Wash your hands.
- Prepare on a clean work surface. Gather all supplies.
- Always keep barrel of syringe intact; do not remove and dump medication into syringe chamber.
- Wipe once with an alcohol wipe on the vial's rubber stopper.
- Enter the needle bevel at a 45° angle to prevent coring of the rubber stopper.
- Release the inherent air in the syringe by pushing the plunger forward prior to loading the syringe.
- When using a large syringe, never push all the air from the syringe into the contrast medium bottle; it will explode. Admit **about** 10 ml at a time and wait for return.
- Retain the vial until the drug is administered.
- Dispose of medical waste appropriately.

Common IV Injection Sites

Forearm

- Ventral veins of the elbow/antecubital
- Basilic/cephalic/median cubital veins

Hand/wrist

- Dorsal metacarpal vein
- Cephalic vein
- Basilic vein

Other IV Injection Sites

- Scalp veins for infants and children
- Feet and legs/superficial veins
- Subclavian/internal and external jugular/ long-term therapy sites

Always have an emergency drug box available at the time of injection and know the location of the closest code cart. Before the injection takes place, ask the patient which arm is easier for accessing blood. Most patients are familiar with their bodies and will tell you immediately which is the best injection site for them.

- Prepare the area of injection; use an alcohol wipe.
- Secure the tourniquet with a slip knot for ease in removal.
- Distend the vein of choice.
- Enter needle, pull back syringe. Check for blood return.
- Tape the needle in place, if required.
- Release the tourniquet.
- Inject.
- Apply pressure and gauze to injection site, postinjection.
- Provide a Band-Aid, if necessary.

Direct IV Injections

These may be of two types:

- Direct bolus: this delivers the entire amount quickly.
- Continuous infusion: this delivers the entire amount at a steady rate over a longer period of time.

Injections may also be delivered through an established line, if one is provided. With this method, the medication is administered directly into the IV line. Blood return must be established, as well as flushing of the site postinjection.

COMPLICATIONS AND REACTIONS
Local and Systemic

- Infiltration/extravasation. This occurs when the needle becomes displaced or the vein has been punctured all the way through. The medication seeps into the surrounding tissue, resulting in redness, pain, and swelling. Stop the injection. Use ice and/or warm compresses to reduce the swelling and increase circulation for distribution of medication away from the site.
- Infection of the site. This will be noted as a red and swollen area at the site. Pain and burning occur. Discontinue the IV and locate another site. Report this to the physician for follow-up care.
- Embolism. A clot that will travel *(move)* throughout the body can develop from improper IV injection management. Remember that a thrombus is a *stationary* clot!
- Phlebitis. This is inflammation of the veins. Symptoms may be pain, edema, and increased skin temperature over the veins. This may be prevented by flushing the vein site with heparinized saline postprocedure. Early ambulation by the patient may also prevent this occurrence. Discontinue the IV and locate it to another site. Report this to the physician for follow-up care.
- Circulation problems. These can manifest when blood volume increases rapidly, by too much fluid entering the system quickly. Symptoms include decreased blood pressure, shortness of breath, rapid breathing, and dilation of the veins. Slow the infusion or discontinue, if possible. Elevate the patient's head, and monitor vital signs.

Reactions

Most contrast media reactions are physiologic or of the *anaphylactic* or *anaphylactoid* variety.

- *Physiologic* reactions are drug and dose dependent. *Example:* warmth, flushing, metallic taste in mouth after iodinated contrast media injection.
- *Anaphylactoid* reactions are independent of drug or dose. They are not true anaphylactic responses because no anticontrast IgE (antibody) is produced, and they may occur in patients without previous exposure to contrast media.
- *Anaphylactic* reactions occur when the patient has been pre-sensitized through previous exposure to a substance and IgE antibodies are present. It is a true histamine reaction. *Example:* Someone is stung by a bee once and does not react; IgE for bee venom is now present. The person is stung a second time and the bee sting is

fatal due to the sensitization to the antigen and the histamine response.

■ *Idiosyncratic* reactions are those that are considered completely unexpected and without explanation. Contrast media reactions do not fall into this category.

Mild Reactions

These will resolve without treatment or with minimal treatment. Observation and reassurance are required.

- Nausea/vomiting
- Dizziness
- Anxiety
- Warmth/flushing
- Sweating
- Unusual taste
- Itching/hives
- Pallor
- Chills/tremors
- Nasal congestion
- Facial edema

Moderate Reactions

These require close observation and treatment to relieve the symptoms.

- Altered heart rate
- Altered blood pressure
- Difficulty in breathing/wheezing
- Laryngospasm/bronchospasm

Severe Reactions

These are life threatening. They require IMMEDIATE treatment and continuous observation to reverse symptoms. They include

- Unresponsiveness
- Convulsions
- Arrhythmia
- Cardiac arrest

Reaction Management—Radiographer's Response

You must get help and stay with the patient. This is not always easy, but manageable. Give a clear and concise report of what has happened to the nurse or physician. Be ready to assist and document. Call an immediate code for cardiac arrest, or 911, if you are in an outpatient facility, if necessary, before obtaining assistance. Generally, if the reaction is mild, simply reassuring the patient and observing appearance and behavior will be enough. Remember to assess vitals pre-

and post-reaction. You will know when a patient is in trouble, most often it happens quickly and generally within twenty minutes. Refer to Chapter 14 for medical emergencies. Should a patient require medication, here is what will correspond to the individual reaction:

Hives

- Diphenhydramine (Benadryl) will be given PO/IM/IV, depending upon the severity of the reaction. The dose will generally start at 50 mg.

Erythema/angioedema or facial edema

- Diphenhydramine, 50 mg IV/IM (with a daily dose of 400 mg), and/or
- Epinephrine: 1:1000 solution SC, 0.2–1 mg. If no relief:
- Epinephrine 1:10,000 solution 0.1–0.25 mg IV (slow)

Laryngeal edema

- Oxygen, 2 to 4 liters/min
- Epinephrine (as above)
- Intubation/code, if no response to medication

Hypotension

- Oxygen (as above)
- Ringer's lactate or normal saline solution
- Dopamine infusion (5–20 mcg/kg/min)
- Code, if no response to medication

Bronchospasm

- Oxygen (as above)
- Albuterol, 2 to 3 inhalations, 2.5 mg (0.5 ml) with 2.5 ml NS in a nebulizer
- Aminophylline, 6 mg/kg in 100–200 ml D5W or NS—do not exceed 25 mg/min.
- Epinephrine (as above)
- Code, if no response to medication

Emergency Box Medications

- *Diphenhydramine* (Benadryl). This is an antihistamine (H-1). It blocks the effects of histamine release. Side effects are drowsiness and thirst. If an outpatient requires this therapy, make sure that someone is available to drive him or her home after the procedure.
- *Epinephrine/adrenaline.* This is the most important medication required to reverse most reactions. This stimulates alpha- and beta-receptors to increase heart rate and blood pressure. It will vasoconstrict and bronchodilate. It may also cause tachycardia, arrhythmia, tremors, and

decreased renal perfusion. Extravasation of this drug may cause necrosis of tissue. It should not be delivered via arterial line.

■ *Atropine*. This reverses bradycardia, increasing the heart rate; it is an anticholinergic drug. It may cause dry mouth, blurred vision, urinary retention, and constipation.

■ *Albuterol*. Bronchodilator, beta-2 agonist. If administered by inhalation, side effects are limited. Relaxes and opens bronchial pathways. In high doses it may cause tachycardia, irritability, and tremors.

■ *Aminophylline*. Bronchodilator; relaxes and enhances diaphragm contractions and opens bronchial pathways. May cause nausea, vomiting, tachycardia, tremors, irritability.

■ *Dopamine*. At low doses, renal blood flow increases; at moderate doses, heart rate increases; at high doses, vasoconstriction occurs. Extravasation causes severe necrosis of the tissue. Tachycardia, hypertension, arrhythmia, nausea, vomiting, and decreased peripheral perfusion are all potential side effects.

■ *Furosemide* (Lasix). A diuretic; aids in the elimination of fluid in cases of pulmonary edema or fluid volume overload.

■ *Methylprednisolone*. A corticosteroid, an anti-inflammatory drug used to lessen or prevent a reaction or the severity of a reaction.

Documentation of Reactions

Accuracy in reporting is the key to understanding the nature and cause of the reaction. It is critical for the patient's future management regarding contrast media. You will be assisting in the treatment of the reaction; most documentation will be the radiographer's responsibility. Complete an incident report, if required.

■ Verify the medical record/chart.
■ Put date and time on all entries.
■ Enter all events in chronologic order.
■ Chart only the events that you were directly involved with.
■ State facts, not opinions.
■ Do not use unapproved abbreviations.
■ Write in blue or black ink, not pencil or colored inks. Use ballpoint pens, not Flair-type markers.
■ Place one line only through errors and initial.
■ If an entry is completely incorrect, make an addendum to it rather than trying to change it.
■ Sign off on every entry.

Adverse Drug Reaction (ADR) Forms

ADRs are standardized forms that **must** be completed on every reaction. They are similar to an incident report, but do not substitute them for that use. They are separate and unique. This form will require information regarding the severity of the reaction and what medium or medication was administered. It is kept on file in the pharmacy department as well as with the patient's medical record. It is useful for statistical tracking and reaction trends.

MedWatch Documentation

This is a program designed by the Food and Drug Administration (FDA) and monitored by the Joint Commission on the Accreditation of Healthcare Organizations (JCAHO). It is a mandatory program in which hospitals report various statistics at a national level. A voluntary program of reportage exists for other medical facilities. The pharmacy department provides all the essential information from the adverse drug reaction (ADR) reports. They report to MedWatch when the following *serious* reactions occur:

■ Death-related reaction
■ Any life-threatening reaction
■ Any reaction that requires the patient to be hospitalized
■ Any reaction that correlates to disability
■ Congenital anomaly outcomes
■ Any reaction that requires intervention to prevent permanent impairment/damage
■ Any reaction to a new product for post-marketing surveillance

It is important to understand that by complying with local requirements, statistical information is being compiled to benefit all potential patients on a national level.

Bibliography

Cohan RH, Leder R, Ellis JH: Treatment of adverse reactions to radiographic contrast media in adults. Advances in Uroradiology I. Radiol Clin North Am 34(5), 1996

Ehrlich RA, McCloskey ED: Patient Care in Radiography. 3rd ed. St. Louis, Mosby–Year Book, 1989

The FDA Desk Guide for Adverse Event and Product Problem Reporting. Rockville, MD, Food and Drug Administration, 1996

Johns HE, Cunningham JR: The Physics of Radiology. 4th ed. Springfield, IL, Charles C Thomas, 1983

Selman J: The Fundamentals of X-Ray and Radium Physics. 6th ed. Springfield, IL, Charles C Thomas, 1980

Tortorici M: Administration of Imaging Pharmaceuticals. Philadelphia WB Saunders, 1996

1. Contrast media are used to:

   A. Limit secondary scatter, affecting contrast outcome
   B. Adjust the gray scale on a video monitor
   C. Enhance visualization of organs or tissue
   D. Increase kVp

2. The atomic interaction that provides visualization of the contrast medium filled organs is:

   A. The Compton effect
   B. The photoelectric effect
   C. Pair production
   D. Characteristic radiation

3. The atomic number of an element refers to the:

   A. Electron configuration
   B. Number of neutrons
   C. Number of protons
   D. Total number of neutrons and protons

4. For photoelectric effect, the kVp selected must render an incident photon with energy equal to or greater than the binding energy of the:

   A. K shell electron
   B. Protons
   C. Nucleus
   D. Redistributed L shell electron

5. Contrast media consisting of elements ranked high on the periodic table would require which of the following for optimal radiographic attenuation?

   A. Low kVp
   B. High kVp
   C. Small focal spot size
   D. Maximum SID

6. Barium sulfate products are:

   1. Water soluble
   2. Suspensions, when mixed with water
   3. Administered enterically

   A. 1, 2, and 3
   B. 1 and 3 only
   C. 2 and 3 only
   D. 2 only

7. Oral iodinated contrast media:

   1. Are water soluble
   2. Do not cause anaphylactoid reactions
   3. Are absorbed and eliminated readily from the body

   A. 1, 2, and 3
   B. 1 and 3 only
   C. 2 and 3 only
   D. 2 only

8. Iodinated contrast medium products used for parenteral injection:

   A. Are chemically configured as monomers, if non-ionic
   B. Are chemically configured as dimers, if non-ionic
   C. May be chemically configured as monomers or dimers, ionic or non-ionic
   D. Are only chemically configured as dimers, if ionic

9. An iodinated contrast medium is rated with a ratio of 3:1. This indicates:

   A. That it is a monomer
   B. That there are three iodine atoms to one particle or ion
   C. That it is a three-sided monomer
   D. That it is a three-sided monomer configured to a dimer

10. The osmolality of the iodinated contrast medium should be similar to:

    A. Plasma
    B. Saline
    C. Lactated Ringer's solution
    D. D5W

11. A toxic response to high osmolality of an iodinated contrast medium would be:

    A. Discomfort
    B. Phlebitis
    C. Nausea
    D. Rigidity of the red blood cells

12. As the iodine concentration of a contrast medium increases, so does the:

    1. Reactivity
    2. Attenuation of radiation
    3. Viscosity

A. 1, 2, and 3
B. 2 and 3 only
C. 1 and 3 only
D. 2 only

13. Non-ionic, low-osmolality iodinated contrast medium MUST be used for:

    A. Hysterosalpingograms
    B. Intravenous pyelograms
    C. Lymphangiograms
    D. Myelograms

14. A radiopaque contrast medium/media is/are:

    1. Barium sulfate
    2. Air
    3. Non-ionic, low-osmolality iodinated products

    A. 1, 2 and 3
    B. 2 and 3
    C. 1 and 3
    D. 2 only

15. A paramagnetic contrast medium is:

    A. Ethiodol
    B. Radiolucent
    C. Gadolinium
    D. A dimer

16. If free air is demonstrated on the erect abdominal radiograph and an upper gastrointestinal series is requested, the contrast medium of choice would be:

    A. Gadolinium
    B. Barium sulfate
    C. Omnipaque or Isovue
    D. Oral iodinated products

17. A pediatric dose of contrast medium is determined by the child's:

    A. Age
    B. Height
    C. Weight
    D. Sex

18. Premedication is helpful in reducing reactions or their severity when given prior to:

    A. Gadolinium injection
    B. Oral iodinated contrast medium
    C. Intravascular ionic iodinated contrast medium
    D. Ethiodol

19. If the laboratory values for the BUN return as 2.5 mg/dl, the iodinated contrast medium would be:

    A. Contraindicated for injection
    B. Used only after the physician assesses all other clinical factors
    C. Administered as an infusion rather than as a bolus
    D. Administered as long as normal creatinine results are available

20. Which diabetic treatment therapy must be withheld for at least 48 hours following injection of an iodinated contrast medium?

    A. Diabinese
    B. Glucophage (metformin)
    C. Pork insulin
    D. Synthetic insulin

21. Select a preprocedural preparation.

    A. Patient education and instruction
    B. Positioning
    C. Exposure factor selection
    D. Proper marker placement

22. An NPO order requires that the patient:

    A. Maintain a light diet
    B. Not take any pills
    C. Take nothing by mouth
    D. May not eat, but may chew gum and drink water

23. Fluid intake should be increased following which procedure(s)?

    1. Barium enema
    2. IVP
    3. Hysterosalpingogram

    A. 1, 2, and 3
    B. 2 and 3 only
    C. 1 and 3 only
    D. 2 only

24. Which drug route administers by injection?

    A. Enteral
    B. Topical
    C. Parenteral
    D. Pulmonary

25. The five rights of medication administration consist of:

   A. Patient, drug, dose, route, time
   B. Patient, drug, day, route, time
   C. Patient, drug, doctor, route, time
   D. Patient, drug, dressing, route, time

26. It is 8 A.M. You are asked to perform an IVP. You go to load a syringe with contrast medium and notice that a syringe is already loaded, but the empty bottle is missing. You would:

   A. Use that preloaded syringe.
   B. Dispose of the preloaded syringe and reload another one.
   C. Try to find the empty bottle of contrast medium and then use the preloaded syringe.
   D. Save the preloaded syringe for the next patient and load a fresh one for now.

27. Another term for infiltration is:

   A. Thrombus
   B. Embolus
   C. Phlebitis
   D. Extravasation

28. An example of a mild reaction is:

   A. Dyspnea
   B. Change in blood pressure
   C. Nausea
   D. Bronchospasm

29. Severe reactions require:

   A. That a cardiac code be initiated
   B. Oxygen administration
   C. An immediate response and continuous patient monitoring
   D. That the patient be sent to the emergency department

30–33. Match the following:

   30. Benadryl
   31. Lasix
   32. Adrenaline
   33. Aminophylline

      A. Epinephrine
      B. Bronchodilator
      C. Diuretic
      D. Diphenhydramine

34. If you make an error in charting, you should:

   A. Erase it; always use pencil.
   B. Use correction fluid.
   C. Remove the entire document.
   D. Place one line through the error and initial it.

35. ADRs and the MedWatch program monitor:

   A. Misadministrations of drugs
   B. Incident reports
   C. Adverse drug reactions and their statistical impact
   D. Adverse drug reactions and the technologists involved

Answers appear at the end of the book.

Section V Questions

1. An unconscious emergency department patient requires skull radiographs. The following will happen:

   A. A relative must sign a consent form.
   B. The procedure will be postponed until the patient resumes consciousness.
   C. Informed consent is legally waived, due to the emergency situation.
   D. The emergency department staff must obtain consent from the county judge.

2. Patients may make specific judgments regarding their own healthcare because of:

   A. Their constitutional rights
   B. HMO policy
   C. The Patient Bill of Rights
   D. The fact that they are paying the bill.

3. Your IVP patient is writhing in pain due to a left-sided kidney stone. You have had to request pain medication for him so that the study may be completed. He asks you to please tell him what is wrong with him. Which of the following would be the *best* answer?

   A. Explain to him that he has a small kidney stone in the left distal ureter.
   B. Tell him it is beyond your scope of practice to tell him anything about his condition.
   C. Explain to him that after the medication takes effect, he will feel much better.
   D. Request that the radiologist or emergency room physician come speak with him.

4. You are radiographing an adolescent girl whose shoulder is dislocated. When she comes into the x-ray room, she begins to cry and tells you that her uncle pulled her arm and slapped her around. She states that he does this every time she is alone with him. You would:

   A. Report this immediately to the physician in charge.
   B. Maintain her confidentiality.
   C. Listen politely, but say nothing.
   D. Obtain the uncle's phone number so that you could speak to him directly.

5. Assault requires that:

   A. Battery accompany it
   B. Physical violence must take place
   C. Only threatened violence take place
   D. Offensive contact be made

6. The major difference between civil and criminal assault and battery is:

   A. There is no difference.
   B. That civil assault and battery requires only unconsensual touch; criminal assault and battery requires actual injury
   C. The amount of financial award to the injured party
   D. That criminal assault and battery never occurs in the workplace

7. Unjustified or threatened restraint of a patient satisfies which of the following torts?

   1. False imprisonment
   2. Assault
   3. Negligence

   A. 1 only
   B. 2 only
   C. 1 & 2
   D. 1, 2, & 3

8. Libel is:

   A. Defamation by unprivileged publication
   B. Defamation by unprivileged speech
   C. Slander
   D. A tort of assault

9. Medical negligence is also referred to as:

   A. Breach of duty
   B. Malpractice
   C. Res ipsa loquitur
   D. Scope of duty tort

10. Your patient bumps his head on the x-ray tube and lacerates his forehead. You would:

    A. Take a PA skull to check for fractures.
    B. Place a Band-Aid on the patient's cut.
    C. Have a nurse or physician check the patient and fill out an incident report.
    D. Do nothing, as long as the cut stops bleeding.

11. TQM and TQI rely on which of the following factors for success?

    A. Measured improvement and outcome tracking
    B. Risk management and quality assurance
    C. Trends and estimates
    D. Anecdotal reporting mechanisms

12. Which of the following is not included in the patient's history?

    A. Chief complaint
    B. Insurance information
    C. Pregnancy status
    D. Date of trauma, duration of condition

13. DNR refers to:

    A. Do not refill prescription
    B. Does not remember, for Alzheimer patients
    C. Do not reimburse, insurance coding
    D. Do not resuscitate, no lifesaving measures for the patient

14. A coil is used in which imaging modality?

    A. Ultrasound
    B. Computed tomography
    C. Nuclear medicine
    D. Magnetic resonance imaging

15. A transducer is used in which of the following imaging modalities?

    A. Ultrasound
    B. Computed tomography
    C. Nuclear medicine
    D. Magnetic resonance imaging

16. Radioisotopes are used for which imaging modality?

    A. Ultrasound
    B. Computed tomography
    C. Nuclear medicine
    D. Magnetic resonance imaging

17. Which of the following imaging modalities cannot be interpreted via soft copy?

    A. MRI
    B. CT
    C. Mammography
    D. Ultrasound

18. The breast can be imaged via the following modalities:

    1. Computed tomography
    2. Ultrasound
    3. Magnetic resonance imaging

    A. 1 only
    B. 2 only
    C. 1 & 2
    D. 2 & 3

19. Your patient requires an IVP, UGI, and BE. They must be scheduled in the following sequence:

    A. IVP, UGI, BE
    B. BE, IVP, UGI
    C. UGI, IVP, BE
    D. IVP, BE, UGI

20. Patient assessment addresses all but the following:

    A. Religious beliefs
    B. Physical impairments
    C. Level of education
    D. Annual income

21. Body mechanics refers to:

    A. Safe movement and transfer of the patient
    B. Physical therapy
    C. Prosthetic devices
    D. Physicians

22. A patient requiring a chest radiograph misplaces her necklace. You would:

    A. Tell her that if you find it, she'll be notified.
    B. Fill out an incident report and report the loss to security.
    C. Tell her that you feel sorry about her loss.
    D. Wonder how she could be so careless

23. Which of the following demonstrates the cycle of infection?

    A. Pathogen, growth, exit, transport, entry, susceptible host
    B. Pathogen, transport, host
    C. Pathogen, growth, host
    D. Pathogen and susceptible host

24. Indirect means of pathogenic transmission include all but the following:

    A. Fomite

B. Nosocomial

C. Vector

D. Airborne

25. An organism that harbors the pathogen without developing the disease but transmits it to another organism is called a:

    A. Fomite

    B. Vortex

    C. Vector

    D. Typhoid Mary

26. In the hospital setting, nosocomial infection is minimized by employing:

    A. Sterility throughout

    B. A "no visitors" policy

    C. Infection control policies

    D. Positive-pressure hospital rooms

27. Medical aseptic technique applies the following concept:

    A. Sterilize all items

    B. Reduce as many microorganisms as possible in a clean environment

    C. Autoclaving as the answer to microbial reduction

    D. Surgical aseptic technique

28. Germicides:

    A. disinfect and destroy pathogenic microbes

    B. inhibit microbial growth

    C. are used in autoclaves

    D. are antiseptics

29. The primary infection control practice is:

    A. Autoclaving

    B. Use of antiseptics

    C. Use of germicides

    D. Hand washing

30. Surgical asepsis is referred to as:

    A. Medical sterility

    B. Sterile technique

    C. Clean technique

    D. Operating room protocol

31. Sterile technique must be utilized under which of the following conditions?

    1. The patient's skin is punctured or opened for a procedure.

    2. The patient's skin is damaged during trauma, burns, or surgery.

    3. Whenever the patient's body is entered by insertion of a device or instrument.

    A. 1 only

    B. 2 only

    C. 1 & 2

    D. 1, 2 & 3

32. When unwrapping a sterile tray, you would first:

    A. Fold back the top flap

    B. Unfold the side flaps

    C. Dump the tray out onto the sterile field.

    D. It doesn't matter in which sequence the tray is opened.

33. The basis of standard (universal) precautions is that:

    A. Every health care worker demand a diagnosis prior to servicing the patient.

    B. Only specific disease processes be protected against.

    C. Every health care worker approach every patient and body specimen as if infected.

    D. All AIDS patients be identified to health care workers.

34. If a health care worker sticks themselves with a dirty needle, he or she must:

    A. Wash the wound out thoroughly, for at least 10 minutes

    B. Receive a tetanus shot

    C. Fill out an incident report and OSHA report and go to employee health or emergency department

    D. Ignore the incident if the wound is only superficial.

35. If a procedure risks splashing or spraying of bodily fluids, the radiographer must wear:

    1. Gloves

    2. Mask/protective eye shields

    3. Gown

    A. 1 only

    B. 2 only

    C. 1 & 2

    D. 1, 2, & 3

36. A patient with active chickenpox may be placed in a(n):

A. positive-pressure room
B. negative-pressure room
C. critical care unit
D. oncology unit

37. Which of the following should not be disposed of in general biohazardous waste containers?

    A. Bloody gauze
    B. Emesis basins
    C. Dirty syringes and used needles
    D. Urine-soaked pads

38. The admitting department informs you that they are sending a patient to radiology who requires an upper GI series. They state that the patient is extremely short of breath. You would:

    A. Have the patient's vital signs assessed prior to the study.
    B. Cancel the patient's procedure.
    C. Proceed as usual.
    D. Take a chest radiograph to determine the patient's problem.

39. If an adult patient has tachycardia, the pulse will be in the following range:

    A. 40 to 60/min
    B. 60 to 80/min
    C. 60 to 100/min
    D. over 100/min

40. Diastolic refers to the _____ number when reading a blood pressure.

    A. Top
    B. Bottom
    C. Lowest
    D. Highest

41. When a patient is cyanotic, the patient's skin:

    A. Will have goosebumps.
    B. Becomes very red.
    C. Takes on a blue tone.
    D. Breaks out into a lacy rash.

42. A cyanotic patient generally has a problem with:

    A. Allergies
    B. Respiration and circulation

C. Elevated temperature
D. The extremities

43. Oxygen administration for most patients is generally:

    A. 1 to 2 liters/min
    B. 2 to 4 liters/min
    C. 6 to 8 liters/min
    D. Over 10 liters/min

44. An E cylinder tank contains 800 psi of oxygen. The patient's flow rate is 4 liters/min. How many minutes of remaining oxygen are there in the tank?

    A. 20 min
    B. 30 min
    C. 40 min
    D. 60 min

45. Heparin locks:

    A. Are used to dissolve blood clots
    B. Are used to secure syringes
    C. Are used as access ports for injectables
    D. Are used only in the pharmacy.

46. You are radiographing the patient and the IMed pump begins to signal a problem. You realize that the IV bag is empty. You:

    A. Unplug the pump and finish the case
    B. Call the unit and alert the nurse, having her replace the required solution.
    C. Replace the IV with D5W and continue with the procedure.
    D. Try to ignore the warning signal and continue with the procedure.

47. Which of the following is *not* a central venous line?

    A. Hickman catheter
    B. Swan-Ganz catheter
    C. Port-O-Cath
    D. Foley catheter

48. During CPR, the compression rate for an adult is:

    A. 80 to 100/min
    B. 60 to 80/min
    C. 50/min
    D. 20 to 40/min

49. After 2 full initial breaths of 1 to 1.5 sec during CPR, how many breaths per minute are required to continue for a child or infant in distress?

    A. 8
    B. 10
    C. 12
    D. 20

50. Abdominal thrusts are used to:

    A. Initiate CPR
    B. Aid in heart compression
    C. Help clear an adult obstructed airway
    D. Prepare the patient for electroshock

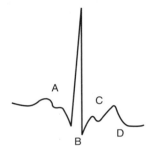

51. The following question refers to the drawing above. Indicate which letter corresponds to the QRS complex.

    A. A
    B. B
    C. C
    D. D

52. The QRS complex represents:

    A. The impulse that causes the atria to contract
    B. The impulse that causes ventricular contraction
    C. The relaxation phase, in preparation for another impulse
    D. The HIS response

53. Gel placed onto the EKG patient's skin prior to electrode placement helps to:

    A. Increase conductivity
    B. Soothe the skin
    C. Prevent burns
    D. Hold the electrodes in place

54. As the nuclear forces increase in an atom:

    A. The number of neutrons decrease.
    B. The atomic weight decreases.

    C. The binding energy of the K shell electron increases.
    D. The attenuation of the incoming radiation decreases.

55. Esophagrams are generally performed using:

    A. Barium paste/suspension
    B. Iodinated contrast media
    C. Ethiodol
    D. Gadolinium

56. The osmolality of human blood is:

    A. 100 mOsm/kg
    B. 150 mOsm/kg
    C. 200 mOsm/kg
    D. 300 mOsm/kg

57. The patient requires an abdominal CT with contrast, a nuclear medicine thyroid uptake scan, and a BE. What is the proper sequence of scheduling?

    A. Abdominal CT, BE, thyroid uptake scan
    B. BE, thyroid uptake scan, abdominal CT
    C. Thyroid uptake scan, abdominal CT, BE
    D. Thyroid uptake scan, BE, abdominal CT

58. Idiosyncratic reactions differ from anaphylactic reactions because:

    A. No IgE antibody is produced from a previous exposure, and it is independent of the drug or dose.
    B. They are not immediate in occurrence.
    C. They do not respond to emergency medications as well.
    D. They are not life threatening.

59. A moving clot that may travel throughout the body is termed:

    A. A thrombus
    B. A varix
    C. A TIA
    D. An embolus

60. MedWatch is a _____ based program.

    A. hospital-
    B. federally
    C. state-
    D. JCAHO-

Answers appear at the end of the book.

Simulated Registry Review—I

1. Which of the following is not an accessory organ of the digestive system?

   A. Liver
   B. Vermiform appendix
   C. Pancreas
   D. Gallbladder

2. At photon energies of 100 keV to 1 Mev, soft tissue absorption of radiation takes place due to:

   A. Pair production
   B. Compton effect
   C. Photoelectric effect
   D. Coherent attenuation

3. Leukemia is termed a:

   A. Linear, nonthreshold response
   B. Nonlinear, nonthreshold response
   C. Linear threshold response
   D. Nonlinear threshold response

4. In fetal circulation, the lungs are bypassed by which of the following?

   1. Interventricular septum
   2. Foramen ovale
   3. Ductus arteriosus

   A. 1 only
   B. 2 only
   C. 1 and 2
   D. 2 and 3

5. Which of the following timers is the most sophisticated and accurate?

   A. Synchronous
   B. Electronic
   C. Mechanical
   D. Spinning top

6. Acute radiation syndrome does not include:

   A. Hematologic death
   B. Gastrointestinal death
   C. Chromosome aberration death
   D. Central nervous system death

7. An intervertebral disc consists of:

   A. Nucleus pulposus and anulus fimbrae
   B. Nucleus fibrosus and anulus fibrosus
   C. Nucleus rugosus and anulus fibrosus
   D. Nucleus pulposus and anulus fibrosus

8. In which projection of the ankle will the intermalleolar plane be placed parallel to the plane of the film?

   A. 30° medial oblique
   B. 45° medial oblique
   C. AP
   D. Lateral

9. Which of the following dislocation and/or fracture(s) occur(s) in the cervical spine?

   1. Jefferson's fracture
   2. Bennett's fracture
   3. Hangman's fracture

   A. 1 only
   B. 2 only
   C. 1 and 2
   D. 1 and 3

10. Referring to the previous question, which fracture occurs at C2 and C3?

    A. Hangman's
    B. Jefferson's
    C. Bennett's
    D. None of the above occur at that location.

11. In the electromagnetic spectrum, which of the following will possess a smaller angstrom measurement than x-radiation?

    1. Gamma radiation
    2. Ultraviolet radiation
    3. Infrared radiation

    A. 1 only
    B. 2 only
    C. 1 and 2
    D. 2 and 3

12. The dose equivalent limit for the occupational radiation worker during a 1 year period is:

    A. 5 mrem
    B. 5000 mrem
    C. 50 mSv
    D. More than one, but not all of the above

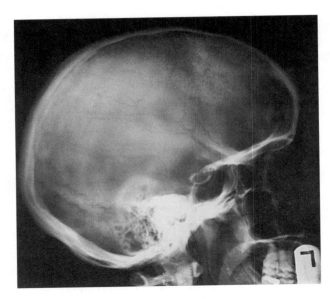

Radiograph 1

Please refer to Radiograph 1 for Questions 13–15.

13. For accurate positioning, the interpupillary line is placed:

    A. Parallel to the plane of the film
    B. Perpendicular to the plane of the film
    C. Perpendicular to the coronal plane
    D. Parallel to the central ray

14. The sinus(es) located directly anterior and inferior to the sella turcica is(are) called the:

    A. Ethmoid air cells
    B. Maxillary sinuses
    C. Sphenoid sinus
    D. Frontal sinus

15. Due to the inherent anatomical composition of the skull, the resultant contrast is normally:

    A. Short scale, high contrast
    B. Long scale, low contrast
    C. Short scale, low contrast
    D. Long scale, high contrast

16. To calculate for geometric unsharpness/penumbra (P), the best formula to use is:

    A. P = SID/SOD
    B. P = FSS × OID/SOD
    C. P = SID × OID/FSS
    D. P = SOD × FSS/OID

17. Exactly how many individual styloid processes exist within the normal adult skeleton?

    A. Six
    B. Eight
    C. Ten
    D. Twelve

18. The law that states that the radiosensitivity of living tissue varies according to the type of cell, the age, the metabolic activity, and the rate of growth is termed:

    A. Ohm's Law
    B. Bergonié and Tribondeau Law
    C. Quality Factor Law
    D. Guerney-Mott Law

19. A hilum exists in which of the following organs?

    1. kidney
    2. lung
    3. spleen

    A. 1 only
    B. 2 only
    C. 1 and 2
    D. 1, 2, and 3

20. When a vertebra is displaced in respect to its inferior vertebrae, it is termed:

    A. Spondylosis
    B. Scoliosis
    C. Spondylolisthesis
    D. Spondylitis

21. The major variance between retrograde and excretory urography is the:

    A. Anatomy visualized
    B. Method of contrast medium administration
    C. Patient preparation
    D. kVp selection

22. The total resistance of a 5-ohm and a 20-ohm resistor in a series circuit is:

    A. 2.5 ohms
    B. 7 ohms
    C. 10 ohms
    D. 25 ohms

23. A 10-ohm and a 5-ohm resistor are placed in a parallel circuit of 120 volts. The circuit current would be:

A. 3.3 amps
B. 5 amps
C. 15 amps
D. 33 amps

24. The superior mesenteric artery supplies blood to the:

    A. Stomach and large intestine
    B. Small intestine and large intestine
    C. Small intestine and spleen
    D. Large intestine only

25. The loss of power due to the rearrangement of magnetic domains is termed:

    A. Eddy currents
    B. Insulation
    C. Hysteresis
    D. Coulomb containment

26. The patella articulates with the:

    A. Femur, tibia, and fibula
    B. Femur and tibia
    C. Tibia and fibula
    D. Femur

27. Which veins join to form the portal vein?

    A. Splenic and superior mesenteric veins
    B. Left renal and splenic veins
    C. Splenic and inferior mesenteric veins
    D. Superior and inferior mesenteric veins

28. An x-ray tube has a heat storage capacity of 155,000 HU. How many rapid sequence films can be made at the following factors, before exceeding the capacity?

    300 mA   34 kVp   4 sec   30″ SID

    A. 2
    B. 3
    C. 6
    D. 12

29. The inverse square law relationship between intensity and distance from a source is based upon:

    A. Scatter
    B. Attenuation
    C. Divergence
    D. Absorption

30. When oxygen therapy is in use, which is not prohibited?

A. Smoking
B. Grounded electrical supplies and equipment
C. Use of aerosols
D. Use of open flame

31. Automatic collimation is also referred to as:

    A. HVL
    B. PBL
    C. AED
    D. VAD

32. Sterile procedure is required for which of the following procedures?

    1. Myelogram
    2. ERCP
    3. Cholecystogram

    A. 1 only
    B. 3 only
    C. 1 and 2
    D. 2 and 3

33. Negligence relies on four basic elements for civil liability. Select the accurate grouping.

    A. Duty, breach, cause, and injury
    B. Torts, consent, breach, and injury
    C. Res ipsa loquitur, breach, cause, and injury
    D. Malpractice, breach, lack of consent, and injury

34. An isotope is an atom that gains or loses a(n):

    A. Electron
    B. Proton
    C. Neutron
    D. Shell

35. You have selected an exposure using 70 kVp. The resultant radiation energy will be:

    A. 50 keV
    B. 70 keV
    C. 90 keV
    D. Polyenergetic

36. The LET of an x-ray or gamma photon is low because of its:

    A. Low energy

B. High penetration
C. Negative charge
D. Positive charge

37. The roentgen is most closely related to which other type of exposure?

    A. Primary radiation
    B. Secondary radiation
    C. Remnant radiation
    D. Off-focus radiation

38. A patient is exposed to 70 rads of alpha-radiation, having a QF (quality factor) of 5. The dose equivalency is:

    A. 75 rads
    B. 250 rads
    C. 350 rads
    D. 12 rads

39. To demonstrate the subacromial bursa, supraspinatus tendon insertion, and greater tubercle of the shoulder joint, which position is best?

    A. AP neutral
    B. AP internal rotation
    C. AP external rotation
    D. The oblique "Y"

40. Which position best demonstrates the apophyseal articulations of the cervical spine?

    A. AP
    B. Lateral
    C. LPO—45°
    D. Open mouth

41. What position will best demonstrate the structural status of the arch of the foot?

    A. Lateral
    B. Stress films
    C. Weight-bearing lateral
    D. Axial calcaneus

42. Radial flexion will best demonstrate the:

    A. Bones of the medial aspect of the wrist
    B. Bones of the lateral aspect of the wrist
    C. Navicular only
    D. Pisiform only

43. To demonstrate the articular facets of the thoracic spine best, the following position is used:

A. Lateral
B. Oblique—70°
C. Oblique—45°
D. AP

44. If you demonstrate the bicipital groove, you will radiograph the:

    A. Skull
    B. Elbow
    C. Humerus
    D. Scapula

45. The term adduction means:

    A. Toward the midline of the body
    B. Away from the midline of the body
    C. At a distance from the film
    D. Away from the head

46. To determine the stability of a spinal fusion in the lumbar region, the following radiographs should be obtained:

    A. AP projections with extension and flexion
    B. Erect AP with lateral bending
    C. Lateral projection with flexion and extension
    D. Obliques

47. Which of the following would best demonstrate the semilunar notch of the elbow?

    A. AP projection
    B. Lateral
    C. 45° medial oblique
    D. 45° lateral oblique

48. To demonstrate esophogeal varices, the following is utilized:

    A. Trendelenburg position
    B. Chassard-Lapine position
    C. Valsalva maneuver
    D. Gas-producing crystals and barium

49. Esophageal varices are generally byproducts of:

    A. Portal hypertension
    B. Dialysis
    C. Carcinoma
    D. Hiatal hernias

50. Varices are actually:

    A. Hernias
    B. Varicose veins
    C. Aneurysms
    D. Dissections

51. Res ipsa loquitur, defined by example, may be:

    A. Surgical instruments remaining in the abdomen after surgery
    B. Restraining the patient without medical order
    C. Publicly announcing the ineptness of a physician
    D. Prescribing medication without a license

52. The primary principle of diagnostic radiation protection is termed:

    A. Time and distance theory
    B. ALARA
    C. MPD
    D. Photoelectric effect

53. The largest sesamoid bone in the body is visualized in which examination?

    A. Skull
    B. Foot
    C. Hip
    D. Knee

54. A sesamoid bone that forms in the popliteal region is termed the:

    A. Patella
    B. Flabella
    C. Osteophyte
    D. Portobella

55. Radiographically, whiplash is usually indicated by:

    A. Muscle spasm, resulting in motion artifacts
    B. Evulsion fractures and dislocations
    C. Decrease in contrast due to ligament tears
    D. Reduction of the lordotic curve of the spine

For Questions 56–61, Refer to the following illustration.

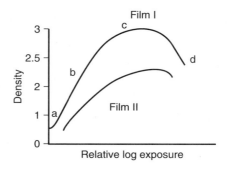

Select Answers Here
1. Toe
2. Shoulder
3. Gamma
4. D-Max
5. Average gradient
6. Base plus fog
7. Solarization
8. Chemical fog

56. The "a" portion represents:

    A. 1 only
    B. 1 and 8
    C. 1 and 6
    D. 8 only

57. The "b" portion represents:

    A. 2 only
    B. 3 only
    C. 3 and 5
    D. 2 and 4

58. The "c" portion represents:

    A. 2 only
    B. 4 only
    C. 5 only
    D. 2 and 4

59. The "d" portion represents:

    A. 2 only
    B. 7 only
    C. 8 only
    D. 3 only

60. Film I plotted indicates that:

    A. Wide exposure latitude is provided.
    B. Narrow exposure latitude is provided.

61. Which film should be used if long-scale contrast is desired?

    A. Film I
    B. Film II

62. Which of the chemical reducing agents affects the shoulder portion of the H&D curve?

    A. Glutaraldehyde
    B. Phenidone
    C. Hydroquinone
    D. Ammonium thiosulfate

63. Your radiographs emerge from the processor in a tacky condition. The most common reason for this is:

    A. Low dryer temperature
    B. Insufficient potassium alum replenishment
    C. Chemical solution temperature is too low.
    D. Roller acceleration during the drying phase

64. When selecting kVp on the control panel, you are actually utilizing the:

    A. Capacitor
    B. Phototimer
    C. Autotransformer
    D. Stator

65. When increasing mA stations sequentially from 50 to 600 on the control panel, you are actually:

    A. Increasing the amperage to the filament
    B. Increasing thermionic emission
    C. Increasing the filament size used
    D. All of the above are true.

66. The anode is:

    A. Always on the negative side of the tube
    B. Always on the right side when facing the tube
    C. Always on the side connected to the high-voltage circuit
    D. Not responsible for the anode-heel effect

67. The *quality* of radiation produced is directly affected by:

    1. kVp selection
    2. EMF
    3. mA selection

    A. 1 only
    B. 1 and 2

C. 2 only
D. 2 and 3

68. The *least* radiosensitive tissue group listed below is the:

    A. Central nervous system
    B. Alimentary tract
    C. Muscular system
    D. Cardiovascular system

69. The linear, nonthreshold curve of radiation dose relationships states that radiation damage is directly proportional to the dose and:

    A. Only high doses are damaging.
    B. Any dose may cause damage.
    C. Damage occurs after a minimum dose.
    D. Many doses must be received prior to damage being caused.

70. The immediate symptoms that occur after an acute radiation exposure are termed:

    A. Latent
    B. Chronic
    C. Prodromal
    D. Prophetic

71. The NCRP recommends that the effective dose equivalent limit to the general public be limited by what percentage of the occupational dose?

    A. 1%
    B. 2%
    C. 10%
    D. 20%

72. The unit of absorbed dose, the rad (gray), is employed in the measurement of:

    A. Alpha- and beta-radiation only
    B. Beta- and gamma-radiation only
    C. Neutrons and alpha-particles only
    D. All forms of radiation

73. Etiology unknown refers to:

    A. Unclear prognosis
    B. Unclear diagnosis
    C. Unclear causation of the disease
    D. Unclear treatment plans

74. TIA refers to:

    A. Total infarct arterial

B. Tortuous infantile arteries

C. Transient ischemic attack

D. Transient idiosyncratic allergies

75. During radiographic exposure, who would be the most likely person to restrain a child?

    A. The technologist
    B. The department secretary
    C. The father
    D. The orderly

76. The only legal "right and left" marking system is(are):

    A. Lead markers placed at time of exposure
    B. Adhesive labels
    C. Permanent ink
    D. More than one, but not all of the above

77. Initial emergency response in the radiology department for cardiopulmonary resuscitation is the responsibility of:

    A. The emergency team
    B. The radiologist
    C. The radiologic technologist
    D. The attending physician

78. Which of the following needles would be the finest and most likely to be used for an infant's injection?

    A. 18-gauge needle
    B. 21-gauge butterfly
    C. 23-gauge butterfly
    D. 25-gauge butterfly

79. Chest tube collection systems and Foley catheter bags should be kept:

    A. Under the stretcher at all times
    B. Below the organ that they are draining
    C. On top of the patient's stretcher
    D. It doesn't matter where they are placed.

80. Which of the following is the most appropriate *measure* of primary radiation quality?

    A. kVp
    B. HVL
    C. mA meter
    D. Densitometer

81. Silver reclamation is critical to the budget of most radiology departments. To which processing element is the reclamation unit attached?

    A. Developer solution section
    B. Fixer solution section
    C. The water drain
    D. The exhaust system

82. Image intensification input phosphor screens are made from which of the following materials?

    A. Zinc cadmium sulfide
    B. Lanthanum
    C. Cesium iodine
    D. Calcium tungstate

83. When utilizing automatic exposure devices, it is best to minimize scatter radiation through tight collimation, use of lead strips, and so on for the following reason:

    A. Increased detail
    B. To prevent premature termination of the exposure device
    C. To prevent radiation exposure to the patient
    D. Decreased contrast

84. A portable grid, cross-table lateral hip radiograph is obtained using the automatic exposure system. The resultant radiograph will be:

    A. Perfectly exposed if the anatomy was positioned properly to the ionization chamber
    B. A lower-contrast radiograph than if manual technique were used
    C. A more detailed radiograph
    D. A completely overexposed radiograph

85. Which of the following yields the longest scale of contrast?

A. 300 mA	1/10 sec	80 kVp	5:1 grid
B. 300 mA	1/5 sec	76 kVp	6:1 grid
C. 300 mA	1/4 sec	70 kVp	12:1 grid
D. 300 mA	1/5 sec	70 kVp	16:1 grid

86. Quantum mottle is increased with the use of:

    1. High-speed screens
    2. High-speed film
    3. High kVp–low mAs exposure factors

A. 1 only
B. 1 and 2
C. 3 only
D. 1, 2, and 3

87. Long wavelength radiation produces:

A. Short-scale contrast
B. Long-scale contrast
C. Poor contrast in low-speed screens
D. Low contrast

88. 16 mm and 35 mm refer to the:

A. Length of the frames of film
B. Line pairs/mm of each frame
C. Width of the frames of film
D. Thickness of the frames of film

89. The BUN laboratory test indicates:

A. How much blood is in the urine
B. Level of kidney function
C. Presence of azotemia
D. More than one, but not all of the above

90. Which of the following pharmaceutical agents is an anticoagulant?

A. Heparin
B. Diphenhydramine
C. Atropine
D. Epinephrine

91. If a diabetic patient on Glucophage (metformin) therapy is scheduled for an iodinated contrast medium procedure, the following must occur:

A. The procedure must be canceled.
B. The Glucophage must be discontinued for at least 48 hours postprocedure and until normal kidney function is assessed.
C. The patient must be placed on insulin until the procedure is over.
D. The patient must receive premedication.

92. Exacerbate refers to:

A. Excision of suderiferous glands
B. Excision of a pus-filled region
C. Drainage of any area
D. Acceleration of symptoms/disease

93. The type of timer that has a minimum exposure time of 1/60 sec and increases in multiples, such as 1/30, 1/20, and so on, is a(n):

A. Electronic timer
B. Mechanical timer
C. Synchronous timer
D. Spinning top timer

94. Which of the following measures the response of a film to exposure and processing?

A. Penetrometer
B. Sensitometer
C. mA meter
D. Densitometer

95. The most efficient type of transformer is the:

A. Air core
B. Open core
C. Closed core
D. Shell type

96. A spinning top test was made with a full-wave rectified, single-phase generator. The test reveals 6 dots. What is the resultant exposure time?

A. 1/60 sec
B. 1/20 sec
C. 1/10 sec
D. 1/5 sec

97. An abdominal radiograph was exposed using the following factors: 20 mAs at 60 kVp. The resultant image is light, due to underpenetration. What percentage of kVp will double the exposure?

A. 5%—add 3 kVp
B. 10%—add 6 kVp
C. 15%–add 9 kVp
D. 20%—add 12 kVp

98. The voltage = 18.
The resistance = 1.8.
What is the current?

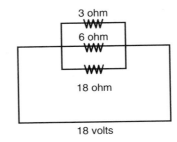

3 ohm
6 ohm
18 ohm
18 volts

A. 10 amps
B. 1.5 amps
C. 2 amps
D. 4 amps

99. Which of these geometric factors affect size distortion the *least*?

    A. SID
    B. FSS
    C. OID
    D. SOD

100. If the circuit has 4 amps of current and 25 ohms of resistance, what is the applied voltage?

    A. 2.5 volts
    B. 21 volts
    C. 50 volts
    D. 100 volts

101. The xiphoid tip of the sternum is the landmark for which anatomy?

    A. The 10th thoracic vertebral body
    B. The cardiac orifice
    C. The carina
    D. More than one but not all of the above

102. Which organ is located in the left hypochondriac region?

    A. The cecum
    B. The left kidney
    C. The spleen
    D. The liver

103. Which of the following organ's physiology is that of an exocrine and endocrine gland?

    A. Thymus
    B. Adrenal
    C. Pancreas
    D. Pineal

104. The longitudinal mucosal folds of the stomach that enable organ expansion and aid in digestion are:

    A. The rugae
    B. The haustra
    C. The serosa
    D. The body

105. The C-shaped duodenum surrounds a portion of which organ?

    A. The pancreas
    B. The spleen
    C. The gallbladder
    D. More than one, but not all of the above

106. You are radiographing a child's knee. Its AP measurement is 7 cm. The exposure factors for this measurement in the Bucky would be:

    mAs: 12   kVp: 62   small focal
    SID: 40″   12:1 Bucky   spot size

    You choose to lower the patient dose by using a screen and tabletop technique. Your new mAs would be:

    A. 10
    B. 7
    C. 5
    D. 3

107. A pediatric follow-up chest examination is ordered. Two days ago another technologist radiographed the child supine at 40″ SID. The following exposure factors were used:

    SID: 40″   kVp: 65
    mAs: 2   screen: nongrid

    You choose to use a 72″ SID and an erect position to obtain a diagnostic study. Your new mAs would be:

    A. 3
    B. 7
    C. 9
    D. 12

108. Photomultipliers, thyratrons, and ionization chambers refer to:

    A. Tomographic units
    B. Automatic exposure devices
    C. Image intensification systems
    D. Personal radiation monitors

109. The loss of hair caused by receiving large doses of radiation is termed:

    A. Epitaxis
    B. Epilation
    C. Erythema
    D. Bromidrosis

110. The most radiosensitive tissue group listed below is the:

    A. Central nervous system
    B. Alimentary tract
    C. Muscular system
    D. Cardiovascular system

111. The amount of energy transferred to a material per unit length of travel is termed:

    A. RBE
    B. REM
    C. LET
    D. DEL

112. Which of the following exposure factors would provide the lowest patient dosage?

    A. 400 mA   1/4 sec   60 kVp   100 speed screens

    B. 400 mA   1/4 sec   80 kVp   100 speed screens

    C. 400 mA   1/8 sec   90 kVp   400 speed screens

    D. 400 mA   1/2 sec   90 kVp   200 speed screens

113. The tomographic movement that affords the thinnest cut is:

    A. Linear
    B. Elliptical
    C. Spiral
    D. Hypocycloidal

114. The condition of telescoping bowel is referred to as:

    A. Volvulus
    B. Intussusception
    C. Enteroclysis
    D. Crohn's disease

115. Perforation of the small bowel would be best diagnosed using the following procedure:

    A. Small bowel series with barium
    B. KUB
    C. Right lateral decubitus
    D. Left lateral decubitus

116. During a double-contrast barium enema procedure, which position or projection would demonstrate air in the lateral aspect of the descending colon?

    A. Left lateral decubitus
    B. Right lateral decubitus
    C. Prone
    D. Left lateral rectum

117. If you have positioned properly for an AP pelvis radiograph, which anatomy would not be visible?

    A. Femoral neck
    B. Femoral head
    C. Greater trochanter
    D. Lesser trochanter

118. Which of the following positions or projections should be used to demonstrate nephroptosis?

    A. Prone and decubitus
    B. RPO and LPO
    C. Supine and erect
    D. Supine and prone

119. Intervertebral foramina are best demonstrated utilizing the following:

    1. Oblique thoracic spine
    2. Oblique cervical spine
    3. Lateral thoracic spine
    4. Oblique lumbar spine

    A. 1 and 2
    B. 2 and 3
    C. 3 and 4
    D. 2 only

120. The ankle mortise is composed of the following articulations:

    A. Tibia and fibula
    B. Cuboid, tibia, and fibula
    C. Navicular, tibia, and fibia
    D. Talus, tibia, and fibula

121. Which anatomical area is most commonly radiographed to determine the patient's bone growth development?

    A. Vertebral column
    B. Hands and wrists
    C. Feet and ankles
    D. Skull

122. A radiograph of the odontoid process via the open mouth projection demonstrates the cranial base superimposed upon the dens. To correct this positioning error, you must:

A. Extend the chin
B. Depress the chin
C. Angle the tube 45° cephalic
D. Angle the tube 45° caudad

123. The parenchyma of the kidneys is called:

    A. Bowman's capsule
    B. The nephrons
    C. The calyces
    D. The renal pyramids

124. The gastrointestinal position/projection that best demonstrates the barium-filled fundus is the:

    A. RAO
    B. Right lateral
    C. LPO
    D. PA

125. A fold of peritoneum between various abdominal organs is termed:

    A. Mesentery
    B. Epithelium
    C. Omentum
    D. Haustra

126. Inspiration/expiration chest radiographs are obtained for the which of the following reasons?

    A. Aspiration of foreign objects
    B. Diaphragm excursion
    C. Pneumothorax
    D. All of the above

127. A medication must be stored at a temperature of 53°F. What would be the *centigrade* storage temperature?

    A. 65°
    B. 5.5°
    C. 25°
    D. 11.7°

128. A ventral decubitus requires that the patient be:

    A. Recumbent, on the left side
    B. Recumbent, on the right side
    C. Supine
    D. Prone

129. A cervical rib is best demonstrated utilizing the following:

A. AP thoracic spine
B. AP cervical spine
C. Oblique rib positioning
D. Oblique cervical spine positioning

Refer to Radiograph 2 for Questions 130–134.

130. The standard optimal exposure factors to obtain this image would be:

    A. Low mA, long exposure time
    B. High mA, short exposure time
    C. Automatic exposure selection
    D. Linear tomography

131. The natural curve of this anatomy is termed:

    A. Lordosis
    B. Kyphosis
    C. Scoliosis
    D. Halitosis

132. This position demonstrates which of the following?

    1. Intervertebral joint spaces
    2. Apophyseal joints
    3. Intervertebral foramina

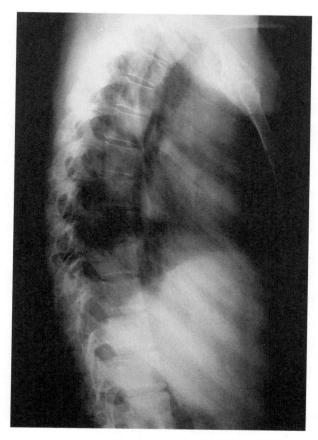

Radiograph 2

A. 1 only
B. 2 only
C. 1 and 2
D. 1 and 3

133. When utilizing this projection on hypersthenic patients, in order to visualize the upper thoracic spine you must:

    A. Roll the patient forward 30°
    B. Angle the tube 10° to 15° cephalic
    C. Utilize tomography
    D. Do a cross-table lateral

134. If you were to utilize the anode-heel effect for this position, the cathode would be placed:

    A. At the head of the table
    B. Over the patient's shoulders
    C. Over the patient's hips
    D. Directly over the midspine

135. A technologist uses a kVp that is too high for the body part being imaged. The resultant image demonstrates unwanted density. This may be attributed to:

    A. Classic scattering
    B. Photoelectric effect
    C. Compton effect
    D. Pair production

136. The output phosphor of an image intensification tube converts:

    A. X-radiation into visible light
    B. Electrons into x-radiation
    C. Visible light into electrons
    D. Electrons into visible light photons

137. A 72″ SID is used during lateral cervical spine radiography to:

    A. Increase OID
    B. Reduce magnification because of increased OID
    C. Magnify the image specifically
    D. Eliminate scatter radiation

138. Standard/universal precautions apply to:

    A. Only patients on precautions
    B. HIV patients
    C. All patients
    D. Patients who are bleeding

139. Forcing a patient to drink barium by threatening him, if he has refused the procedure, may be considered:

    A. Assault
    B. Battery
    C. False imprisonment
    D. Negligence

140. Rectification may be defined as:

    A. The process of modifying alternating current to pulsating direct current
    B. Thermionic emission
    C. Wave tail cut-off
    D. Timer modification

141. The milliammeter is located:

    A. In the filament circuit
    B. In the secondary, high-voltage circuit
    C. In the primary, low-voltage circuit
    D. In the x-ray tube

142. Indicate which statement(s) is(are) true regarding the primary coils of the step up transformer.

    1. The number of turns is directly proportional to the secondary voltage increase.
    2. They are located in the primary circuit.
    3. They operate on the principle of electromagnetic self-induction.

    A. 1 only
    B. 1 and 2
    C. 1 and 3
    D. 1, 2, and 3

143. Which of the following operates on the principle of electromagnetic self-induction?

    A. The autotransformer
    B. The circuit breaker
    C. Primary coils of the step up transformer
    D. Rectifiers

144. Indicate which of the following is true regarding a rheostat.

    1. It operates on AC or DC current.
    2. It is located in the filament circuit.
    3. It decreases voltage and increases amperage.

    A. 1 only
    B. 1 and 2

C. 2 and 3

D. 1, 2, and 3

145. Quantum mottle may be reduced by:

A. Increasing screen speed

B. Increasing mA

C. Increasing kVp

D. Increasing SID

146. Indicate which of the following transform visible light into a video signal.

A. Cathode ray tube

B. Vidicon tube

C. Plumbicon tube

D. More than one, but not all of the above

147. The greatest radiation exposure to the patient occurs with which of the following imaging formats?

A. 35-mm film

B. 70-mm film

C. 105-mm chip film

D. 9 × 9 spot film cassette

148. Image intensification tubes operate at which current?

A. 0.5 to 5.0 mA

B. 5 to 10 mA

C. 120 kVp

D. 140 kVp

149. Ohm's law is expressed as:

A. I = V/R

B. R = V/I

C. V × R = I

D. More than one, but not all of the above

150. Which material provides diagnostic range photons postelectron bombardment?

A. Molybdenum

B. Rhenium

C. Tungsten

D. Copper

151. Which of the following would not aid in limiting patient motion?

A. Short time exposure

B. Patient preparation

C. Pro-Banthine injection

D. Low mA station

152. Using adhesive tape for immobilization on a child's skull that leaves residual tape burns on the child's skin could be construed as:

A. Assault

B. Battery

C. Negligence

D. Malpractice

153. Which of the following is considered regulated medical waste?

1. A used, but empty, syringe

2. A used bedpan

3. Blood-soaked gauze

A. 1 only

B. 3 only

C. 1 and 3

D. 1, 2, and 3

154. A tort is defined as:

A. A breach of contract

B. A civil wrong, other than a breach of contract

C. Malpractice

D. Operating outside of your scope of practice

155. When the health care facility is in equal responsibility with the technologist for negligence, the term that applies is:

A. Res ipsa loquitur

B. Respondeat superior

C. Suit equality

D. Co-malpractice

156. An incident report would be required for which of the following?

A. An examination is canceled.

B. The patient refuses a procedure.

C. The patient's head bumps the x-ray tube housing.

D. The patient refuses to pay for a procedure.

157. After an acute radiation exposure, the time in which it takes the initial effects to be seen is termed the:

A. Postdromal period

B. Postexposure period

C. Latent period

D. Pre-effectual period

158. The dose at which a biologic effect can be attributed to radiation is termed the:

    A. Effectual dose
    B. Biologic dose
    C. Radiation dose
    D. Threshold dose

159. Indicate which of the following is most radiosensitive.

    A. Neuron
    B. Erythrocyte
    C. Lymphocyte
    D. Ovum

160. A pocket dosimeter does not contribute to the following:

    A. Accurate results
    B. Permanent radiation record
    C. Portable radiation monitoring
    D. Speed in monitoring results

161. A 500-rad exposure equals which of the following?

    A. 500 gray
    B. 50 gray
    C. 5 gray
    D. 0.5 gray

162. An inaccurate radiation reading is threatened from the film badge if which of the following occur?

    A. The badge has been exposed to multiple radiation exposures.
    B. The badge is worn out of the department.
    C. The badge is laundered.
    D. The badge is exposed to fluorescent lighting.

163. Which exposure will present with the highest dose equivalency?

    A. 6 gray of x-radiation
    B. 6 rads of x-radiation
    C. 6 gray of beta-radiation
    D. 6 gray of alpha-radiation

164. Indicate which of the following would be utilized for personnel radiation monitoring.

    A. Ionization chamber
    B. Thermoluminescent dosimeter

C. Geiger-Müller counter
D. Scintillation counter

165. Personalized film badges are used in conjunction with a _____ to measure for accurate results.

    A. Control badge
    B. Dosimeter
    C. Geiger counter
    D. Annual blood sampling

166. The total dose equivalent limit for fetal exposure is:

    A. 0.5 rem
    B. 50 mSv
    C. 5 rem
    D. 500 mSv

167. Maintenance of the cumulative radiation dose records for each radiation worker is the responsibility of the:

    A. Radiation worker
    B. Contracted monitoring company
    C. Radiation safety committee
    D. Institution

168. The first arterial branch off the aorta is the:

    A. Carotid arteries
    B. Pulmonary arteries
    C. Coronary arteries
    D. Vertebral arteries

169. A transformer will operate on which of the following?

    A. Alternating current only
    B. Direct current only
    C. Alternating and direct current
    D. Batteries only

170. To convert electrical energy into mechanical energy, which of the following is essential?

    A. Generator
    B. Motor
    C. Transformer
    D. Choke coil

171. The only device that can change current in an electrical circuit by using either alternating or direct current is the:

A. Transformer
B. Solenoid
C. Rheostat
D. Induction coil

172. Which of the following is an advantage to using solid state rectification?

    A. Less heat production
    B. Utilization of less space
    C. Elimination of filaments
    D. All of the above are correct.

173. Which of the following would not reduce radiation exposure to the patient?

    A. High-speed screens
    B. Utilization of collimation
    C. Use of a grid
    D. Utilization of highest kVp possible

174. The primary function of added filtration in the diagnostic x-ray tube is to:

    A. Reduce contrast on the resultant radiograph
    B. Reduce skin dosage
    C. Reduce scatter
    D. Increase the x-ray beam wavelength

175. A radiographic film with a high average gradient will demonstrate:

    A. A wide range of latitude
    B. A narrow range of latitude
    C. A shallow slope
    D. Long-scale contrast on the resultant radiograph

176. The size of the object is 7″. The SID is 40″. The OID is 9″. What is the resultant size of the image?

    A. 3.4″
    B. 5.4″
    C. 9.03″
    D. 10.4″

177. Find the GU (geometric unsharpness) for the following factors: A chest radiograph is taken at 72″ SID, 80 kVp, 8 mAs, and a 6″ OID. The FSS is 0.3.

    A. 0.27
    B. 1.27
    C. 12.7
    D. 127

178. If 30 mAs were used at 40″ SID and the distance was then changed to 60″ SID, what new mAs would be required to maintain density?

    A. 35 mAs
    B. 45 mAs
    C. 55 mAs
    D. 68 mAs

179. An AP shoulder is radiographed at 36″ SID using 1/8 of a second. If the new SID is 72″, what new time would be required?

    A. 1/10 sec
    B. 1/2 sec
    C. 3/4 sec
    D. 1 sec

180. To maintain film density when increasing the kVp by 15%, the mAs must be:

    A. Increased by 25%
    B. Increased by 50%
    C. Decreased by 25%
    D. Decreased by 50%

181. Dark treelike or lightning-like images appear on your freshly developed radiograph. They are most probably:

    A. Light fog artifacts
    B. Chemical fog artifacts
    C. Static electricity artifacts
    D. Improper film-handling artifacts

182. In reference to question 181, what could you do to prevent these from continuing to occur?

    A. Increase humidity
    B. Raise the safe light
    C. Change the chemistry
    D. Store the film boxes upright

183. An increase in the screen speed may be obtained by:

    A. Using a thinner crystal layer
    B. Selecting a phosphor with a high conversion factor
    C. Adding dye enhancement
    D. Using smaller crystals

184. The silver halogen used in the manufacture of most radiographic film is called:

A. Silver tungsten
B. Silver bromide
C. Silver phosphate
D. Silver iodide

185. The conversion of silver halogen into black metallic silver requires a(n):

A. Alkaline solution
B. Acid solution
C. Potassium-laden solution
D. Sodium-laden solution

186. If a radiographic exposure produced 110 mr at 72″ SID, what would the output be at 18″ SID?

A. 220 mr
B. 420 mr
C. 840 mr
D. 1760 mr

187. An acceptable abdominal radiograph was taken at 40″ SID with a 10:1 Bucky grid ratio. A second exposure is made, with the only change being the use of a 5:1 stationary grid. This second radiograph will exhibit the following:

1. Greater density
2. Higher contrast
3. Longer scale of contrast

A. 1 only
B. 1 and 2
C. 2 and 3
D. 1 and 3

188. To see a visible difference in density, what percentage increase is required in mAs selection?

A. 5%
B. 15%
C. 25%
D. 30%

Refer to the following Radiograph 3A and B for Question 189.

189. Your initial attempt to obtain a Waters' parietocanthal projection is *A*. To obtain the results shown in *B*, you must correct the repeat positioning by:

A. Elevating the patient's chin
B. Depressing the patient's chin
C. Angling the tube
D. Angling the film

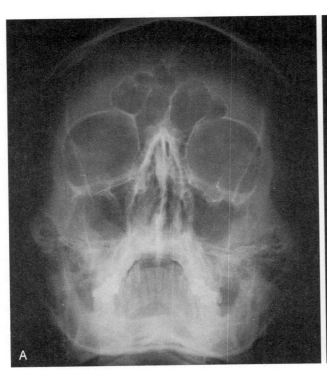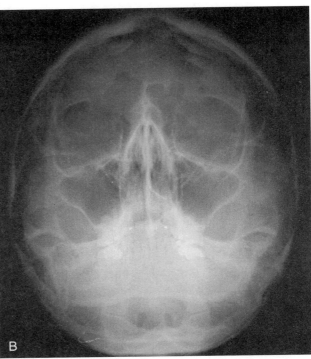

Radiograph 3

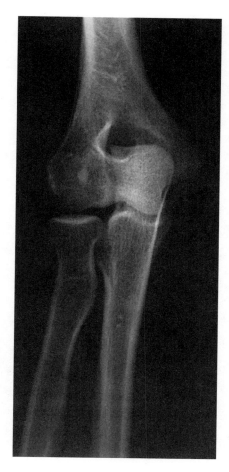

Radiograph 4

Refer to Radiograph 4 for Questions 190–192.

190. To obtain this projection of the elbow joint, the patient assumed which of the following positions?

   A. The arm was extended for a true AP.
   B. External oblique position
   C. Internal oblique position
   D. AP projection in flexion

191. If the patient were unable to assume the required position, in which direction and at how many degrees would you angle the tube to provide the same information?

   A. The central ray would be directed medially at 25°.
   B. The central ray would be directed medially at 45°.
   C. The central ray would be directed laterally at 25°.
   D. The central ray would be directed laterally at 45°.

192. The opposite position of the one depicted would best demonstrate the:

   A. Olecranon process
   B. Coranoid process
   C. Radial tuberosity
   D. Coracoid process

193. The position that best demonstrates an abdominal aortic aneurysm is the:

   A. Lateral recumbent
   B. Ventral decubitus
   C. Erect AP
   D. Left lateral decubitus

194. Which bone forms most of the medial wall of the orbit?

   A. Ethmoid
   B. Sphenoid
   C. Frontal
   D. Lacrimal

195. Name the obvious projection of bone that extends above the perpendicular plate of the ethmoid bone.

   A. Sella turcica
   B. Crista galli
   C. Pterion
   D. Bregma

196. For an AP projection of the forearm, which portion of the forearm will be affected if the hand is pronated?

   A. Distal third
   B. Proximal third
   C. The ulna and radius will cross directly in the middle.
   D. The forearm will remain unaffected.

197. A rib that is attached to the sternum indirectly is referred to as:

   A. A floating rib
   B. A true rib
   C. A false rib
   D. An articulated rib

198. Scoliosis patients must have which of the following included on their radiographs?

   A. Cervical body 7, lumbar body 5, and iliac crests
   B. Thoracic body 12, lumbar body 5, and iliac crests

C. Lumbar body 5, the sacrum, and iliac crests

D. Only the portion of the spine that is curved

199. Scoliosis patients are generally radiographed at 72″ SID. For what reason?

A. Increased contrast
B. Decreased contrast
C. Increased magnification
D. Decreased magnification

200. You are requested to obtain an AP and lateral spot film of lumbar body 4. You would place the central ray at the level of:

A. The xiphoid
B. The umbilicus
C. The ASIS (anterior superior iliac spine)
D. The symphysis pubis

Simulated Registry Review—II

1. The exposure switch design for fluoroscopic equipment must be:

   A. Remote control
   B. Dead-man
   C. Terminating
   D. Magnetic

2. Inherent filtration consists of:

   A. Aluminum—0.5 mm
   B. Aluminum—1.5 mm
   C. Aluminum—2.5 mm
   D. Pyrex glass and oil

3. Lead gloves and aprons must contain a minimum of:

   A. 0.25 mm Pb equivalent
   B. 1.25 mm Pb equivalent
   C. 2.0 lead
   D. 2.5 lead

4. Indicate which of the following is not an SI unit:

   A. Gy
   B. Sv
   C. C/kg
   D. Ci

5. The first symptom of acute radiation exposure is:

   A. Epilation
   B. Erythema
   C. Nausea
   D. Dysuria

6. Which one of the following is an example of the ASRT's Code of Ethics?

   A. Professional confidentiality
   B. Troubleshooting equipment problems
   C. Measuring each patient with calipers and recording that information
   D. Understanding radiographic interpretation

7. Competency reviews for radiographers are now required by the JCAHO for which of the following?

   A. Age-specific procedures
   B. Radiologic interpretation
   C. Minor surgical procedures
   D. Issuing of prescriptions

8. COPD is the abbreviation for:

   A. Congestive output pulmonary distress
   B. Chronic obstructive pulmonary disease
   C. Coronary obstructive pleural disease
   D. Cerebral obstructive plexus disease

9. One milliliter is equivalent to:

   A. 1 cubic centimeter
   B. 1 tablespoon
   C. 1 teaspoon
   D. More than one, but not all of the above

10. Indicate which of the following is not a parenteral drug route:

    A. Intramuscular (IM)
    B. Intravenous (IV)
    C. Subcutaneous (SC)
    D. By mouth (PO)

11. To demonstrate polyps of the intestine, the following procedure is ordered:

    A. Single-contrast barium enema
    B. Double-contrast barium enema
    C. Gastrointestinal motility series
    D. An obstruction abdominal series—AP and erect

12. When checking the tomography scout for renal tomography, the anatomy used as a check for proper fulcrum selection is:

    A. Body of the spine
    B. Spinous process
    C. Pedicles of the spine
    D. Renal parenchyma

13. When a technologist is performing a verticosubmental projection of the skull, the central ray enters at:

    A. The external auditory meatus
    B. The mental point
    C. The nasion
    D. The vertex of the skull

14. The patient's chest measures 23 cm in the AP dimension. Tomos are to be performed in an AP projection of a questionable lesion 3 cm posterior to the anterior chest wall. The fulcrum must be set:

    A. 3 cm from the tabletop
    B. 23 cm from the tabletop
    C. At the midline
    D. 20 cm from the tabletop

15. The position of the grid for a translateral hip should be:

    A. Parallel to the central ray
    B. Perpendicular to the femoral neck
    C. Parallel to the femoral neck
    D. Perpendicular to the femur shaft

16. Which of the following set of exposure factors will produce the optimum recorded detail?

	mAs	kVp	Grid Ratio	Screen Speed	Focal Spot Size
A.	60	80	8:1	medium	2 mm
B.	50	70	5:1	detail	1 mm
C.	70	85	5:1	medium	1 mm
D.	80	65	8:1	detail	2 mm

17. The straight line portion of a characteristic curve is also referred to as:

    A. The gamma portion
    B. The toe
    C. The shoulder
    D. The beta

18. Solarization insures that given additional exposure, the radiograph will demonstrate:

    A. Greater density
    B. Less density
    C. Greater detail
    D. Less detail

Use the following factors for Questions 19–21.

	mA	Seconds	kVp	Focal Spot	Screen
I.	400	1/4	70	large	high-speed
II.	25	4	70	small	detail
III.	50	2	70	small	medium
IV.	100	1	70	small	detail

19. Indicate which selection would provide the greatest density.

A. I
B. I and II
C. III and IV
D. All would provide the same density

20. Indicate which selection would be used for an autotomographic sternum examination.

A. I
B. II
C. III
D. None of the above

21. Indicate which would provide the least recorded detail.

A. I
B. II
C. III
D. More than one, but not all of the above

22. A prereading kVp meter measures the EMF:

A. Of the filament circuit
B. Of the primary side of the autotransformer
C. Between the autotransformer and the primary side of the step up transformer
D. Of the primary of the step up transformer

23. The two energy interactions that occur during diagnostic range x-radiation production are:

A. Characteristic and Compton
B. Bremsstrahlung and characteristic
C. Coherent and characteristic
D. Pair production and bremsstrahlung

24. The cathode is connected to which of the following?

A. High-voltage circuit
B. Filament circuit
C. Primary side of the secondary circuit
D. More than one, but not all of the above

25. Which of the following statements is(are) correct regarding the anode?

    1. It is the positive pole.
    2. The electron cloud forms here.
    3. It may be stationary or rotating.

A. 1 only
B. 2 only

C. 1 and 2

D. 1 and 3

26. The allowable heat units for a single-phase unit are 33,600. Use the following exposure factors to determine the maximum amount of rapid sequence exposures that may be made without damage:

300 mA   70 kVp   0.20 sec

A. 2

B. 4

C. 6

D. 8

27. Minification gain occurs when:

A. Electrons from the input screen converge on the output screen.

B. The overall boost of image intensification is measured.

C. The conversion efficiency of the output phosphor is measured.

D. The automatic brightness control is measured.

28. During tomography, the distance that the tube travels during the exposure is termed:

A. Linear travel

B. Amplitude

C. Arc travel

D. Film-tube travel

29. Which of the following statements is inaccurate regarding x-radiation?

A. X-radiation may cause ionization of matter.

B. X-radiation may be focused.

C. X-radiation may cause certain elements to illuminate.

D. X-radiation does not carry a charge.

30. The energy interaction that occurs in the diagnostic range and allows for variations in tissue contrast is termed:

A. Coherent

B. Compton

C. Photodisintegration

D. Photoelectric

Refer to Radiograph 1 for Questions 31–35.

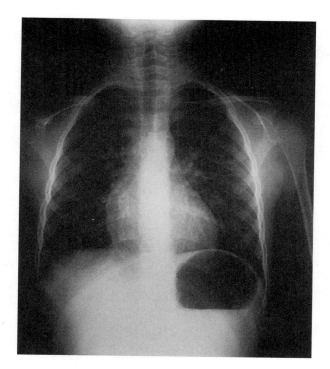

Radiograph 1

31. The right diaphragm is higher than the left; this is due to:

A. The location of the heart

B. The location of the liver

C. The amount of inspiration

D. The rotation of the patient

32. The bony thorax consists of:

A. The sternum, vertebrae, and ribs

B. The sternum, ribs, and shoulder girdle

C. The sternum and ribs only

D. The sternum and vertebrae only

33. The kVp selected was optimal. You realize this by:

A. Observing the lung tissue

B. Observing that the area surrounding the chest anatomy is exposed sufficiently

C. Observing that the mediastinum is penetrated adequately

D. Observing the soft tissue neck

34. The position for this examination was erect, with the central ray parallel to the floor. This is ascertained by:

A. Observing the air-fluid level in the fundus

B. The full expiration
C. The shape of the heart
D. The size of the heart

35. The primary reason that chest radiographs are exposed at 72″ SID is:

    A. To reduce contrast
    B. To obtain the most accurate heart size
    C. To increase OID
    D. To reduce radiation to the patient

36. Another name for the body of the sternum is:

    A. Ensiform
    B. Angle of Louis
    C. Gladiolus
    D. Carina

37. The greatest number of joints in the body is considered:

    A. Synarthrodial
    B. Diarthrodial
    C. Gliding
    D. Hinged

38. Intermittent claudication is:

    A. Angina
    B. A thrombus
    C. A stent placement
    D. Pain in the lower extremities upon exertion

39. The articulation between the frontal, sphenoid, parietal, and temporal bones on the lateral aspect is known as the:

    A. Bregma
    B. Inion
    C. Lambda
    D. Pterion

40. Loss of smell will occur if there is a fracture of the:

    A. Cribriform plate
    B. Petrous portion
    C. Perpendicular plate
    D. Sella turcica

41. Lymphangiograms can assess which of the following conditions?

    A. Lymphatic obstruction
    B. Hodgkin's disease

C. Reticulum cell carcinoma
D. All of the above

42. Why should the rubber stopper of a pharmaceutical be swabbed only once with the alcohol wipe prior to loading the contents into the syringe?

    A. So that the stopper is not recontaminated
    B. It saves time.
    C. Bacteria will be sterilized in one application.
    D. Actually, it should be swabbed more than once.

43. Asepsis must be employed:

    A. For all procedures
    B. Whenever the skin is broken or an invasive procedure takes place
    C. When known pathogenic organisms are present
    D. When the patient requests it

44. Hypotension is indicated by which of the following symptoms?

    A. Flushed face
    B. Epistaxis
    C. Dizzy/lightheaded
    D. Febrile

45. An emergency patient requires skull and cervical spine radiographs. The patient is anxious, with cool and moist skin, a low blood pressure, and tachycardia. It is evident that the patient is in:

    A. Cardiovascular collapse
    B. Neurogenic shock
    C. Hypovolemic shock
    D. Septic shock

46. If CPR were required on the patient experiencing cervical spine trauma, to initiate an airway you would use the following maneuver:

    A. Head tilt—lift chin
    B. Pinch nose and completely cover the patient's mouth with yours
    C. Jaw thrust
    D. Perform a tracheotomy

47. Compression-to-breath ratio for a two-rescuer save is:

A. 5:1
B. 10:1
C. 15:1
D. 15:2

48. Which of the following patient conditions would not preclude an iodinated contrast medium injection?

A. Pheochromocytoma
B. Azotemia
C. Multiple myeloma
D. Diabetes, insulin therapy

49. The most common injection site is the:

A. Basilic vein
B. Antecubital vein
C. Cephalic vein
D. Scalp vein

50. A common bronchodilator pharmaceutical is:

A. Diphenhydramine
B. Valium
C. Aminophylline
D. Lasix

51. An ADR (adverse drug reaction) form is used whenever there is a:

A. Severe reaction to medication
B. Moderate reaction to medication
C. Mild reaction to medication
D. All of the above

52. If grid lines appear on your resultant radiograph from the reciprocating Bucky, it may be due to:

A. An errant lead marker stuck in the Bucky mechanism
B. The Bucky was not pushed in.
C. The table was tilted.
D. The central ray was angled.

53. An IUD would be considered what type of artifact?

A. Anatomical
B. Processing-related
C. Internal
D. External

54. Which of the following tissues is not considered radiosensitive?

A. Thyroid
B. Eyes
C. Gonads
D. Brain

55. PACS is:

A. Photo Access and Communication System
B. Picture Archive and Communication System
C. Processing and Communication System
D. Pixel and Computerized System

56. If the technologist using automatic exposure selected the outer chambers for positioning an AP lumbar spine, the resultant radiograph would be:

A. Overexposed
B. Underexposed
C. Completely exposed
D. Not exposed at all

57. A radiographic unit that requires an oscilloscope to detect voltage waveform irregularities would be:

A. A full-phase, 3-pulse unit
B. A single-phase, half-wave unit
C. A single-phase, 6-pulse unit
D. A 3-phase, 12-pulse unit

58. To reduce safelight fogging, which would be the best measure to take?

A. Replace bulb with lower wattage bulb.
B. Paint the walls black.
C. Raise the safelight distance from the work area.
D. Remove the light.

59. Grid efficiency is based upon which of the following factors?

1. Grid ratio
2. Grid selectivity
3. Grid frequency

A. 1 only
B. 1 and 2
C. 1 and 3
D. 1, 2, and 3

60. Grid ratio is expressed as:

A. $r = h/d$
B. $r = d/h$

C. r = h/n
D. r = d/n

61. The general population is allowed a DEL (dose equivalent limit) that is _____ of the occupational radiation worker.

    A. 1/5
    B. 1/10
    C. 1/20
    D. 1/100

62. When radiation interacts with a cell of living tissue, which of the following is not feasible?

    A. The radiation passes without damage.
    B. Temporary damage may occur, but the cell repairs itself.
    C. The cell is damaged.
    D. The cell dies and may revive to normal function.

63. Human tissue that optimally attenuates low-energy radiation would be:

    A. Fat
    B. Muscle
    C. Bone
    D. Nerve

64. A film badge device can measure which type of radiation?

    A. X-radiation
    B. Beta-radiation
    C. Gamma-radiation
    D. All of the above

65. If high-intensity radiation requires monitoring, the following would be the best choice:

    A. Thermoluminescent dosimeter
    B. Victoreen chamber
    C. Geiger counter
    D. Cutie pie

66. A portable radiographic unit must have an exposure cord that is:

    A. Three pronged
    B. 6′ in length
    C. Retractable
    D. More than one, but not all of the above

67. The central ray is angled 5° to 7° cephalic for knee studies because it:

    A. Elongates the patella
    B. Minimizes the magnification of the femoral condyles and allows better joint visualization
    C. Places the central ray above the apex of the patella for better joint visualization
    D. Aids in the anode heel effect for better penetration

68. When the hand is pronated, the thumb assumes which natural position?

    A. It rests on the medial surface.
    B. It pronates.
    C. Oblique
    D. It supinates.

69. The stomach, liver, spleen, and pancreas receive arterial blood from the first branch of the abdominal aorta, called the:

    A. Celiac artery
    B. Mesenteric artery
    C. Portal artery
    D. Superior epigastric artery

70. The astragalus is also known as the:

    A. Calcaneus
    B. Cuneiform
    C. Talus
    D. Cuboid

71. Which of the following facial bones is not paired?

    A. Maxilla
    B. Malar
    C. Palatine
    D. Vomer

72. A barium enema should not be performed in cases of:

    A. Internal bleeding
    B. Acute appendicitis
    C. Diverticulitis
    D. Acute irritable bowel syndrome

73. During a barium enema, the hepatic flexure of the colon is best demonstrated in which of the following?

    1. LPO
    2. RPO
    3. RAO

A. 1 only
B. 2 only
C. 1 and 3
D. 2 and 3

74. Bile is produced in the _____ and stored in the _____.

    A. Liver, gallbladder
    B. Gallbladder, liver
    C. Common bile duct, gallbladder
    D. Gallbladder, spleen

75. The innominate bone is formed by the:

    1. Ischium
    2. Ilium
    3. Pubis

    A. 1 only
    B. 1 and 2
    C. 2 and 3
    D. 1, 2, and 3

76. Which of the following is not part of the female reproductive system?

    A. Epididymis
    B. Fimbrae
    C. Infundibulum
    D. Fallopian tubes

77. Cerebrospinal fluid is produced in the:

    A. Subarachnoid space
    B. Choroid plexus
    C. Dura mater
    D. Diploë

78. The lateral Sims' position is used for:

    A. Catheter placement for retrograde urography
    B. Tip placement for a barium enema
    C. A hysterosalpingogram
    D. Diagnosing congenital club feet

79. A patient c/o right posterior axillary rib pain. Visualization of that area would be best using the:

    A. AP
    B. PA
    C. RPO
    D. LAO

80. Positioning for an AP projection of the humerus requires that the epicondyles be:

A. Placed parallel with the film
B. Perpendicular to the film
C. Obliqued medially, 45° to the film
D. None of the above

81. Short-scale contrast is derived by using the following radiation:

    A. Low kVp, long waves
    B. Low kVp, short waves
    C. High kVp, short waves
    D. High kVp, long waves

82. When radiographing for a foreign body, all the following criteria are used except:

    A. Low kVp
    B. A localizer
    C. Fast speed film-screen combination
    D. Small focal spot size

83. X-ray film base is composed of:

    A. Cellulose
    B. Polyester
    C. Recycled plastic
    D. Gelatin

84. In reference to the curve designed by Hurter and Driffield, how are latitude and contrast related?

    A. Directly proportional to the square of the average gradient
    B. Indirectly proportional
    C. Directly proportional
    D. Inversely proportional

85. The thickness of the tomographic section is determined by:

    A. Objective plane
    B. Exposure angle
    C. Amplitude
    D. More than one, but not all of the above

86. Subtraction film is primarily used in:

    A. Angiography
    B. Mammography
    C. Urography
    D. Copying radiographs

87. Almost all the scattered radiation produced during diagnostic radiography originates from:

    A. Photoelectric effect

B. Compton effect

C. Coherent scattering

D. Pair production

88. The Compton effect is characterized by:

   A. No transfer of energy upon collision

   B. Part transfer of energy upon collision

   C. Total transfer of energy upon collision

   D. The absence of secondary radiation

89. Which type of grid has lead strips placed horizontally and longitudinally?

   A. Cross-hatch

   B. Rhombic

   C. Focused

   D. Linear

90. Which of the following would produce the greatest density?

	mA	Seconds	SID	Grid Ratio
A.	200	3/8	74″	6:1
B.	150	1/2	70″	8:1
C.	50	1/5	72″	12:1
D.	200	1/2	72″	16:1

91. The phases, in order, of a cell's division are:

   A. Metaphase, prophase, anaphase, telophase

   B. Prophase, anaphase, metaphase, telophase

   C. Prophase, metaphase, anaphase, telophase

   D. Anaphase, metaphase, prophase, telophase

92. Gamma and x-radiation are the same in every way except:

   A. Both have no mass or charge.

   B. Both travel at the speed of light.

   C. Both have the same origin.

   D. Both are electromagnetic ionizing radiation.

93. The technologist is standing 2 feet from the source for 15 min and receives 300 mr. Which of the following will reduce the technologist's exposure?

   A. Stand 6′ away for 30 min

   B. Stand 3′ away for 45 min

   C. Stand 18″ away for 91 min

   D. Stand 4′ away for 90 min

94. At 50 to 70 kVp, the total filtration of the useful beam shall be:

   A. 1.0 mm Al

   B. 1.5 mm Al

   C. 2.0 mm Al

   D. 2.5 mm Al

95. For mobile equipment, the source-to-skin distance shall be not less than:

   A. 12″

   B. 15″

   C. 18″

   D. 24″

96. The expenditure of 1 joule of work in 1 sec would describe the:

   A. Watt

   B. Volt

   C. Coulomb

   D. Amp

97. The turns ratio of a high-voltage transformer is 1:800, and the supply voltage is peaked at 120 volts. What is the secondary voltage supplied to the x-ray tube?

   A. 96 volts

   B. 96 kV

   C. 92 volts

   D. 92 kV

98. A coil of wire, induced with current, wrapped around a magnetic material such as iron, is a(n):

   A. Transformer

   B. Rheostat

   C. Electromagnet

   D. Magnet

99. The left hand generator rule refers to:

   A. The direction of the magnetic field

   B. The motion of the conductor

   C. The flow of induced current

   D. All of the above

100. All the following are true regarding the x-ray circuit except:

   A. The rectifier is located on the

secondary side of the high voltage transformer and the tube.
B. A transformer operates on mutual induction.
C. The autotransformer serves only as the primary winding coil.
D. The choke coil is used to vary voltage and current.

101. A patient at the wall Bucky experiences syncope. You would:

A. Administer CPR.
B. Ease the patient onto the floor, elevate the legs, determine status of pulse and respiration, then call for assistance.
C. Put a cool cloth on the patient's head.
D. Provide the patient with smelling salts, while preventing a fall.

102. When radiographing a patient with an obvious fracture, which of the following should never be done?

A. Remove the splint to obtain a better radiograph.
B. Lift the fractured limb uniformly with two hands.
C. Use positioning variation to obtain optimal images.
D. Refuse to radiate the patient, if he or she hasn't any name ID band.

103. What is the most important factor to keep in mind prior to beginning a procedure?

A. Leave the patient alone in the room until you are all set up.
B. Refrain from conversing with the patient; it may slow you down.
C. Explain the procedure to the patient; entertain questions.
D. Remove the patient's gown to better visualize the anatomy.

104. Which of the following pharmaceuticals is(are) considered a bronchodilator and cardiac stimulant?

1. Diphenhydramine
2. Adrenaline
3. Epinephrine

A. 1 only
B. 1 and 2

C. 1 and 3
D. 2 and 3

105. "Log rolling" is required if the patient has:

A. A spinal injury
B. A skull fracture
C. Pelvic fractures
D. More than one, but not all of the above

106. A radioactive source has a half-life of 5 hours. How many hours are required to reduce a 100-millicurie-hr dose to a level of 6.25 millicuries/hr?

A. 5 hours
B. 10 hours
C. 15 hours
D. 20 hours

107. A fixed exposure switch is designed to:

A. Lower patient exposure
B. Confine the technologist to the exposure booth
C. Terminate the exposure after 2 minutes
D. More than one, but not all of the above

108. Fluoroscopic cumulative timers are preset for _____-minute intervals.

A. 3
B. 5
C. 15
D. 30

109. The exposure dose to the patient and the procedural dose to the technologist are:

A. Inversely proportional
B. Inversely squared
C. Directly proportional
D. The exact same amount

110. Which of the following devices does not reduce radiation to the patient?

A. A grid
B. Collimation
C. Filtration
D. Lead shielding

111. A controlled radiation area would be:

A. The waiting room
B. The nuclear medicine hot laboratory
C. A radiation decay storage room
D. More than one, but not all of the above

112. A technologist should not wear the film badge during which of the following?

    A. A fluoroscopic procedure on a patient
    B. A portable chest procedure
    C. The annual chest screening
    D. While visiting another radiation department in the facility, such as nuclear medicine

113. The intensifying screen's primary advantage over direct exposure film is:

    A. Increased detail
    B. Reduced patient dose
    C. Increased latitude
    D. More than one, but not all of the above

114. Exposure reproducibility testing must be carried out:

    A. Annually
    B. Biannually
    C. Monthly
    D. Weekly

115. The integrity of the lead gloves and aprons must be tested:

    A. Annually
    B. Semiannually
    C. Monthly
    D. Weekly

116. When performing sensitometry testing for QA purposes and a new control box with a new emulsion number of film needs to be used, the following must take place:

    A. Five films must be developed from the old emulsion number and five from the new control number on a single day to establish proper sensitometric compliance.
    B. When the old box is running low, begin with the new film whenever it is convenient.
    C. Both the old film and the new film must match exactly, sensitometrically, to insure compliance.
    D. Run one of the new films and see whether it is within the acceptable sensitometric range.

117. Intensifying screens are cleaned with:

    A. Alcohol
    B. Soap and water
    C. Manufacturer's screen cleaner
    D. Ammonia

118. The image of cineradiography is obtained from the:

    A. Television camera
    B. Output screen of the image intensifier
    C. Input of the image intensifier
    D. Video signal

119. Tungsten is used for anode construction due to its:

    A. High melting point
    B. Low atomic weight
    C. Highly insulative qualities
    D. Malleable characteristics

120. The force that initiates the flow of electric current is termed:

    A. Wattage
    B. Amperage
    C. Voltage
    D. Resistance

121. The first law of electrostatics states that:

    A. Only positive charges move through a conductor.
    B. Like charges attract.
    C. Like charges repel.
    D. Electric charges reside only on the inside of the conductor.

122. The proper developer temperature is:

    A. 35°C
    B. 95°C
    C. 35°F
    D. 105°F

123. If the developer temperature is excessive, the resultant radiograph will demonstrate:

    A. Decreased density, increased contrast
    B. Increased density, decreased contrast
    C. Green streaks
    D. Light fog

124. The effective focal spot dimensions may be measured with a:

    A. Cutie pie
    B. Densitometer
    C. Pinhole camera
    D. Caliper

125. Focal spot resolution may be measured with a:

    A. Penetrometer
    B. Wire mesh test
    C. Pinhole camera
    D. Star test pattern

126. The following factors represent which of the following?

    25 mA at 4 sec
    100 mA at 1 sec
    200 mA at 1/2 sec

    A. Ohm's law
    B. The law of Tribondeau and Bergonié
    C. The reciprocity law
    D. The mAs equivalency law

127. If the "tube side" of the grid is not facing the tube during a radiograph, it will demonstrate:

    A. Complete unexposure
    B. Complete overexposure
    C. Severe peripheral cut-off
    D. An adequate radiograph without gridlines

128. Grid frequency refers to:

    A. The height of the lead strips divided by the distance between them
    B. The number of lead strips or lines per inch
    C. The SID range that may safely be used with the grid
    D. More than one, but not all of the above

129. The tomographic movement that will present streaking and ghostlike shadowing is:

    A. Linear
    B. Spiral
    C. Circular
    D. Hypocycloidal

130. Zonography is obtained by using:

    A. Breathing technique
    B. A long amplitude
    C. A high fulcrum setting
    D. A small exposure arc

131. What is the magnification of the resultant image using the following factors? The object measures 15″. The OID is 10″. The SID is 40″.

    A. 5″
    B. 10″
    C. 20″
    D. 30″

132. If the radiation intensity at 60″ is 10 R/min, what will the intensity be at 20″?

    A. 30 R/min
    B. 60 R/min
    C. 90 R/min
    D. 120 R/min

133. Which of the following crystals continue to glow after cessation of radiation?

    A. Fluorescent crystals
    B. Phosphorescent crystals
    C. Quartz crystals
    D. Calcium crystals

134. Using a wire mesh test, a warped cassette will demonstrate which of the following?

    A. Increased contrast
    B. Increased detail in certain areas
    C. Blurred, blotchy, dark areas
    D. Static artifacts

135. The photographic effect refers to:

    A. Chemical processing of radiographs
    B. Focusing the x-rays
    C. The afterglow of phosphorescent crystals
    D. Radiographic density (98%) being attributable to visible light, not radiation

136. Duplitized film refers to:

    A. Double-emulsion film
    B. Duplicating film
    C. Subtraction film
    D. Cine film

137. The primary function of gelatin in film construction is:

    A. For stability
    B. To suspend silver halide crystals
    C. To soften the illuminative quality of the film
    D. To increase latitude

138. To limit the graininess of the resultant image, which would be most appropriate to do?

    A. Use a film with large crystals.
    B. Use a film with small crystals.
    C. Use high-speed film.
    D. Use a thicker-base film.

139. The basic reward of air-gap technique, improved contrast, relies on the following principle:

    A. Due to increased OID, the angle of the scatter will miss the film.
    B. Divergence of the beam
    C. Anode heel effect
    D. Ohm's law

140. Sensitometric density on an unexposed film postprocessing is due to:

    A. Chemical fog
    B. Poor storage design
    C. Blue tint in the film base
    D. High developer temperature

141. If a 15% increase in kVp occurs, the result will be:

    A. Improved penetration
    B. Increased contrast
    C. Increased overall density
    D. More than one, but not all of the above

142. Lead foil placed on the back lid of the cassette is used for:

    A. Increasing screen speed
    B. Prevention of back scatter radiation
    C. Stability
    D. Grids only

143. In the automatic processing cycle, which of the following prevent(s) developer from being transported into the fixer solution, contaminating it?

    A. Squeegee rollers
    B. Stop bath
    C. Rinse water
    D. Guideshoes

144. To decrease object magnification, use which of the following?

    A. Increased SID
    B. Decreased SID
    C. Large focal spot
    D. High-speed cassette

145. To enhance contrast between an organ and the surrounding tissue, which of the following is utilized?

    1. Contrast media
    2. Low kVp
    3. Short SID

    A. 1 only
    B. 2 only
    C. 1 and 2
    D. 1, 2, and 3

146. A humerus tomogram presents with streaks and ghostlike images. This is most likely due to:

    A. The humerus being parallel with the tube movement
    B. The humerus being perpendicular to the tube movement
    C. The effects of spiral tomography
    D. Patient movement

147. The Bucky tray slot must be covered with _____ during fluoroscopy.

    A. Plastic protective drape
    B. 0.25 mm Pb equivalent protection
    C. A sheet
    D. Disposable paper toweling

148. Below 50 kVp, the total filtration must be:

    A. 0.5 mm Al
    B. 1.0 mm Al
    C. 1.5 mm Al
    D. 2.5 mm Al

149. If a female patient is pregnant and requires a radiographic procedure, the best time to perform it is:

    A. The first trimester
    B. The second trimester
    C. The third trimester
    D. It doesn't matter.

150. Effective gonadal radiation protection during chest radiography includes:

    A. Collimation
    B. High kVp technique
    C. Erect positioning
    D. Low mAs

151. Filtration affects all but the following:

    A. Radiation wavelength
    B. Penetrability of the beam
    C. Exposure rate
    D. Electron cloud formation

152. Biologic half-life is a measure of:

    A. A radionuclide's effectiveness in the body
    B. A radionuclide's physical atomic decay
    C. The length of time it takes for a radionuclide to decrease its maximum activity by half in a body or organ
    D. Physical and effective half-life, in hours

153. Which represents the correct order of tissue from most to least radioresistant?

    A. Lymphocyte, gonadal, serous, muscle, nerve
    B. Gonadal, nerve, muscle, lymphocyte, serous
    C. Serous, nerve, muscle, gonadal, lymphocyte
    D. Nerve, serous, muscle, gonadal, lymphocyte

154. Which of the following represents the correct ascending order of subdivision of matter?

    A. Compound, element, molecule, atom
    B. Element, atom, molecule, compound
    C. Atom, element, molecule, compound
    D. Atom, molecule, element, compound

155. A natural magnet is:

    A. Selenium
    B. The Earth
    C. A nuclear reactor
    D. Electromagnet

156. If a magnet is broken, a phenomenon occurs. It is that:

    A. It no longer functions as a magnet.
    B. Each piece retains a north and south pole.
    C. It will now attract aluminum.
    D. All its lines of flux reverse their direction.

157. Potential energy refers to:

    A. Stored energy
    B. Energy in motion
    C. Work = force × distance
    D. Kinetic energy

158. Sodium's location on the periodic table of elements is lower than mercury's. From this information you can deduce the following:

    A. Sodium has fewer protons than mercury.
    B. The mass number of mercury is greater than that of sodium.
    C. The weight of sodium is less than that of mercury.
    D. All of the above are true.

159. The K shell orbit in atomic formation is able to contain only:

    A. 2 protons
    B. 2 electrons
    C. 2 neutrons
    D. 4 electrons

160. Ionization requires that:

    A. An electron be added or removed from a neutral atom
    B. A proton be added to the nucleus
    C. Iodine atoms interact with the neutral atom.
    D. Radiation interacts with the atom.

161. Myelography is still clinically utilized in addition to CT and MRI studies of the spine because:

    A. It is less expensive.
    B. It is a dynamic study.
    C. It is easier to do.
    D. It makes the other examination easier to format.

162. The cauda equina is positioned at which of the following levels?

    A. T12
    B. L1
    C. L3
    D. L4

163. Myelography must be performed using which of the following contrast agents?

    A. Gadolinium
    B. Ionic, iodinated, water-soluble contrast media

C. Non-ionic, low-osmolar, iodinated, water-soluble contrast media

D. Ethiodol

164. Mammography requires imaging soft tissue that is basically homogeneous. Adequate contrast is obtained by which of the following?

A. Low kVp
B. Low mAs
C. Image intensification
D. Contrast media use

165. Hysterosalpingography visualizes:

A. The vagina, uterus, ovaries
B. The uterus, fallopian tubes, ovaries
C. The uterus and the fallopian tubes
D. The ovaries only

166. Arthrography is still a viable procedure despite the onset of CT and MRI because:

A. It is a dynamic study.
B. It provides more accurate information.
C. It can be done as an outpatient procedure.
D. All of the above are correct.

167. Interventional radiography may provide the following:

A. Diagnosis only
B. Treatment only
C. Diagnosis and treatment
D. Angiography only

168. Utilizing ERCP, the physician is capable of evaluating/performing which of the following?

A. Duct patency
B. Stent placement
C. Gallstone removal
D. All of the above

169. If there is a question of discrepancy in leg length, the following procedure would be ordered:

A. Scanogram
B. Bone age study
C. Scoliosis survey
D. Bone survey

170. Which of the following is considered a retrograde procedure(s)?

1. Hysterosalpingogram
2. Cystogram
3. Intravenous cholangiogram

A. 1 only
B. 2 only
C. 1 and 2
D. 1, 2, and 3

171. The kidneys are situated anatomically so that they are:

A. Retroperitoneal, upper pole most anterior
B. Retroperitoneal, lower pole most anterior
C. Contained within the peritoneum, lower pole anterior
D. Contained within the abdomen, upper pole most anterior

172. In studies of the ankle, a rupture of the lateral ligament would be noticeable in which position?

A. Inversion stress
B. Eversion stress
C. Medial oblique
D. All of the above

173. A joint that moves freely is termed:

A. Synarthrodial
B. Amphiarthrodial
C. Diarthrodial
D. Gliding

174. The correct obliquity for an LAO of the chest, when the heart and great vessels are of interest, is:

A. 30°
B. 45°
C. 60°
D. 75°

175. The _____ is located at the end of the bone and is responsible for children's bone growth.

A. Epiphysis
B. Diaphysis
C. Growth center
D. Epiphyseal plate

176. A condition that requires a reduction in exposure factors is:

A. Pneumonia
B. Paget's disease
C. Osteomalacia
D. Congestive heart failure

177. An incomplete dislocation is referred to as a:

  A. Fracture
  B. Slipped epiphysis
  C. Subluxation
  D. Sprain

178. A fracture of the distal radius, displacing the hand outward and backward, is termed:

  A. Pott's
  B. Colles'
  C. Barton's
  D. Bennett's

179. The normal oxygen therapy for most patients is:

  A. 1 to 2 liters/min
  B. 2 liters/min
  C. 2 to 4 liters/min
  D. 4 to 6 liters/min

180. A lithotomy position is used for which of the following procedures?

  1. Hysterosalpingogram
  2. Cystoscopy
  3. ERCP

  A. 1 only
  B. 2 only
  C. 1 and 2
  D. 1, 2, and 3

181. A 24-hour, portable ECG monitor is termed a:

  A. Port-a-G
  B. Holter monitor
  C. VAD
  D. Oximeter

182. If a patient's tympanic temperature reading is 37°C, it would indicate:

  A. That the patient is febrile
  B. That the patient is in shock
  C. That it is normal
  D. That the patient is deceased

183. The equipment necessary to determine blood pressure is:

  A. Thermometer and sphygmomanometer
  B. Wrist watch, stethoscope, and sphygmomanometer
  C. Wrist watch and sphygmomanometer
  D. Stethoscope and sphygmomanometer

184. Which is not considered to be a vascular access device?

  A. Swan-Ganz
  B. Hickman
  C. Miller-Abbott
  D. Port-A-Cath

185. Which stoma location may not require a bag?

  A. Ileostomy
  B. Transverse colostomy
  C. Sigmoid colostomy
  D. All require bags

Refer to Radiograph 2 for Questions 186–190.

186. To visualize this area in the AP axial projection, you must:

  A. Angle the central ray caudad 10°
  B. Angle the central ray caudad 30° to 35°
  C. Angle the central ray cephalic 30° to 35°
  D. Use a vertical beam.

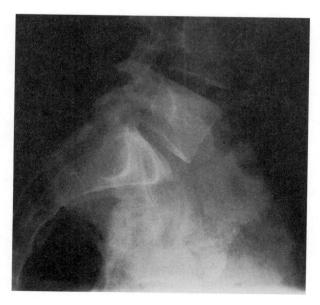

Radiograph 2

187. The central ray enters between which two bony landmarks for this position?

    A. The iliac crest and symphysis pubis
    B. The iliac crest and the greater trochanter
    C. The ASIS and the symphysis pubis
    D. The ASIS and the iliac crest

188. If your lateral lumbar spine exposure factors provided you with an optimal radiograph, what would you need to do to those same factors prior to obtaining this particular position?

    A. Decrease the kVp, to obtain a shorter scale of contrast
    B. Increase the kVp, due to increased collimation
    C. Use a longer time, to utilize autotomography
    D. No changes are required, the original technique will be used.

189. If the patient requires angulation of the central ray due to the spine not being parallel with the film plane, how much angulation is required?

    A. 30° to 35° caudad
    B. 5° to 8° caudad
    C. 30° to 35° cephalic
    D. 5° to 8° cephalic

190. Which plane is centered on the table for this projection?

    A. Mid sagittal
    B. Transverse
    C. Coronal
    D. Horizontal

191. An example of a saddle joint is:

    A. The thumb
    B. The knee joint
    C. The temporomandibular joint
    D. The elbow joint

192. If barium will not flow through the duodenal bulb during a gastrointestinal study, what will help move it along?

    A. Placing the patient into a right lateral position.
    B. Have the patient imagine eating the foods that they enjoy.

    C. If possible, have the patient walk around.
    D. All of the above are correct.

193. How does a cardiac esophagram differ from a routine esophagram?

    A. It must be done at 72″ SID.
    B. Oral iodinated contrast medium must be used.
    C. It must be done with cine.
    D. It must be done with a full stomach.

194. The Y shoulder position is best used to rule out:

    A. Humeral head fractures
    B. Humeral head subluxations or dislocation
    C. Distal humerus subluxations or dislocation
    D. Clavicular fractures

195. Most humeral head dislocations are displaced:

    A. Posteriorly
    B. Laterally
    C. Anteriorly
    D. Dorsally

196. One of the advantages of utilizing the Y position rather than the transthoracic shoulder position is:

    A. That the patient receives less radiation
    B. That the patient can be radiographed erect or recumbent
    C. That the patient can breathe throughout the exposure
    D. That the patient can move the injured arm

197. The greater trochanter is in the same transverse plane as the:

    A. Coccyx
    B. Ischial spine
    C. Iliac crest
    D. Symphysis pubis

198. A patient is placed on the left side with a horizontal beam directed to the median sagittal plane and a grid cassette. This position is:

    A. Ventral decubitus

B. Lateral abdomen
C. Right lateral decubitus
D. Left lateral decubitus

199. A decubitus is necessary to visualize:

A. Polyps
B. Air-fluid levels
C. Tuberculosis
D. Barium in the fundus

200. The skull position that best demonstrates the foramen magnum, foramen spinosum, and foramen ovale is:

A. The acanthoparietal projection
B. The submentovertical projection
C. The AP axial projection
D. A true lateral

Chapter **Answers**

Chapter 1

1. C—p 4	8. D—p 7	15. D—p 9	22. D—p 10	29. C—p 13
2. C—p 4	9. B—p 5	16. C—p 9	23. B—p 11	30. B—p 13
3. A—p 4	10. B—p 7	17. B—p 10	24. B—p 11	31. B—p 13
4. D—p 4	11. C—p 7	18. C—p 10	25. A—p 11	32. A—p 14
5. B—p 5	12. A—p 7	19. D—p 10	26. D—p 11	33. A—p 11
6. D—p 5	13. A—p 8	20. A—p 10	27. B—p 12	34. D—p 14
7. D—p 5	14. C—p 9	21. C—p 10	28. C—p 12	35. B—p 15

Chapter 2

1. A—p 22	5. C—p 22	9. D—p 22	13. C—p 23	17. D—p 24
2. B—p 22	6. D—p 22	10. A—p 22	14. A—p 23	18. C—p 24
3. D—p 22	7. C—p 22	11. B—p 22	15. A—p 23	19. D—p 24
4. D—p 22	8. B—p 22	12. A—p 22	16. D—p 23	20. B—p 24

Chapter 3

1. C—p 28	7. D—p 28	13. C—p 30	19. B—p 32	25. B—p 33
2. D—p 28	8. B—p 28	14. A—p 30	20. B—p 32	26. D—p 33
3. C—p 28	9. D—p 28	15. B—p 30	21. C—p 32	27. B—p 34
4. C—p 28	10. B—p 28	16. D—p 30	22. C—p 32	28. A—p 34
5. B—p 28	11. A—p 28	17. A—p 30	23. D—p 32	
6. A—p 28	12. C—p 28	18. A—p 32	24. A—p 32	

Chapter 4

1. D—p 54	8. A—p 60	15. C—p 63	22. B—p 66	29. C—p 68
2. D—p 55	9. B—p 60	16. C—p 63	23. B—p 66	30. B—p 69
3. C—p 55	10. B—p 61	17. B—p 63	24. B—p 67	31. A—p 69
4. C—p 55	11. A—p 61	18. D—p 63	25. A—p 66	32. B—p 69
5. A—p 57	12. B—p 61	19. B—p 63	26. D—p 68	33. B—p 69
6. A—p 58	13. B—p 61	20. D—p 65	27. D—p 68	34. A—p 72
7. B—p 59	14. A—p 62	21. C—p 66	28. B—p 66	35. D—p 72

Chapter 5

1. C—p 78	6. A—p 79	11. A—p 80	16. D—p 81	21. B—p 82
2. C—p 78	7. C—p 80	12. D—p 80	17. B—p 81	22. D—p 82
3. B—p 78	8. A—p 80	13. B—p 80	18. C—p 81	23. B—p 82
4. B—p 78	9. D—p 80	14. B—p 81	19. B—p 82	24. C—p 83
5. C—p 79	10. B—p 80	15. D—p 81	20. B—p 82	25. C—p 83

Chapter 6

1. C—p 104	16. A—p 105	30. A—p 107	45. B—p 109	59. B—p 119
2. D—p 104	17. C—p 105	31. C—p 107	46. C—p 110	60. B—p 120
3. C—p 104	18. A—p 105	32. B—p 107	47. C—p 110	61. D (A & C)
4. D—p 104	19. C—p 105	33. B—p 108	48. B—p 111	—p 120
5. C—p 104	20. A—p 106	34. A—p 108	49. A—p 111	62. A—p 120
6. B—p 104	21. C—p 106	35. D—p 108	50. A—p 112	63. D—p 120
7. B—p 104	22. B—p 106	36. A—p 108	51. B—p 113	64. D—p 120
8. C—p 104	23. B—p 106	37. A—p 108	52. C—p 113	65. C—p 121
9. D—p 104	24. C—p 106	38. D—p 108	53. D (B & C)	66. A—p 122
10. A—p 104	25. D (A & C)	39. A—p 108	—p 114	67. C—p 123
11. C—p 104	—p 106	40. C—p 109	54. C—p 114	68. C—p 123
12. A—p 104	26. A—p 106	41. D—p 109	55. B—p 116	69. D—p 124
13. A—p 105	27. D—p 106	42. B—p 109	56. A—p 117	70. A—p 124
14. B—p 105	28. B—p 106	43. D—p 109	57. A—p 119	
15. B—p 105	29. D (A & B)	44. C—p 109	58. A—p 119	
	—p 106			

Chapter 7

1. D (A & B)—	5. A—p 134	10. C—p 135	15. B—p 138	20. B—p 139
p 134	6. C—p 134	11. B—p 136	16. D—p 138	
2. D—p 134	7. D—p 135	12. A—p 136	17. D—p 138	
3. D—p 134	8. A—p 135	13. D—p 136	18. B—p 139	
4. C—p 134	9. B—p 135	14. C—p 138	19. B—p 139	

Chapter 8

1. C—p 144	4. D—p 145	7. C—p 145	10. A—p 146	13. B—p 147
2. A—p 146	5. A—p 145	8. B—p 145	11. C—p 146	14. C—p 147
3. C—p 144	6. D—p 145	9. B—p 146	12. D—p 146	15. D—p 147

Chapter 9

1. D—p 162	4. B—p 164	7. F—p 163	10. A—p 163	13. A—p 164
2. C—p 162	5. D—p 164	8. E—p 163	11. A—p 165	14. C—p 164
3. C—p 164	6. B—p 163	9. C—p 163	12. D—p 164	15. D—p 165

Chapter 11

1. C—p 236	7. A—p 237	12. D (A & B)	16. D—p 239	22. C—p 239
2. D—p 236	8. A—p 237	—p 239	17. B—p 239	23. B—p 240
3. A—p 236	9. C—p 237	13. C—p 238	18. D—p 239	24. A—p 240
4. B—p 236	10. D—p 237	14. B—p 238	19. C—p 239	25. D—p 240
5. C—p 236	11. C—p 237	15. D—p 238	20. C—p 239	
6. C—p 237			21. A—p 239	

Chapter 12

1. C—p 246	6. B—p 246	12. A—p 247	18. C—p 249	24. A—p 249
2. B—p 246	7. D—p 247	13. A—p 247	19. C—p 249	25. B—p 249
3. C—p 246	8. B—p 246	14. C—p 246	20. C—p 249	
4. D—p 246	9. A—p 247	15. A—p 248	21. B—p 249	
5. C—p 247	10. B—p 246	16. B—p 249	22. C—p 249	
	11. A—p 247	17. A—p 248	23. C—p 249	

Chapter 13

1. B—p 256	7. A—p 256	13. A—p 256	19. D—p 257	25. B—p 260
2. C—p 256	8. C—p 257	14. D (A & C)	20. D—p 258	26. B—p 256
3. C—p 256	9. A—p 257	—p 256	21. D—p 258	27. A—p 256
4. D—p 256	10. C—p 257	15. B—p 256	22. D—p 259	28. B—p 256
5. A—p 256	11. B—p 256	16. C—p 256	23. C—p 259	
6. D—p 256	12. B—p 256	17. C—p 256	24. A—p 260	
		18. B—p 257		

Chapter 14

1. C—p 266	5. B—p 266	9. C—p 266	13. B—p 267	17. B—p 268
2. B—p 266	6. C—p 266	10. D—p 267	14. A—p 267	18. D—p 268
3. D—p 266	7. B—p 266	11. C—p 267	15. A—p 267	19. C—p 268
4. A—p 266	8. D—p 266	12. A—p 267	16. C—p 268	20. D—p 269

Chapter 15

1. C—p 280	8. C—p 280	15. C—p 282	22. C—p 283	29. C—p 286
2. B—p 280	9. B—p 281	16. D—p 282	23. A—p 283	30. D—p 287
3. C—p 280	10. A—p 281	17. C—p 282	24. C—p 284	31. C—p 287
4. A—p 280	11. D—p 281	18. C—p 284	25. A—p 285	32. A—p 287
5. B—p 280	12. A—p 281	19. B—p 283	26. B—p 285	33. B—p 287
6. C—p 280	13. D—p 282	20. B—p 283	27. D—p 285	34. D—p 288
7. B—p 280	14. C—p 282	21. A—p 283	28. C—p 286	35. C—p 288

Section **Answers**

1. B—p 4	29. B—p 10	56. B—p 22	83. D—p 28	109. C—p 32
2. C—p 4	30. C—p 10	57. B—p 22	84. B—p 28	110. D—p 32
3. D—p 4	31. A—p 10	58. D (B & C)	85. A—p 28	111. D (A & B)
4. A—p 5	32. C—p 11	—p 22	86. C—p 28	—p 32
5. C—p 5	33. D—p 11	59. B—p 22	87. D—p 28	112. C—p 32
6. B—p 5	34. D—p 11	60. D—p 22	88. C—p 28	113. D—p 32
7. D—p 5	35. B—p 11	61. D—p 22	89. B—p 28	114. B—p 32
8. A—p 5	36. A—p 12	62. D—p 22	90. C—p 28	115. D—p 32
9. C—p 6	37. C—p 12	63. D—p 22	91. B—p 28	116. B—p 33
10. A—p 6	38. A—p 12	64. A—p 22	92. D (B & C)	117. C—p 32
11. B—p 6	39. A—p 12	65. B—p 22	—p 28	118. D—p 32
12. A—p 6	40. D—p 12	66. B—p 22	93. D (B & C)	119. D—p 32
13. D—p 6	41. A—p 13	67. A—p 22	—p 28	120. C—p 33
14. C—p 6	42. D—p 13	68. C—p 22	94. C—p 28	121. C—p 33
15. C—p 7	43. D—p 13	69. B—p 22	95. A—p 28	122. C—p 33
16. A—p 8	44. D—p 13	70. D—p 22	96. A—p 28	123. C—p 33
17. D—p 8	45. A—p 14	71. C—p 23	97. C—p 28	124. B—p 34
18. C—p 8	46. A—p 14	72. C—p 23	98. C—p 28	125. D—p 33
19. B—p 8	47. D—p 14	73. C—p 23	99. A—p 28	126. C—p 33
20. B—p 9	48. D—p 14	74. C—p 23	100. D—p 28	127. D—p 24
21. B—p 9	49. C—p 14	75. D—p 23	101. C—p 30	128. B—p 33
22. C—p 9	50. B—p 15	76. C—p 24	102. A—p 30	129. B—p 33
23. D—p 9	51. D—p 15	77. A—p 24	103. C—p 30	130. B—p 24
24. C—p 9	52. D—p 4	78. B—p 24	104. A—p 30	
25. B—p 9	53. C—p 22	79. C—p 24	105. B—p 30	
26. C—p 10	54. D (A & B)	80. A—p 28	106. B—p 32	
27. C—p 10	—p 22	81. B—p 28	107. C—p 32	
28. C—p 10	55. C—p 22	82. A—p 28	108. A—p 32	

Section II

1. D—p 54	31. C—p 56	61. D—p 60	91. C—p 67	121. A—p 80
2. D—p 54	32. D—p 56	62. B—p 60	92. D—p 67	122. A—p 80
3. A—p 54	33. B—p 57	63. C—p 60	93. D—p 68	123. D—p 80
4. D—p 54	34. C—p 56	64. C—p 60	94. D—p 68	124. A—p 80
5. C—p 54	35. B—p 56	65. B—p 61	95. D—p 68	125. D—p 80
6. C—p 54	36. C—p 57	66. D—p 61	96. B—p 68	126. B—p 80
7. B—p 54	37. A—p 57	67. D—p 61	97. C—p 69	127. C—p 80
8. A—p 54	38. B—p 57	68. B—p 61	98. A—p 69	128. C—p 80
9. D—p 54	39. B—p 57	69. B—p 61	99. C—p 69	129. C—p 81
10. B—p 54	40. C—p 57	70. D—p 62	100. C—p 69	130. B—p 81
11. C—p 54	41. D—p 57	71. C—p 63	101. C—p 69	131. D—p 81
12. C—p 54	42. D—p 57	72. D—p 63	102. D—p 70	132. C—p 81
13. C—p 54	43. D—p 57	73. D—p 63	103. B—p 70	133. D—p 82
14. B—p 55	44. C—p 58	74. C—p 63	104. B—p 70	134. D—p 82
15. A—p 55	45. B—p 58	75. B—p 63	105. A—p 70	135. B—p 82
16. C—p 55	46. A—p 58	76. A—p 63	106. B—p 71	136. C—p 82
17. D—p 55	47. C—p 58	77. A—p 64	107. B—p 71	137. C—p 82
18. B—p 55	48. D—p 58	78. D—p 64	108. C—p 71	138. D—p 82
19. A—p 56	49. C—p 59	79. B—p 65	109. D—p 71	139. D—p 79
20. C—p 56	50. B—p 59	80. C—p 65	110. A—p 72	140. D—p 81
21. B—p 55	51. B—p 59	81. B—p 66	111. D—p 73	141. A—p 83
22. C—p 57	52. C—p 59	82. C—p 67	112. C—p 73	142. A—p 83
23. B—p 57	53. B—p 60	83. D—p 67	113. A—p 78	143. B—p 83
24. B—p 57	54. D—p 60	84. B—p 67	114. C—p 78	144. C—p 83
25. C—p 57	55. A—p 60	85. B—p 66	115. D—p 78	145. A—p 83
26. D—p 55	56. D—p 60	86. A—p 66	116. A—p 78	146. C—p 80
27. B—p 55	57. A—p 60	87. D—p 67	117. B—p 78	147. D—p 83
28. D—p 55	58. D—p 60	88. B—p 67	118. D—p 79	148. A—p 55
29. B—p 55	59. B—p 60	89. C—p 66	119. C—p 79	149. B—p 67
30. A—p 56	60. C—p 60	90. B—p 66	120. B—p 80	150. D—p 67

Section III

1. D—p 104	17. A—p 104	34. A—p 111	49. B—p 135	64. D (B & C) —p 139
2. C—p 104	18. A—p 107	35. D—p 118	50. D—p 137	65. C—p 139
3. A—p 104	19. B—p 107	36. C—p 118	51. A—p 137	66. D—p 145
4. D—p 104	20. A—p 108	37. C—p 119	52. D—p 137	67. D (A & B) —p 145
5. C—p 104	21. C—p 108	38. A—p 119	53. A—p 137	68. C—p 145
6. A—p 104	22. C—p 108	39. D—p 119	54. A—p 137	69. C—p 146
7. B—p 104	23. C—p 108	40. A—p 119	55. A—p 137	70. D—p 146
8. A—p 104	24. A—p 109	41. D—p 119	56. B—p 137	71. A—p 146
9. B—p 104	25. C—p 109	42. C—p 122	57. C—p 137	72. D—p 147
10. B—p 104	26. B—p 109	43. D (A & C) —p 123	58. C—p 137	73. D—p 145
11. D—p 105	27. B—p 109	44. A—p 124	59. D (B & C) —p 138	74. B—p 147
12. A—p 105	28. B—p 110	45. C—p 134	60. B—p 138	75. C—p 147
13. D—p 106	29. A—p 110	46. D—p 134	61. A—p 138	
14. C—p 106	30. C—p 110	47. B—p 134	62. C—p 139	
15. A—p 106	31. B—p 110	48. D (A & C) —p 135	63. C—p 139	
16. D (B & C) —p 106	32. B—p 110			
	33. C—p 111			

Section IV

1. D—p 171	22. D—p 185	43. A—p 189	64. A—p 200	84. C—p 211
2. B—p 171	23. A—p 185	44. B—p 194	65. B—p 200	85. C—p 211
3. D—p 172	24. D—p 181	45. C—p 189	66. A—p 200	86. D—p 210
4. C—p 172	25. B—p 182	46. B—p 189	67. D—p 201	87. C—p 211
5. B—p 172	26. C—p 182	47. B—p 189	68. C—p 205	88. C—p 218
6. D—p 173	27. D—p 183	48. D—p 189	69. A—p 205	89. C—p 218
7. D—p 177	28. A—p 185	49. A—p 190	70. B—p 205	90. B—p 216
8. A—p 177	29. C—p 187	50. C—p 190	71. B—p 205	91. A—p 216
9. B—p 177	30. A—p 183	51. B—p 190	72. C—p 206	92. B—p 216
10. A—p 173	31. D—p 183	52. A—p 191	73. C—p 206	93. D—p 216
11. C—p 173	32. D—p 187	53. D—p 191	74. C—p 207	94. A—p 216
12. B—p 178	33. A—p 188	54. B—p 192	75. C—p 207	95. C—p 213
13. C—p 178	34. B—p 186	55. D—p 192	76. D—p 207	96. C—p 213
14. B—p 175	35. D—p 187	56. D—p 197	77. B—p 207	97. B—p 216
15. C—p 174	36. A—p 187	57. C—p 197	78. B—p 211	98. D—p 219
16. A—p 179	37. C—p 187	58. C—p 202	79. D—p 217	99. D—p 214
17. C—p 179	38. B—p 187	59. D—p 202	80. D (B & C) —p 211	100. A—p 219
18. D—p 175	39. D—p 188	60. B—p 198	81. A—p 210	
19. D—p 179	40. C—p 188	61. C—p 202	82. D—p 211	
20. B—p 180	41. C—p 188	62. B—p 199	83. C—p 217	
21. C—p 185	42. D—p 189	63. C—p 200		

Section V

1. C—p 236
2. C—p 237
3. D—p 237
4. A—p 237
5. C—p 238
6. B—p 238
7. C—p 238
8. A—p 239
9. B—p 239
10. C—p 239
11. A—p 240
12. B—p 246
13. D—p 246
14. D—p 246
15. A—p 247
16. C—p 247
17. C—p 247
18. D—p 247
19. D—p 248
20. D—p 248
21. A—p 248
22. B—p 249
23. A—p 256
24. B—p 256
25. C—p 256
26. C—p 256
27. B—p 256
28. A—p 257
29. D—p 257
30. B—p 257
31. D—p 257
32. A—p 257
33. C—p 258
34. C—p 258
35. D—p 258
36. B—p 259
37. C—p 260
38. A—p 266
39. D—p 266
40. B—p 266
41. C—p 267
42. B—p 267
43. B—p 267
44. D—p 268
45. C—p 268
46. B—p 268
47. D—p 268
48. A—p 271
49. D—p 271
50. C—p 271
51. B—p 273
52. B—p 273
53. A—p 273
54. C—p 280
55. A—p 280
56. D—p 281
57. C—p 283
58. A—p 286
59. D—p 286
60. B—p 288

Simulated Registry Review I **Answers**

1) B Vermiform appendix is attached to the cecum but does not aid in the digestive process.

2) B Compton interactions begin to occur at 100 keV.

3) A Leukemia is a type of cancer; all cancer responds to radiation in a stochastic, linear, nonthreshold response.

4) D The foramen ovale and the ductus arterious allow most of the blood flowing into the heart to bypass the pulmonary trunk and supply fetal systemic circulation.

5) B Electronic timers allow for very short exposure times (milliseconds) with a high level of accuracy.

6) C The three types of radiation syndromes are hematopoietic, gastrointestinal, and central nervous system.

7) D Intervertebral discs consist of a soft, jelly-like material, nucleus pulposus, covered with a tough, fibrous material, anulus fibrosus.

8) C Proper positioning will align a plane passing through the medial and lateral malleoli parallel to the plane of the film.

9) D Jefferson's is a bursting fracture of C1, atlas; Hangman's is a fracture of the posterior components of C2, usually with dislocation of C2 and C3; Bennett's fracture is a fracture with dislocation of the first metacarpal of the hand.

10) A Hangman's fracture involves C2 and C3.

11) A Gamma radiation has a higher frequency than ultraviolet or infrared radiation.

12) D (B & C) The guidelines established by the NCRP state that the effective dose limit annually is 50 mSv. 50 mSv are equal to 5000 mrem.

13) B To ensure a true lateral projection, the interpupillary line must be perpendicular to the plane of the film.

14) C The sphenoid sinus is located inferior and anterior to the sella turcica.

15) A The skull is basically composed of bone and nerve tissue; therefore, the radiographic contrast will be short scale, high contrast.

16) B The formula to calculate penumbra is:

$$FSS \times \frac{OID}{SOD} = P$$

17) B Eight styloid processes: two radial; two ulnar; two temporal; two fibular.

18) B The law of Bergonié and Tribondeau states that tissue radiosensitivity is determined by mitotic activity, differentiation, and oxygen content.

19) D The kidneys, lungs, and spleen all have a hilum, the depression that allows for the passage of blood vessels and nerves.

20) C Spondylolisthesis is forward displacement of one vertebra over another, most frequently occurring at L4–L5 or L5–S1. It is usually due to a developmental defect of the pars interarticularis.

21) B In a retrograde examination, the contrast medium is forced to flow back into a structure rather than from the structure, as in excretion.

22) D Resistance formula for a series circuit: $R_1 + R_2 + R_3 = R_T$; therefore, 5 ohms + 20 ohms = 25 ohms.

23) A Resistance formula for a parallel circuit: $1/R_1 + 1/R_2 + 1/R_3 = C_T$: $1/C_T = R_T$; therefore, $1/10 + 1/5 = 3/10$ $C_T = 10/3$ $R_T = 3.33$.

24) B The superior mesenteric artery originates from the abdominal aorta and supplies a portion of the small and large intestine.

25) C Hysteresis loss, lagging loss, is a loss of current within a transformer due to the rapidly changing electrical currents.

26) D The patella articulates with the femur only.

27) A The splenic and superior mesenteric veins join to form the portal vein, which transports blood to the hepatic sinusoid.

28) B Calculate the HU for one exposure: mA × time × kVp × 1 = HU. 300 × 4 × 34 × 1 = 40,800 HU. Then divide the HU into the thermal capacity of the anode (155,000) to determine the number of rapid exposures that can safely be made; 40,800/155,000 = 3.799; therefore, three exposures can be made without exceeding the heat limit.

29) C The inverse square law is based upon the divergence of the beam; the beam will cover four times the area if the distance is doubled; therefore the intensity will be one fourth of the original intensity.

30) C Oxygen is extremely flammable; therefore smoking, an open flame, or electrical equipment may ignite a fire.

31) B The abbreviation for automatic collimation is PBL—positive beam limitation.

32) C Sterile technique is required for a myelogram and an ERCP.

33) A The elements of negligence include duty, breach, cause, and injury.

34) C An isotope is created by the addition or subtraction of a neutron.

35) D Polyenergetic. Photons produced will range from 0 to 70 keV.

36) B Because of the high energy level, most of the radiation will pass through the structure rather than becoming attenuated by the structure; therefore, the linear energy transfer is low.

37) A The roentgen is the unit of measure used to describe primary radiation in air.

38) C 70 rads × 5 QF = 350 rads.

39) C External rotation of the humerus will allow the visualization of the greater tubercle.

40) B The apophyseal articulations are visible in the lateral projection.

41) C Weight-bearing lateral feet studies are performed to evaluate the structural status of the foot.

42) A Radial flexion is used to evaluate the medial aspect of the wrist.

43) B The apophyseal articulations of the thoracic spine are visible in a 70° oblique position.

44) C The bicipital groove is located on the head of the humerus.

45) A Adduction is a motion toward the midline of the body.

46) A A lateral projection with flexion and extension will evaluate spinal fusion.

47) B The semilunar notch of the elbow is best visualized in the lateral position.

48) C The Valsalva maneuver (bearing-down pressure) will increase blood pressure and will expand esophageal varices, allowing them to be visualized.

49) A Esophageal varices can be caused by hypertension of the portal circulation, which strains the veins of the esophagus, weakening their vascular walls.

50) B Varices is another name for varicose veins.

51) A Res ipsa loquitur is grossly obvious negligence; leaving surgical instruments in a patient's abdomen would be obvious negligence.

52) B ALARA—As low as reasonably achievable.

53) D The largest sesamoid bone is the patella.

54) B Flabella is a sesamoid bone that may be found in the popliteal region.

55) D A whiplash injury will cause the cervical spine to lose its lordotic curvature due to muscle spasms.

56) C The toe portion demonstrates the film's minimum density; density of the base plus fog.

57) C Average gradient or gamma portion will demonstrate the film's latitude.

58) D The shoulder portion of the curve will demonstrate the maximum density that the film is able to record, also called D-Max.

59) B The solarization portion of the curve will demonstrate additional exposure. Once the film has reached D-Max, the film will lose density.

60) B Film I demonstrates narrow latitude because the average gradient responds faster when compared with film II.

61) B Film II responds to exposures much slower than film I; therefore, the scale of contrast is longer.

62) C Hydroquinone is a developer agent that is responsible for the shoulder portion of the H&D curve.

63) B Potassium alum is a hardening agent found in the fixer that is responsible for hardening the emulsion layer; insufficient replenishment may result in tacky films exiting from the processor.

64) C The autotransformer allows the technologist to select a predetermined amount of kVp.

65) D An increase in mA will result in an increase in amperage to the filament, increase the amount of thermionic emission, and increase the filament size from small to large.

66) C The anode is always connected to the high-voltage circuit.

67) B EMF (electromotive force) and kVp are interchangeable terms, and both are responsible for the quality or penetrating ability of the beam.

68) A According to the law of Bergonié and Tribondeau, nerve tissue is the least radiosensitive because it is highly specialized.

69) B A linear, nonthreshold dose response states that any dosage is damaging and will increase proportionally as the dosage increases.

70) C The prodromal period is the first stage that will occur after an acute radiation exposure.

71) C Occupational annual dose limit = 5000 mrem. Limits for the general public annual limit = 50 mrem : 5000/500 = 10%.

72) D Rad (gray) may be used for any type of radiation exposure.

73) C Etiology is defined as the study of all factors that may contribute to the disease process.

74) C TIA is an abbreviation for transient ischemic attack (stroke), most commonly caused by carotid atherosclerotic disease, with secondary causes being cardiac emboli or intracranial atherosclerosis.

75) C Whenever possible, a family member should be used to restrain a pediatric patient.

76) A The only type of radiographic markings considered legal are markers that are exposed onto the film at the time of the exposure.

77) C The technologist should be educated in CPR as a health care provider.

78) D The smallest needle would be used: 25 gauge. The higher the number of the gauge, the smaller the needle is.

79) B The drainage bag should always be kept below the organ it is draining to facilitate drainage with gravity and help prevent backflow and possible infection.

80) B Half value layer is the most common method of measuring the quality of the radiation beam.

81) B The highest concentration of silver available to be reclaimed is in the fixer solution.

82) C The input phosphor of the image intensification tube is cesium iodine.

83) B The ion chambers may terminate prematurely if excess scatter radiation is detected. Ion chambers are unable to distinguish between remnant and scatter radiation.

84) A If the hip study was performed with a portable grid, the exposure would last as long as the back-up time set, since little or no radiation reaches the ion chamber. It would read only scatter that reached it; therefore, the radiograph would be grossly overexposed.

85) A With the highest effective kVp and the lowest grid ratio, the radiographic contrast will be low, long-scale contrast.

86) D The chance of having quantum mottle increases with high kVp–low mAs techniques and fast imaging systems (screens and film). Quantum mottle is the grainy or patchy appearance of a radiograph, caused by insufficient radiation to create a uniform image.

87) A Long wavelength radiation would be low kVp, this decreases the penetrating ability of the beam; this would result in a short scale, high contrast film.

88) C 16mm and 35mm describe the film frame size.

89) D (B & C) BUN (blood urea nitrogen) gives an approximate idea of kidney function and the kidney's ability to eliminate nitrogen in the form of urea, which in excess may cause uremia (azotemia).

90) A Heparin is an anticoagulant or anticlotting agent.

91) B Glucophage is contraindicated for use with intravascular iodinated contrast media as it may induce renal failure and exacerbate lactic acidosis, which could prove fatal.

92) D Exacerbation is the acceleration or increase in the seriousness of symptoms or the disease process.

93) C A synchronous timer is able to provide exposure times only in multiples of 1/60 sec (1/30, 1/20, 1/5), with the shortest exposure time of 1/60 sec.

94) D A densitometer is a device that measures the density recorded on the radiograph.

95) D The shell type of transformer is the most efficient type of transformer.

96) B 1/20 sec. Formula: (# of dots) $\times$ 1/120 = exposure time; 6 dots $\times$ 1/120 = 1/20 sec.

97) C To double the density and to increase penetration, use the kVp 15% rule: 60 kVp + 15% (9 kVp) = 69 kVp.

98) A Ohm's law: I = V/R, therefore 18/1.8 = 10 amps.

99) B SID, OID, and SOD will affect size distortion to a much greater degree when compared with FSS.

100) D Ohm's law: V = I $\times$ R, therefore 4 $\times$ 25 = 100 volts.

101) D The xiphoid process is at the same level as the 10th thoracic vertebra and the cardiac orifice.

102) C The spleen is located in the left hypochondriac region.

103) C The pancreas is both an exocrine and endocrine gland. An exocrine gland secretes substances into a duct or onto a surface. An endocrine secretes substances directly into the blood stream.

104) A Rugae are one of the four layers of the stomach wall. They are best demonstrated with a contrast procedure.

105) A The duodenum, or duodenal sweep, surrounds the head of the pancreas.

106) D mAs/grid formula:

$$\frac{mAs_1}{mAs_2} = \frac{GCF_1}{GCF_2} \quad \frac{12}{X} = \frac{4}{1} \quad X = 3 \text{ mAs}$$

107) B mAs/distance formula:

$$\frac{mAs_1}{mAs_2} = \frac{(D_1)^2}{(D_2)^2} \quad \frac{2}{X} = \frac{(40)^2}{(72)^2}$$

$$\frac{2}{X} = \frac{1600}{5184} \quad X = 6.48 \text{ (7 mAs)}$$

108) B Photomultipliers, thyratrons, and ionization chambers are all components of automatic exposure devices.

109) B Epilation is a condition of the hair falling out; it may be temporary or it may be permanent.

110) B The alimentary tract is the most radiosensitive according to Tribondeau and Bergonié because the lining cells of the alimentary tract are rapidly dividing, highly oxygenated, and unspecialized.

111) C LET (linear energy transfer) is defined as the amount of energy deposited per unit of tract length.

112) C The technical factors (400 mA, ⅛ sec, 90 kVp) that have the highest kVp and the lowest mAs will provide the lowest patient dosage. In this particular case, the imaging speed does not contribute to dosage.

113) D A hypocycloidal movement will provide the thinnest cut, the most tomographic movement, the longest exposure time, most heat unit production, and greatest patient exposure.

114) B Intussusception is a condition of one portion of the bowel telescoping into itself, most often in children, but it does occur in adults.

115) D A left lateral decubitus or an erect abdomen will demonstrate free air within the abdomen; barium should never be used if intestinal perforation is suspected.

116) B A right lateral decubitus will allow the air to fill the lateral aspect of the descending colon.

117) D 15° internal rotation of the legs will rotate the lesser trochanter behind the femoral neck.

118) C Nephroptosis is the drooping or downward placement of the kidney; therefore, supine and erect positions will demonstrate any kidney movement.

119) B The intervertebral foramina are visible in an oblique cervical spine and a lateral thoracic spine.

120) D The mortise joint of the ankle is composed of the talus (inferior), tibia (superior and medial), and fibula (lateral).

121) B The hands and wrists are the most common areas to be radiographed for a bone survey to determine growth.

122) B Depression of the chin will move the cranial base superior to the dens, eliminating the overlap. Extension of the chin would be used if the teeth were overlapping the dens.

123) B A nephron is the smallest functional unit of the kidney. Parenchyma is the smallest functional unit of an organ.

124) C LPO (left posterior oblique). The position of the stomach within the body is with the fundus and pylorus most posterior; therefore, in an LPO the barium will gravitate toward the fundus and pylorus, leaving the body air filled.

125) C The omentum is an extension of the peritoneum that surrounds one or more nearby organs.

126) D Inspiration and expiration chest radiographs can be used for evaluation of a pneumothorax (lung markings), diaphragm excursion (diaphragm movement), and foreign objects (to show the object's movement).

127) D Fahrenheit/centigrade conversion formula:

$$C° = 5/9(F° - 32) \text{ or } F° = 9/5(C° + 32)$$
$$5/9(53 - 32) = 11.7C°$$

128) D For a ventral decubitus, the patient would be prone, with the beam horizontal to the body.

129) B An AP projection of the cervical spine will demonstrate the presence of a cervical rib, a rib attached to C7.

130) A A low mA and long exposure time will best depict the anatomy of the lateral thoracic spine by using a breathing technique and blurring the lung markings and overlying ribs.

131) B The thoracic spine's normal curvature is kyphotic, convex posteriorly.

132) D A lateral thoracic spine will demonstrate the intervertebral joint spaces and the intervertebral foramina; the apophyseal joints would be visible in a 70° oblique.

133) B Direct the central ray 10° to 15° cephalic to allow the shoulder farthest from the film to be projected above the thoracic spine.

134) B Over the shoulders; the cathode should be placed over the thickest part of the anatomy.

135) C Scatter radiation within the diagnostic range most often is Compton scatter; this is characterized by ejection of an outer shell electron (recoil electron) and a photon that is able to cause additional ionizations.

136) D The output screen of the image intensification tube converts electrons into visible light photons. This becomes the image the user will view.

137) B The SID is increased to minimize the OID because of the shoulders.

138) C Standard/universal precautions should be used with all patients, without exception.

139) A Assault is the intentional threat of injury to a patient with force.

140) A The process converts alternating current into pulsating direct current.

141) B The milliammeter is located in the secondary, high-voltage circuit.

142) B The primary coils of the step up transformer: the primary and secondary side of the step up transformer are directly proportional. Transformers operate on the principle of electromagnetic mutual induction.

143) A The autotransformer operates on the principle of electromagnetic self-induction.

144) D A rheostat can operate on AC or DC, is located in the filament circuit, and functions to decrease voltage and increase amperage.

145) B Quantum mottle can be reduced by making more radiation available to expose the film; therefore, increasing the mA will help reduce it.

146) D (B & C) Vidicon and plumbicon tubes both convert visible light into a video signal.

147) D Spot films use the most radiation to record an image; it is a direct exposure system.

148) A The mA used in image intensification is between 0.5 and 5 mA; this is due to the long exposure times and the heat units created.

149) D (A & B) Ohm's law can be expressed as $V = I/R$; $I = V/R$; $R = V/I$

150) C The atomic number of tungsten provides the appropriate frequency of radiation used in the diagnostic range.

151) D A low mA station will require an increase in time to maintain density; long times do not limit patient motion.

152) B Battery, because physical harm was inflicted upon the child.

153) C Only a used syringe and a blood-soaked gauze pad are considered medical waste.

154) C Malpractice is a civil liability.

155) B Respondeat superior, meaning "Let the master answer."

156) C An incident report should be filled out whenever the patient is injured.

157) C The time necessary for the effects to manifest is the latent period.

158) D A threshold dose is a dosage that would be great enough to cause a specific response.

159) C Lymphocytes rapidly divide and are highly oxygenated, which makes them one of the most radiation-sensitive tissues, as described by the law of Tribondeau and Bergonié.

160) B A pocket dosimeter does not provide a long-term record of radiation exposures.

161) C 500 rad = 5 gray.

162) C If the badge is laundered (wet) and dried (high temperature), this will add an extreme amount of density on the radiographic film of the film badge.

163) D Alpha-radiation has the highest LET, with a quality factor of 20, therefore 6 gray of alpha-radiation is equal to 180 gray of x-radiation.

164) B A thermoluminescent dosimeter would be the only personnel-monitoring device.

165) A A control badge will account for background radiation. The personal film badges will be compared with the control badge to calculate the dosage received.

166) A 0.5 rem, as established by the NCRP.

167) D The institution that employs the technologist is responsible for maintenance of cumulative exposure records.

168) C The coronary arteries feeding the heart are the first branch from the aorta.

169) A Transformers operate only on alternating current.

170) B A motor converts electrical energy into mechanical energy.

171) C A rheostat will operate on alternating or direct current.

172) D The advantages of solid state rectifiers include less heat production and elimination of filaments, and they occupy less space compared with valve tube rectifiers.

173) C The use of a grid would increase the patient exposure because the mAs would need to be increased to maintain density.

174) B Filtration will filter out low-energy photons that would not otherwise contribute to the image but would be absorbed by the patient.

175) B The H&D curve would have a steep slope, allowing for only a narrow latitude, high or short scale contrast.

176) C The magnification formula: SID/SOD = magnification − 40/31 = 1.29. Multiply the magnification factor by the object size to get the projected image size: 7 × 1.29 = 9.03.

177) A The penumbra/geometric unsharpness formula: FSS × OID/SOD = Penumbra − 3 × 6/66 = 0.27 Penumbra = 0.27.

178) D The mAs/distance formula:

$$\frac{mAs_1}{mAs_2} = \frac{(D_1)^2}{(D_2)^2} \qquad \frac{30}{X} = \frac{(40)^2}{(60)^2}$$

$$\frac{30}{X} = \frac{1600}{3600} \qquad X = 67.50 \qquad 68\ mAs$$

179) B The time factor would have the same relationship as the mAs factor; therefore, the mAs/distance formula would be used to calculate:

$$\frac{T_1}{T_2} = \frac{(D_1)^2}{(D_2)^2} \qquad \frac{0.125}{X} = \frac{(36)^2}{(72)^2}$$

$$648 = 1296X \qquad X = 0.50\ or\ 1/2\ sec$$

180) D kVp 15% rule: If the kVp is increased by 15%, decrease mAs by half, or 50%.

181) C This type of artifact is caused by an electrical discharge, usually because the humidity is too low; also called tree branch artifact.

182) A To correct this problem, raise the humidity; this will reduce the amount of static discharges occurring within the darkroom.

183) B Selecting a phosphor that has a high conversion efficiency will increase the intensifying screen speed.

184) B Silver bromide is used in the emulsion layer of the radiographic film.

185) A The formation of black metallic silver is performed by the developer chemicals, an alkaline solution.

186) D Use the inverse square to calculate:

$$\frac{I_1}{I_2} = \frac{(D_2)^2}{(D_1)^2} \qquad \frac{110}{X} = \frac{324}{5184}$$

$$X = 1760\ mr$$

187) D By using a less efficient grid, the density and scatter reaching the film will increase; therefore, the scale of contrast will be longer.

188) D A 30% change in mAs is the minimum necessary to see a visible difference in the finished radiograph.

189) A By raising the patient's chin, the petrous ridges will not be projected in the maxillary sinuses.

190) B The patient position is external oblique.

191) D The central ray would be directed 45° laterally.

192) B The opposite position is internal oblique, used to evaluate the coranoid process.

193) A The lateral recumbent (dorsal decubitus) would best depict an aortic aneurysm.

194) A The ethmoid bone forms the medial aspect of the orbit.

195) B The superior projection of the perpendicular plate is the crista galli.

196) B The radius and ulna will cross each other in the proximal third.

197) C The false ribs are attached to the sternum via costal cartilage.

198) A An AP projection for scoliosis should include C7, L5, and both iliac crests.

199) D Scoliosis series are generally performed at 72″ SID to decrease magnification to include as much anatomy as possible and achieve a more accurate measurement of a possible curvature.

200) B The topographic landmark for L4 is the umbilicus.

1) B Dead-man switch will prevent overexposure; as soon as the user releases the switch, the radiation ceases to be produced.

2) D Inherent filtration is the Pyrex glass and the oil. The amount depends upon the type of construction and is determined by the manufacturer.

3) A According to the NCRP recommendation, protective gloves should be at least 0.25 mm Pb equivalent.

4) D Ci is the abbreviation for curie, which is a traditional unit of measure that measures radioactivity.

5) C The first symptom in a radiation-induced illness/syndrome is nausea.

6) A Professional confidentiality is found in the ASRT code of ethics.

7) A Age-specific procedures are clinical competencies that are specific to the patient's age, from young infants to elderly people. They are required by the JCAHO.

8) B COPD is the abbreviation for chronic obstructive pulmonary disease.

9) A One milliliter is equivalent to 1 cubic centimeter.

10) D Parenteral drugs are given by injection, not by mouth.

11) B A double-contrast barium enema will coat the mucosal lining of the large intestines, allowing polyps to be better visualized.

12) C The pedicles of the lumbar spine lie in the same transverse plane as the renal pelvis.

13) D The projection of the central ray enters the vertex (top) of the skull and exits from the base.

14) D The patient is 23 cm thick AP and the lesion is located 3 cm from the anterior wall of the chest; therefore, the fulcrum should be set at 20 cm from the tabletop to align with the questionable lesion.

15) C The grid and film should be placed parallel to the femoral neck, to minimize the foreshortening of the femoral neck.

16) B The slowest screen speed and the smallest focal spot size will afford the greatest amount of recorded detail.

17) A The straight line portion of the H&D or characteristic curve is referred to as the gamma portion.

18) B Once a radiographic film has reached D-Max, any additional exposure will cause the film to become lighter, not darker due to the downward slope of the resultant sensitometric curve or solarization.

19) A The technical factors for I would provide the greatest density because of the high-speed screen.

20) B The technical factors with the longest time would be used for an autotomographic procedure (breathing technique).

21) A The technical factors with the fastest screen speed and largest focal spot size would have the least recorded detail.

22) C The prereading kVp meter is located after the autotransformer and before the step-up transformer.

23) B Bremsstrahlung and characteristic interactions occur at the target when radiation is produced within the diagnostic range.

24) D (A & B) The cathode is connected to the high voltage circuit and the filament circuit.

25) D The anode is the positive pole of the x-ray tube, and it may be rotating or stationary.

26) D Calculate heat units for a single-phase unit: $kVp \times mA \times time = HU$; $300 \times 0.20 \times 70 = 4200$ HU; then divide HU by the tube limit, $33,600/4200 = 8$, therefore 8 rapid exposures can safely be made.

27) A Minification gain will occur as a result of electrons being forced to converge from a large input screen to a smaller output screen.

28) B The amplitude is the total distance that the tube will travel during a tomographic examination.

29) B X-radiation is manmade radiation that diverges in a straight line from its point of origin. It cannot be focused or made to converge.

30) D The amount of photoelectric interactions determines the amount of tissue contrast that will be recorded on the radiograph.

31) B The right hemidiaphragm is located higher than the left because of the position of the liver immediately inferior to the diaphragm.

32) A The bony thorax is composed of the sternum, ribs, and thoracic vertebrae.

33) C kVp is responsible for the penetrating ability of the beam; a quality chest radiograph requires that the dense heart and mediastinum be penetrated, while maintaining radiographic visualization of the lung parenchyma.

34) A An air-fluid level is visualized in the fundus of the stomach; this is indicative of an erect position with a perpendicular central ray.

35) B Chest radiography is performed at 72″ SID to minimize the magnification of the heart and great vessels.

36) C Another name for the body of the sternum is the gladiolus.

37) B Diarthrodial joints are freely moveable joints; this type outnumbers all other types of joints.

38) D Intermittent claudication is pain or cramping in the lower legs, usually associated with poor circulation. It is relieved by rest.

39) D The pterion is the junction of the frontal, sphenoid, parietal, and temporal bones.

40) A The loss of smell may occur with a fracture in the cribriform plate because the olfactory nerves (of smell) pass through it.

41) D All these disease processes involve the lymphatic system; obstruction, Hodgkin's disease, and reticulum cell carcinoma.

42) A Swabbing the rubber stopper will decontaminate it: by doing this more than once the rubber stopper will become recontaminated.

43) B Asepsis or clean technique will prevent transmission of body fluids from one person to another.

44) C Dizziness and lightheadedness are symptoms of hypotension (low blood pressure).

45) B Neurogenic shock is caused by trauma to the central nervous system, which causes blood vessel dilation, hypotension, and tachycardia.

46) C A patient with suspected cervical trauma cannot have the neck manipulated; therefore, the jaw thrust technique would be used to obtain an airway, as described by the American Heart Association.

47) D The compression-to-breath ratio for a two-person rescue is 15:2, as described by the American Heart Association.

48) D A diabetic patient on insulin therapy is not at risk with intravascular iodinated contrast media injections, unless the BUN and creatinine levels are out of normal limits. The other conditions are contraindicated for intravascular iodinated contrast-medium injection.

49) B The most common injection site is the antecubital vein because of its accessibility and reliability.

50) C Aminophylline is a bronchodilator medication that is given to patients experiencing bronchospasms.

51) D Whenever a patient has any type of reaction to a contrast medium, an ADR form must be filled out, as required by the JCAHO.

52) A If a marker is stuck in the Bucky tray, it may prevent the grid from reciprocating; therefore, grid lines will be visible on the radiograph.

53) C An IUD (intrauterine device) would be an internal artifact, because it is within the patient. A pacemaker on a chest radiograph would be considered the same.

54) D Nervous tissue does not have a high degree of radiosensitivity as described by Tribondeau and Bergonié. Nerve tissue is highly specialized and does not divide.

55) B The acronym PACS stands for Picture Archive and Communication System. This system allows images to be acquired digitally and transmitted to distant locations and is the future of radiology.

56) B The radiograph would be underexposed because the AEC would terminate early. The density of the abdomen is much less than that of the lumbar spine.

57) D A 3-phase, 12-pulse unit would require an oscilloscope to determine current changes and voltage waveform accuracy within the x-ray circuit.

58) C Raising the distance of the safelight to the work station will reduce the amount of safelight fog because of the decrease in the light intensity at the level of the work station. Inverse square law states that as the distance increases, the intensity decreases.

59) C Grid efficiency is determined by grid frequency and grid ratio.

60) A The formula used to determine grid ratio is h/d = grid ratio. h = height of the opaque material, d = distance between the opaque material, the interspace.

61) B The general population's DEL (dose equivalent limit) is 1/10 that of a radiation worker. Radiation worker: 5 mrem/year and general population: 0.5 mrem.

62) D If cell damage occurs, the cell may repair itself, but if cellular death occurs, the cell will not revive.

63) C Bone tissue has a higher atomic number compared with fat, muscle, and nerve; therefore, bone will absorb low energy radiation. The other tissues may scatter the radiation rather than absorb it.

64) D Film badges are designed with filters to detect x-radiation, gamma-radiation, and beta-radiation.

65) D A cutie-pie ion chamber is a survey instrument used for exposure levels from 1 mr/hr to several thousand mr/hr. For low-level exposures under 100 mr/hr, a Geiger-Müller counter may be used.

66) B The portable exposure cord must be at least 6′ in length.

67) B By angulation of the central ray, the joint space will be better visualized because the femoral condyles will not overlap the joint space because of magnification, especially of the lateral femoral condyle.

68) C When the hand is pronated, the first digit (thumb) will assume an oblique position.

69) A The celiac artery provides arterial blood flow to the liver, spleen, and stomach.

70) C The talus bone of the ankle is also known as the astragalus.

71) D The vomer bone is a facial bone that is not paired.

72) B A barium enema should not be performed on a patient with appendicitis because of the possibility of the appendix rupturing or the possible need for surgical intervention.

73) C LPO and RAO will minimize the overlap of the hepatic flexure, allowing better visualization. LPO and RAO are considered corresponding positions.

74) A Bile is produced in the liver and stored in the gallbladder. Bile is used in digestion for fat emulsification.

75) D The formation of the innominate bone is the junction of the pubis, ilium, and ischium to form one half of the pelvic girdle.

76) A The epididymis is one of a pair of tightly coiled tubes that carry sperm from the testicles to the penis.

77) B The choroid plexus is located in the lateral ventricles in the brain and is responsible for making cerebrospinal fluid.

78) B The lateral Sims' position is used for insertion of the enema tip for a barium enema. The lateral Sims' will position the rectum so as to allow for easier insertion of the enema tip.

79) C The RPO (right posterior oblique) position will best demonstrate the axillary posterior ribs.

80) A To achieve a true AP projection of the humerus, the epicondyles must be parallel with the plane of the film.

81) A A short scale of contrast will result from using a low kVp technique; low kVp is less penetrating; its energy is depicted as a long wavelength.

82) C A detail film-screen combination should be used when performing a foreign body study.

83) B The base material of radiographic film is polyester. Polyester allows for good light transmission and is dimensionally stable; it resists shrinking and stretching.

84) D Latitude and contrast are inversely proportional when plotted on the H&D (Hurter and Driffield) curve, therefore as latitude increases, contrast decreases, and as latitude decreases, contrast increases.

85) D (B & C) The thickness of the tomographic slice will be determined by the exposure angle and the amplitude of the tube motion.

86) A Subtraction film is used for angiographic procedures; subtraction is used to subtract out the anatomy and allow for better visualization of the blood vessels. Most subtraction studies are now imaged digitally.

87) B Most of the scatter production that occurs within the diagnostic range is through Compton interactions.

88) B Compton interactions are characterized by an incoming photon, which deposits enough energy in an outer shell electron to eject it (recoil). The remainder of energy will continue on and may cause additional interactions.

89) D A cross-hatched grid has lead strips placed horizontally and longitudinally, forming squares.

90) B B has the shortest distance, with an 8:1 grid ratio; although D has a high mAs value, it also has a longer distance and a higher grid ratio; therefore, the recorded density would be lower than that of B.

91) C The proper order of cell division is prophase, metaphase, anaphase, telophase.

92) C Gamma-radiation is emitted from an unstable radioactive source (isotope); x-radiation is manmade.

93) A If the technologist receives 300 mr for 15 min at 2 feet, he or she would receive 20 mr per min at 2 feet. With the inverse square law, it can be calculated that by standing 6 feet away for 30 min, the technologist would receive less exposure.

$$\frac{20}{X} = \frac{(6)_2}{(2)_2}$$

$$80 = 36X : X = 2.22 \text{ mr/min} : 2.22 \text{ mr} \times 30 \text{ min} = 66 \text{ mr total exposure}$$

94) B The total filtration required for a diagnostic unit operating at 50 to 70 kVp is 1.5 mm Al equivalent.

95) A The minimum SSD (source-to-skin distance) for portable units is 12 inches. This includes image intensification units such as C-arms. The collimator/tube housing generally measures 12 inches to insure this minimum SSD.

96) A A watt is 1 amp of current flowing through an electrical potential of 1 volt. A volt is 1 joule of work done on 1 coulomb of charge.

97) B 96 kV. This is described by the transformer law:

$$\frac{V_1}{V_2} = \frac{W_1}{W_2} \qquad \frac{120}{X} = \frac{1}{800}$$

$$X = 96,000$$

98) C A coil of wire with an electrical current in the wire, coiled around a ferrous material such as iron, is an electromagnet.

99) D The left hand generator rule describes the motion of the conductor (thumb), direction of the magnetic field (index finger), and flow of the induced current (middle finger).

100) C The autotransformer operates on electromagnetic self-induction and has only one coil of wire, with a large iron core that varies voltage through various tap-off points.

101) B Always help the patient down, never try to hold the patient up, then assess the patient and get help.

102) A A splint should never be removed from a patient with an obvious fracture. Alter imaging techniques to obtain optimal films without manipulating the fracture site.

103) C Patients may have experienced a trauma or may be very unfamiliar with hospital procedure, therefore the technologist should make every effort to make the patient comfortable. One way of doing this is to explain the procedure thoroughly, and leave time for questions throughout the procedure.

104) D Adrenaline and epinephrine are both bronchodilators and cardiac stimulants.

105) D (A & C) Log rolling is required for any patient with a suspected or known pelvic or spinal injury who has to be turned. This will prevent additional acute trauma to pelvic organs, vascular structures, and the spinal cord.

106) D The half-life of this isotope is 5 hours; therefore, for every 5 hours the radioactivity is reduced by half: 5 hours = 50 millicurie; 10 hours = 25 millicurie; 15 hours = 12.5 millicurie; 20 hours = 6.25 millicurie.

107) B The exposure switch is located so as to prevent the technologist from accidentally exposing the self.

108) B The fluoroscopic timer is preset for 5 min. At this time an alarm will sound, but the exposure will not stop. The alarm will inform the user of the length of time the radiation beam has been "on."

109) C The dosage delivered to the patient is directly proportional to the dosage that the technologist may receive.

110) A The use of a grid will not reduce the dosage delivered to the patient. In fact, with the use of a grid the patient will receive more exposure. The patient will receive more back scatter, and the exposure factor must be increased over a screen technique to maintain the radiographic density.

111) D (B & C) The radiology waiting room should not be located in a radiation area; the nuclear medicine hot lab (storage and preparation of radioactive isotopes) and the radiation decay room (an area used to reduce isotopes to a safe level so they may be disposed of) are both radiation-controlled areas.

112) C Personnel monitoring devices should be worn only during occupational exposures. An annual chest radiograph is not an occupational exposure.

113) B The use of an intensifying screen greatly reduces the exposure dose that the patient receives.

114) A An exposure reproducibility test must be carried out annually, according to the NCRP guidelines.

115) A Protective gloves, along with all other protective apparel, should be tested annually. This is a visual and fluoroscopic examination.

116) A These guidelines are established as a total quality management program for mammography by the Mammography Quality Standards Act and the American College of Radiology, but they may be applied to all film wet processing.

117) C Intensifying screen should be cleaned only with a screen cleaner approved by the manufacturer; this is to insure that the screen is not damaged by the cleaner.

118) B In cineradiography or direct exposure films, the radiation used to expose the film is emitted from the output screen of the image intensification tube.

119) A The heat that is produced on the anode's focal track requires that it be made of a material with a high melting point. The melting point of tungsten is 3410°C.

120) C Voltage is the force that moves electrical charges across a conductor.

121) C The first law of electrostatics is repulsion-attraction, which states that like charges repel and unlike charges attract.

122) A The developer chemical mixture is very temperature dependent. If consistent results are to be expected, the developer mixture should be maintained at 35°C, or 95°F.

123) B If the developer temperature is excessive, the resultant radiographs will demonstrate excessive density and decreased contrast due to overdevelopment.

124) C A pinhole camera allows for the dimensions to be measured to determine the effective focal spot size but not resolution of the focal spot size.

125) D A star test pattern or line pair test pattern will allow for evaluation of recorded detail but not the size of the focal spot.

126) C These factors represent the relationship between mA and time, where different mA and time factors will be adjusted to yield the same mAs. This is the reciprocity law.

127) C If a focused grid is used upside down, the resulting radiograph will demonstrate decreased density on both edges of the film, because of the divergence of the x-ray beam and the angulation of the lead strips.

128) B The frequency of the grid is determined by the number of lead strips per inch.

129) A The tomographic motion that results in streaking or ghosting artifacts is a linear motion. This occurs because the tube motion is unidirectional.

130) D Zonography is another name for tomography with very thick slices, usually due to a very small arc.

131) C Use the magnification formula SID/SOD = Mag. First you must solve for SOD; SID − OID = SOD; therefore, 40 − 30 = 10 (SOD); 40/30 = 1.33 (magnification factor). Multiply the object by the MF − 15 × 1.33 = 19.95 projected image size.

132) C Use the inverse square formula:

$$\frac{I_1}{I_2} = \frac{(D_2)^2}{(D_1)^2} \qquad \frac{10}{X} = \frac{(20)^2}{(60)^2}$$

$$36{,}000 = 400X \qquad X = 90 \text{ mr/h}$$

133) B Phosphorescent crystals will continue to illuminate after the exposure has ceased. This does not make these types of crystals a good choice for intensifying screens.

134) D The blotchy or blurry areas would be due to the increase in the distance between the intensifying screen and the film.

135) D The photographic effect occurs because the conversion efficiency of the intensifying screens is very high; a very small amount of radiation can form the entire image.

136) A Duplitized film refers to film that has two emulsion layers, one on either side of a base material, making it sensitive to radiation on both sides.

137) B The gelatin in the film serves to suspend the silver halide crystals. They must be distributed perfectly evenly over the surface of the film in order to obtain even density across the film.

138) B The parallax effect is the graininess effect of the radiograph; the film with the smallest crystals would minimize this effect.

139) A The primary reason why an increase in contrast is seen with an air-gap technique is that most of the scatter occurring within the patient will miss the film due to the increased OID and the angle of the scatter.

140) C Any density recorded on an unexposed film that is evident postprocessing is the tint of the base material (usually blue) and any fog that may have affected the film (may be due to environmental radiation).

141) D (A & C) As described by the kVp 15% rule, an increase in kVp of 15% will result in a higher overall beam energy (penetrability) and double the recorded density on the radiograph.

142) B The thin lead foil that is placed in the back of radiographic cassettes functions to absorb photons that may otherwise backscatter and cause an increased fog on the radiograph.

143) A The squeegee rollers or cross-over rollers will help prevent cross-contamination of the developer into the fixer.

144) A To decrease the amount of magnification that is recorded on the radiograph, a long SID should be used. If the SID is reduced, an increase in magnification will occur. Film/screen combination and focal spot size will not affect the amount of magnification recorded on the film.

145) C To increase the contrast between adjacent structures, a decrease in kVp may be used (this will provide a shorter scale of contrast), and a specially designed material with a high atomic number (for positive contrast) or a low atomic number (for negative contrast) will increase the contrast between structures.

146) A A streaky, ghostlike artifact with unidirectional tomographic units. Any structure that is parallel to the tube movement will be streaked.

147) B The lead equivalent required for the Bucky slot is 0.25 mm PB Eq according to the NCRP guidelines.

148) A Diagnostic units that operate under 50 kVp would require 0.5 mm Al Eq according to the NCRP guidelines.

149) C The best time to radiograph a pregnant patient is after she gives birth, but if the procedure is absolutely necessary, the best time would be the third trimester. This is because the fetus is allowed to mature. The cells will become more specialized, but they will still be rapidly dividing and have a relatively high oxygen content, which will increase the radiosensitivity.

150) A Gonadal shielding would include collimation when performing chest radiography.

151) D A change in filtration will change the exposure rate exiting from the tube, overall beam energy, and the wavelengths of the photons exiting from the tube, but filtration will not affect the formation of the electron cloud.

152) C The biologic half-life is the length of time necessary for a radionuclide to be reduced to half its original intensity within the body.

153) A According to the laws of Tribondeau and Bergonié, the tissues' radiosensitivity from most to least is lymphocytes, germ, epithelium, muscle, and nerve.

154) D The ascending order of the subdivision of matter is atom, molecule, element, compound.

155) B The earth is the largest natural magnet.

156) B If a permanent magnet is broken into two pieces, they both will become magnets on their own.

157) A Potential energy is stored energy: ability to do work by virtue of position.

158) D Sodium has fewer protons, less mass, and less atomic weight than mercury.

159) B The K shell of an atom is able to hold two electrons.

160) A The process of ionization requires the addition or subtraction of an electron.

161) B The major advantage of a myelographic procedure is that it provides a dynamic study.

162) B The cauda equina is located at the level of L1.

163) C The contrast used for myelography is ionic or non-ionic, water-based, low osmolar, with a very small incidence of adverse reactions.

164) A A low kVp technique is used to increase the contrast in a tissue that has very little tissue contrast (such as a breast).

165) C A hysterosalpingogram is a contrast examination of the female reproductive organs: uterus and fallopian tubes.

166) A An arthrography examination will not only show the joint structure but also the joint function, because the radiologist is able to manipulate the joint under fluoroscopy.

167) C Interventional radiology may be used for diagnosis (occluded vessel) and treatment (balloon angioplasty).

168) D While performing an ERCP, the doctor can diagnose and treat many conditions, including removal of stones, placement of stents, and the opening of occluded ducts.

169) A A scanogram is a radiologic procedure that utilizes a radiopaque ruler to measure long bone length.

170) C In a retrograde procedure, the contrast is introduced in the opposite direction of normal physiologic flow.

171) D The position of the kidneys within the abdominal cavity is retroperitoneal, with the lower pole more anterior than the upper pole.

172) A A rupture of the lateral ligament of the ankle would be demonstrated with an inversion stress view. This will show an abnormal opening of the joint space on the lateral side of the ankle.

173) C A freely movable joint is termed diarthrodial. This type of joint is also identified by its synovial joint capsule.

174) C The correct obliquity for chest radiography when the cardiac and great vessels are of interest is 60° LAO.

175) A The epiphysis is located at the end of a bone and is responsible for bone formation in children.

176) C Osteomalacia is a destructive disease that is characterized by bone softening secondary to the loss of calcium.

177) C A subluxation is defined as a partial dislocation.

178) B Colles' fracture is characterized by a distal radial fracture and posterior displacement of the hand.

179) C The most common prescription for oxygen therapy is 2–4 L/min.

180) C The lithotomy position is characterized by the patient supine, the pelvis and hips fully flexed, and the legs held in stirrups. This position would be used for hysterosalpingograms and cystograms.

181) B A Holter monitor is used to record a 24-hour ECG. This monitor is capable of recording transient or occult cardiac arrhythmias in relation to the patient's activity level.

182) C The tympanic temperature is taken in the ear and is normally 37°C or 98.6°F.

183) D The equipment necessary to take a blood pressure is a stethoscope (to listen for the pulse) and a sphygmomanometer (blood pressure cuff).

184) C Miller-Abbott is a double-lumen nasogastric (NG) tube.

185) C A sigmoid colostomy stoma is usually just irrigated.

186) C The proper angulation for an AP spot radiograph of L5–S1 is 30° to 35° cephalic.

187) D The central ray for this position is midway between the ASIS and the iliac crest.

188) B An increase in kVp would compensate for the decrease in density, because of the collimation.

189) B A 5° to 8° caudad angulation will usually overcome the angle of the lumbar spine.

190) C The patient is in a lateral position; therefore, a coronal plane passing through the spine would be aligned to the center of the table.

191) A The thumb is a saddle joint. It allows for a diverse amount of movement. The first carpometacarpal joint is another example of a saddle joint.

192) D Placing the patient in a right lateral position or an erect position will cause the duodenal bulb to fill with barium and through an increase in peristalsis will help it empty. Having the patient imagine eating favorite food may increase peristalsis and aid in the emptying of the duodenal bulb.

193) A An esophagogram that is performed for cardiac structures must be performed at 72″ to minimize the magnification of the heart and great vessels.

194) B The Y view is performed primarily on patients with suspected dislocations. This projection will best demonstrate the position of the humeral head in relation to the articulating surface of the scapula.

195) C Most shoulder dislocations are dislocated anterior and inferiorly.

196) A A Y view affords better radiation protection over a transthoracic shoulder, because the exposure factors for a transthoracic are considerably higher compared with a Y view of the scapula.

197) D The greater trochanter is located at the same level as the symphysis pubis.

198) D The patient placed on the left side with a horizontal beam passing through the body is in a left lateral decubitus; the position is described by which side of the patient is down (left or right). The projection is a decubitus because a horizontal beam is used.

199) B One of the most common indications for a decubitus projection is to demonstrate air-fluid levels.

200) B The submentovertical projection will best demonstrate the foramen magnum, foramen spinosum, and foramen ovale.

APPENDIX A: Glossary of Terms

General Positioning Terminology

Anterior– the front of the body
Posterior– the back of the body
Lateral– toward the side of the body
Medial– toward the middle of the body
Superior– toward the head
Inferior– toward the feet
Proximal– toward the point of origin
Distal– away from the point of origin
Dorsal– toward the back
Ventral– toward the front
Supine– patient lying face up
Prone– patient lying face down
Erect– patient standing with feet on the floor

Body Planes (Figure A–1)

Coronal– divides the body into front and back portions; *mid coronal* or *mid axillary* divides the body into equal anterior and posterior halves
Axial– divides the body into superior and inferior portions
Sagittal– divides the body into right and left portions; *mid sagittal* divides the body into equal right and left halves

Bodily Divisions

Four Quadrants (Figure A–2)

RUQ– right upper quadrant
LUQ– left upper quadrant
RLQ– right lower quadrant
LLQ– left lower quadrant

Nine Regions (Figure A–3)

Right hypochondriac region
Epigastric region
Left hypochondriac region
Right lateral abdominal region
Umbilical region
Left lateral abdominal region
Right iliac (inguinal) region
Hypogastric region
Left iliac (inguinal) region

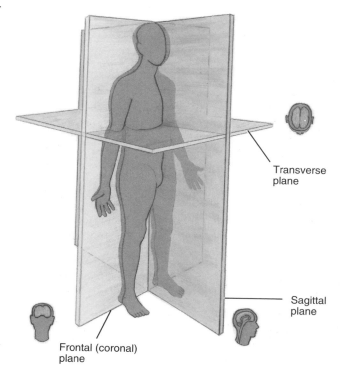

Figure A–1 ■ Planes of the body. (From Applegate EJ: The Anatomy and Physiology Learning System. Philadelphia: WB Saunders; 1995, p 14.)

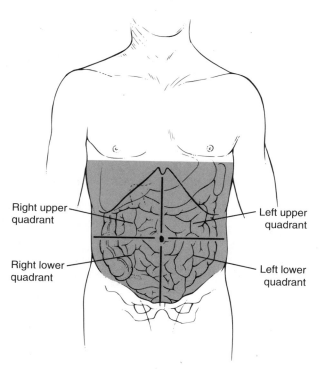

Figure A–2 ■ Quadrants of the abdomen. (From Swartz MH: Textbook of Physical Diagnosis. Philadelphia, WB Saunders, 1989, p 320.)

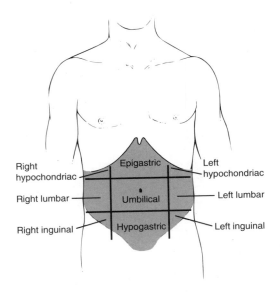

Figure A-3 ■ Regions of the abdomen. (From Swartz MH: Textbook of Physical Diagnosis. Philadelphia, WB Saunders, 1989, p 320.)

Body Habitus

Hypersthenic– a very large build with wide shoulders

Sthenic– an average build that comprises 50% of the population

Hyposthenic– a hybrid between sthenic and asthenic; a slightly below average build but does not fit into the category of very slender

Asthenic– a very slender build, with long limbs and an angular profile and prominent muscles or bones

Topographical Anatomy (Figure A–4)

Cervical Region

C1– mastoid tip; hard palate
C2, C3– mandibular angle; hyoid bone
C4, C5– thyroid cartilage
C7– vertebral prominence

Thoracic Region

T2, T3– sternal notch; superior margin of the scapula
T4, T5– junction of the manubrium and body of the sternum; sternal angle
T9, T10– xiphoid process of the sternum

Lumbar Region

L1– transpyloric plane
L3– costal margin

L3, L4– umbilicus
L4– top of the iliac crest

Pelvic/Sacral Region

S1– ASIS (anterior superior iliac spine)
Coccyx– symphysis pubis; greater trochanter

Standard Terminology for Positioning and Projection*

Radiographic view– describes the body part as seen by the x-ray film or other recording medium, such as a fluoroscopic screen. Restricted to the discussion of a *radiograph* or *image*

Radiographic position– refers to a specific body position, such as supine, prone, recumbent, erect, or Trendelenburg. Restricted to the discussion of the *patient's physical position*

Radiographic projection– restricted to the discussion of the entrance and exit *path of the central ray.*

Positioning Terminology

Lying Down

Supine– lying on the back
Prone– lying face downward
Decubitus– lying down with a horizontal x-ray beam
Recumbent– lying down in any position

Erect or Upright

Anterior position– facing the film

- **Left anterior oblique–** body rotated, with the left anterior portion closest to the film
- **Right anterior oblique–** body rotated with the right anterior portion closest to the film

Posterior position– facing the radiographic tube, with the back of the body closest to the film.

*©1995 The American Registry of Radiologic Technologists. The ARRT does not review, evaluate, or endorse publications. Permission to reproduce ARRT copyrighted materials within this publication should not be construed as an endorsement of the publication by the ARRT.

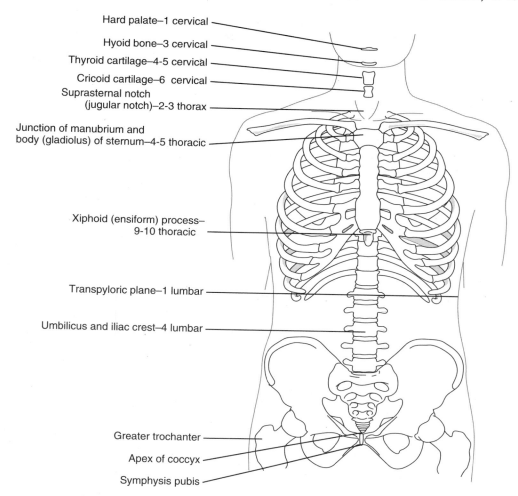

Hard palate–1 cervical

Hyoid bone–3 cervical

Thyroid cartilage–4-5 cervical

Cricoid cartilage–6 cervical

Suprasternal notch
(jugular notch)–2-3 thorax

Junction of manubrium and
body (gladiolus) of sternum–4-5 thoracic

Xiphoid (ensiform) process–
9-10 thoracic

Transpyloric plane–1 lumbar

Umbilicus and iliac crest–4 lumbar

Greater trochanter

Apex of coccyx

Symphysis pubis

Figure A-4 ■ Topographic anatomy.

- **Left posterior oblique**– body rotated, with the left posterior portion closest to the film
- **Right posterior oblique**– body rotated, with the right posterior portion closest to the film

Oblique position– (erect or lying down)

Basic Radiographic Projection
(Figure A–5)

Anteroposterior (AP)– from the front of the body to the back of the body

Posteroanterior (PA)– from the back of the body to the front of the body

Superoinferior (Craniocaudal) (Verticosubmental)– from the head toward the feet

Submentovertical– from the inferior mandible (mental point) toward the superior head (vertex)

Mediolateral– from the medial aspect to the lateral aspect

Lateromedial– from the lateral aspect to the medial aspect

Axial– describes an angled central ray through the body part, longitudinally

Tangential– describes a central ray that skims over or through a body part, to place that body part in profile without superimposition

Decubitus– describes a horizontal beam that passes across the patient

Joints Classification

Functional classification– joints classified by the amount of movement they allow:

- **Synarthrosis**– an immovable joint, such as a suture of the skull
- **Amphiarthrosis**– a slightly movable joint, such as a vertebra

ANTEROPOSTERIOR PROJECTION

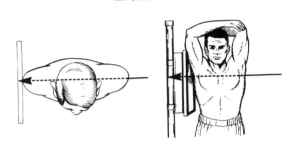

POSTEROANTERIOR PROJECTION

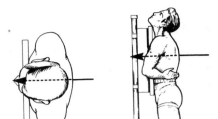

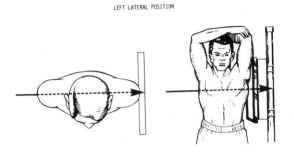

RIGHT LATERAL POSITION

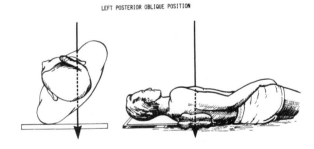

LEFT LATERAL POSITION

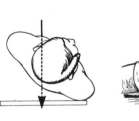

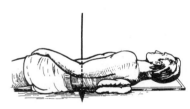

LEFT POSTERIOR OBLIQUE POSITION

RIGHT POSTERIOR OBLIQUE POSITION

LEFT ANTERIOR OBLIQUE POSITION

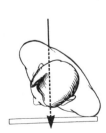

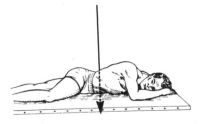

RIGHT ANTERIOR OBLIQUE POSITION

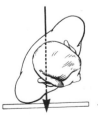

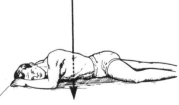

Figure A–5 ■ Basic radiographic projections. (From American Registry of Radiologic Technologists: Conventions Specific to the Radiography Examination. St. Paul, MN, ARRT, © 1995. The ARRT does not review, evaluate, or endorse publications. Permission to reproduce ARRT copyrighted materials within this publication should not be construed as an endorsement of the publication by the ARRT.)

- **Diarthrosis**– a freely moveable joint, such as the shoulder

Structure classification– joints classified by the manner they are held together:

- **Fibrous**– Strong connective tissue fibers extend from one bone to the other, tightly holding them together without a joint cavity, such as sutures and gomphoses (joints that hold the teeth in); these joints are usually immovable.
- **Cartilaginous**– The bones are held together by a piece of cartilage between them and fastened to each by strong connective tissue, such as symphysis pubis and the vertebrae; these joints are usually slightly moveable.
- **Synovial**– The bones are held together by ligaments, and the joint space has a joint capsule that is filled with a lubricating fluid, called synovial fluid. The ends of the bones are covered with articular cartilage. These joints are always freely moveable joints, such as the knee, hip, or shoulder.

NCRP Shielding Recommendation for Protective Devices

Contact shields– 0.25 mm lead equivalent
Aprons– 0.25 mm (up to 1.00 mm) lead equivalent
Eyeglasses– 0.35 mm (up to 0.50 mm) lead equivalent
Thyroid shield– 0.50 mm lead equivalent
Protective gloves– 0.25 mm lead equivalent
Bucky slot cover– 0.25 mm lead equivalent
Fluoro drape– 0.25 mm lead equivalent
Primary barriers– 1/16″ or 1.6 mm

Secondary barriers– 1/32″ or 0.8 mm
Tube housing– the thickness of lead or equivalent necessary to reduce the leakage radiation to less than 100 mr/hr at 1 meter

H and D Curve (Figure A–6)

Base plus fog (A)– the density recorded on the film that is inherent to the film before being used. This density arises from the tints and dyes in the base material. Any number of agents, such as chemical fumes, natural background radiation, and x-radiation may cause the fog. The fog may also be caused by processing methods, such as excessive temperature and hyperactivity of the developer solution. The base plus fog is normally between 0.10 OD and 0.22 OD.

Toe portion (B)– where the film begins to demonstrate density owing to radiation exposure, which is recorded above the base plus fog. This portion of the curve is responsible for the fine gray tones. The toe portion of the curve is controlled by the developer chemical phenidone.

Straight line or gamma portion (C)– the region of optimal diagnostic densities. This portion is usually fairly straight because the film is responding to the radiation exposure in a linear fashion. It demonstrates inherent latitude of film. Densities within the straight line portion range between 0.25 OD and 3.0 OD.

Shoulder portion (D)– the heavy black tones and point where almost all of the silver halide crystals are exposed. The shoulder portion of the curve is controlled by the developer chemical hydroquinone.

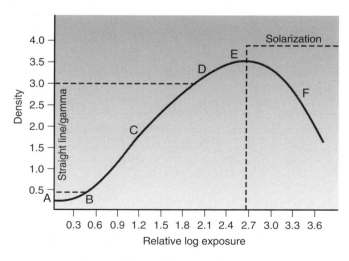

Figure A-6 ■ Characteristic curve.

D_{max} **(E)**– represents the maximum density that the film is able to demonstrate. At this exposure level all of the silver halide crystals are completely bound by silver atoms. With additional exposure to radiation the recorded density would not increase, rather it would decrease causing solarization of the radiographic film.

Solarization (F)– the process of reducing the density on a radiograph that is at D_{max}; the basis for duplication film. When radiographic film reaches D_{max} all of the silver halide crystals are bound by silver atoms and are unable to receive any additional atoms. With additional exposure to radiation the atoms become ionized, reversing the charge of the silver atoms, thereby repelling them from the silver halide crystals. Duplication film is pre-exposed or solarized. As additional exposure occurs, the resultant image becomes lighter or less dense rather than darker. The second or declining half of the sensitometric bell curve demonstrates this process.

Content Category	Percent of Test	Number of Questions
A. Radiation Protection	15%	30
B. Equipment Operation and Maintenance	15%	30
C. Image Production and Evaluation	25%	50
D. Radiographic Procedures	30%	60
E. Patient Care	15%	30
	100%	200

A. RADIATION PROTECTION (30)

I. Patient Protection (12)
A. Biological Effects of Radiation
   1. dose-effect relationships
   2. long-term effects
      a. cancer (including leukemia)
      b. cataracts
      c. life-span shortening
   3. somatic effects
      a. embryonic and fetal effects
      b. bone marrow
      c. thyroid
      d. skin
   4. genetic effects
      a. genetically significant dose (GSD)
      b. genetic effects
   5. relative tissue radiosensitivities
B. Minimizing Patient Exposure
   1. exposure factors
      a. kVp
      b. mAs
      c. single-phase, 3-phase, and high-frequency generators
   2. shielding
      a. rationale for use
      b. types of protective devices
      c. placement of protective devices
   3. beam restriction
      a. purpose of primary beam restriction
      b. effect on secondary (scatter) radiation
      c. types (collimators, cones, aperture diaphragms)
   4. filtration
      a. effect on skin and organ exposure
      b. effect on average beam energy
      c. NCRP recommendations
   5. patient positioning (i.e., PA versus AP)
   6. film, screens, and film-screen combinations
   7. grids; air-gap techniques
   8. automatic exposure control

II. Personnel Protection (9)
A. Sources of Radiation Exposure
   1. exposure to primary x-ray beam
   2. secondary radiation
   3. leakage radiation
B. Basic Methods of Protection
   1. time
   2. distance
   3. shielding
C. NCRP Recommendations for Protective Devices
D. Special Considerations
   1. portable (mobile) units
   2. fluoroscopy
      a. protective drapes
      b. protective Bucky slot cover
      c. cumulative timer
   3. guidelines for fluoroscopy and portable units (NCRP, CFR-21)

III. Radiation Exposure and Monitoring (9)
A. Basic Properties of Radiation
B. Units of Measurement
   1. rad (gray)
   2. rem (sievert)
   3. roentgen (C/kg)
C. Dosimeters (types, proper use)
D. NCRP Recommendations for Personnel Monitoring

1. ALARA and dose equivalent limits
2. evaluation of cumulative dose records
3. maintenance of cumulative dose records

B. EQUIPMENT OPERATION AND MAINTENANCE (30)

I. Radiographic Equipment (21)

A. Components of Basic Radiographic Unit
   1. operating console
   2. x-ray tube
      a. tube construction
      b. warm-up procedures
      c. tube rating charts
   3. automatic exposure control
      a. radiation detectors (e.g., ionization chamber, photomultiplier tube)
      b. back-up timer
   4. exposure controls
   5. beam restriction devices
B. X-Ray Generator, Transformers, and Rectification System
   1. basic principles
   2. phase and pulse
C. Fluoroscopic Unit
   1. image intensifier
   2. viewing systems (e.g., TV monitor)
   3. recording systems (e.g., videotape)
   4. automatic brightness control
D. Types of Units
   1. stationary
   2. portable (mobile)
   3. specialized or dedicated units

II. Evaluation of Radiographic Equipment and Accessories (9)

A. Equipment Calibration
   1. kVp
   2. mA
   3. time
B. Beam Restriction
   1. light field to radiation field alignment
   2. central ray alignment
C. Recognition of Malfunctions
D. Screens and Cassettes
   1. construction
   2. handling
   3. artifacts
   4. maintenance
E. Shielding Accessories (e.g., lead apron testing)

C. IMAGE PRODUCTION AND EVALUATION (50)

I. Selection of Technical Factors (26)

A. Density
   1. mAs
   2. kVp
   3. distance
   4. film-screen combinations
   5. grids
   6. filtration
   7. beam restriction
   8. anatomical and pathologic factors
   9. anode heel effect
B. Contrast
   1. kVp
   2. beam restriction
   3. grids
   4. filtration
   5. anatomic and pathologic factors
C. Recorded Detail
   1. OID
   2. SID
   3. focal spot size
   4. film-screen combinations
   5. motion
D. Distortion
   1. size
   2. shape
E. Film, Screen, and Grid Selection
   1. film characteristics
      a. film contrast
      b. film latitude
      c. exposure latitude
   2. film-screen combination
      a. phosphor type
      b. relative speed
      c. single-versus double-emulsion film
      d. special applications (e.g., detail, latitude)
   3. conversion factors for grids
F. Technique Charts
   1. caliper measurement
   2. fixed versus variable kVp
   3. anatomical considerations
      a. tissue density
      b. part thickness
   4. special considerations (e.g., casts, pathology, pediatrics, contrast media)
   5. automatic exposure control
G. Manual Versus Automatic Exposure Control
   1. effects of changing exposure factors on radiographic quality
   2. selection of ionization chamber or photocell

3. alignment of part to ionization chamber or photocell

II. Film Processing and Quality Assurance (12)

A. Film Storage
   1. pressure artifacts
   2. fog (e.g., age, chemical, radiation, temperature, safelight)
B. Cassette Loading
   1. matching film and screens
   2. film-handling artifacts (e.g., static, crinkle marks, fog)
C. Radiographic Identification
   1. methods (e.g., photographic, radiographic)
   2. legal considerations (e.g., patient data, examination data)
D. Automatic Film Processor
   1. processor chemistry
   2. components and systems
      a. transport
      b. replenishment
      c. temperature regulation
      d. recirculation
      e. dryer
   3. maintenance
      a. start-up and shut-down procedure
      b. removal and cleaning of cross-over assembly
      c. sensitometric monitoring
   4. system malfunction
      a. observable effects (e.g., artifacts, fluctuations in density, contrast, fog)
      b. possible causes (e.g., improper temperature, contamination, roller alignment, replenishment, water flow)

III. Evaluation of Radiographs (12)

A. Criteria for Diagnostic Quality Radiographs
   1. radiographic density
   2. radiographic contrast
   3. recorded detail
   4. distortion
   5. artifacts
   6. grid alignment
   7. proper demonstration of anatomical structure
   8. identification markers (e.g., anatomical, patient, date)
B. Causes of Poor Radiographic Quality
   1. technical factors (e.g., kVp, mAs, distance, filtration, film-screen combination, grids)

2. positioning (e.g., OID, SID, tube-part-film alignment)
   3. patient considerations (e.g., pathologic conditions, motion)
   4. processing (e.g., fog, contamination, temperature)
   5. artifacts
C. Improvement of Suboptimal Image

D. RADIOGRAPHIC PROCEDURES (60)

I. General Procedural Considerations (6)

A. Patient Preparation (e.g., explaining procedures, removal of radiopaque objects)
B. Equipment Capabilities
C. Positioning Terminology
D. Patient Respiration and Motion Control
   1. instruction for the examination
   2. effect on radiographic quality
   3. adapting to patient's cooperative ability (e.g., mA and time adjustments)
   4. immobilization devices and techniques
E. Technique and Positioning Variations (e.g., for trauma or pediatric patients; adapting to patient's body habitus)

II. Specific Imaging Procedures (54) (including POSITIONING, TECHNICAL FACTORS, ANATOMY, PHYSIOLOGY, and PATHOLOGY)

A. Thorax (6)
   1. chest
   2. ribs
   3. sternoclavicular joints
   4. sternum
B. Abdomen and GI Studies (10)
   1. abdomen
   2. esophagus
   3. upper GI series
   4. small bowel series
   5. barium enema, single-contrast
   6. barium enema, double-contrast
   7. operative cholangiography
   8. T-tube cholangiography
   9. Cholecystography
   10. ERCP (endoscopic retrograde cholangiopancreatography)
C. Urologic Studies (4)
   1. cystography
   2. cystourethrography
   3. intravenous urography
   4. retrograde urography
   5. retrograde urethrography

D. Extremities (16)
1. toes
2. foot
3. os calcis
4. ankle
5. tibia, fibula
6. knee
7. patella
8. femur
9. fingers
10. hand
11. wrist
12. forearm
13. elbow
14. humerus
15. shoulder
16. scapula
17. clavicle
18. acromioclavicular joints
19. bone survey
20. long bone measurement
21. bone age
22. soft tissue

E. Spine and Pelvis (8)
1. cervical spine
2. thoracic spine
3. scoliosis series
4. lumbosacral spine
5. sacrum
6. sacroiliac joints
7. coccyx
8. pelvis
9. hip

F. Head and Neck (7)
1. skull
2. mastoids, temporal bones
3. facial bones
4. mandible
5. zygomatic arch
6. temporomandibular joints
7. nasal bones
8. optic foramina
9. orbit
10. paranasal sinuses
11. soft tissue neck

G. Other (3)
1. tomography
2. arthrography
3. myelography
4. venography
5. hysterosalpingography

E. PATIENT CARE (30)

I. Legal and Professional Responsibilities (6)

A. Scheduling and Sequencing Examinations
B. Legal Aspects of Radiology

1. request to perform examination
2. patient rights (e.g., confidentiality, consent)
3. professional liability

C. Patient Identification (e.g., wrist band, questioning)
D. Verification of Requested Examination
1. clarification of terminology
2. comparison of request to clinical indications (e.g., left arm injured, but right arm requested)
3. evaluation of need for additional projections
4. modification of routine projection

II. Patient Education, Safety, and Comfort (4)

A. Communication with Patients
1. review of patient history
2. explanation of current procedure
3. respond to inquiries about other imaging procedures (basic concepts of mammography, CT, MRI, sonography, nuclear medicine)

B. Assessment of Patient Condition (e.g., motor control, severity of injury, support equipment)
C. Proper Body Mechanics for Patient Transfer
D. Patient Privacy, Safety, and Comfort

III. Prevention and Control of Infection (6)

A. Transmission of Infection
B. Universal Precautions
C. Disinfection and Sterilization; Asepsis and Sterile Technique
D. Handling of Biohazardous Materials
E. Isolation Procedures
1. types (e.g., respiratory, protective, reverse)
2. radiography of isolation patients

IV. Patient Monitoring (9)

A. Routine Monitoring
1. equipment (e.g., stethoscope, sphygmomanometer)
2. vital signs (e.g., blood pressure, pulse, respiration, temperature)
3. physical signs and symptoms

B. Support Equipment (e.g., IV tubes, chest tubes, catheters)
C. Common Medical Emergencies (e.g., seizure, cardiac arrest, loss of consciousness, bleeding)
D. Management of Common Medical Emergencies (e.g., CPR, hemostasis)

V. Contrast Media (5)

A. Types and Properties (e.g., iodinated, water-soluble, barium, ionic versus non-ionic)
B. Appropriateness of Contrast Medium to Examination and Patient Condition (e.g., perforated bowel, patient age, patient weight)
C. Contraindications
D. Patient Education
   1. instructions regarding preparation, diet, and medications
   2. postexamination instructions
E. Administration
   1. routes (e.g., venous, rectal, oral)
   2. supplies (e.g., enema kits, needles)
   3. venipuncture
F. Complications/Reactions
   1. local effects (e.g., extravasation, phlebitis)
   2. systemic effects
      a. mild (e.g., flushing, hives, nausea)
      b. severe (e.g., shock, hypotension)
   3. radiographer's response (e.g., first-aid, documentation)

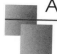

APPENDIX C: Blood Chemistry, Blood Counts, and Abbreviations

Normal Blood Chemistry: Laboratory Test and Range

Glucose– 65–115 mg/dl
Potassium (K)– 3.5–5.3 mg/dl
Sodium (Na)– 135–147 mEq/l
Chloride (C)– 95–105 mEq/l
Phosphorus (P)– 2.5–4.5 mg/dl
Creatinine (Cr)– 0.5–1.5 mg/dl
Copper (Cu)– 100–200 μg/dl
Iron (Fe)– 35–180 μg/dl
Magnesium (Mg)– 1–2 mg/dl
Sulfate– 0.5–1.5 mEq/l
Uric acid– 3.5–8 mg/dl
Blood urea nitrogen (BUN)– 8–25 mg/dl
Protein (total)– 6–8 g/dl
  Albumin– 3.5–5 g/dl
  Globulin– 1.5–3.5 g/dl
Cholesterol (total)– 150–200 mg/dl
  HDL cholesterol– Male: 30–75 mg/dl
                       Female: 40–90 mg/dl
  LDL cholesterol– <130 mg/dl
Carbon dioxide (CO$_2$)– 22–32 mEq/l

Complete Blood Count: Laboratory Test and Range

Red blood cells (RBC)– 4–6 μl
Hemoglobin (Hgb or Hb)– 12–17 g/dl
Hematocrit (Hct)– 35%–54%
White blood cells (WBC)– 4500–10,000 μl
  Neutrophils– 2500–7000 μl
  Eosinophils– 100–300 μl
  Basophils– 40–100 μl
  Monocytes– 200–600 μl
  Lymphocytes– 1700–3500 μl
Platelets– 150,000–400,000 μl

Common Medical Abbreviations

C/O– complains of . . .
CC– chief complaint . . .
Dx:– diagnosed with . . .
Hx:– history of . . .
Abd– abdomen
ADH– antidiuretic hormone
Ad lib– as desired
AIDS– acquired immunodeficiency syndrome
AKA– above the knee amputation
ALL– acute lymphocytic leukemia
Angio– angiography

Aq– water
ASD– atrial septal defect
ASHD– arteriosclerotic heart disease
Au– Gold
BaE/BE– barium enema
b.i.d.– twice a day
BKA– below the knee amputation
BM– bowel movement
BP– blood pressure
BUN– blood urea nitrogen
Bx– biopsy
c̄– with
Ca– cancer
CABG– coronary artery bypass graft
CAD– coronary artery disease
CBC– complete blood count
CCU– coronary care unit
  ICU– intensive care unit
  SICU– surgical intensive care unit
  PICU– pediatric intensive care unit
  NICU– neonatal intensive care unit
CHF– congestive heart failure
COPD– chronic obstructive pulmonary disease
CPR– cardiopulmonary resuscitation
CSF– cerebrospinal fluid
CVA– cerebral vascular accident
C/W– compare with
CXR– chest x-ray
D/C– discontinue
DM– diabetes mellitus
DOA– dead on arrival
DOB– date of birth
DSA– digital subtraction angiography
DVT– deep vein thrombosis
ECG (EKG)– electrocardiogram
EEG– electroencephalogram
EMG– electromyogram
IVDA– intravenous drug abuse
p.c.– post cibum (after meals)
PD– peritoneal dialysis
PDA– patent ductus arteriosus
p.o.– per os (by mouth)
PM– post mortem
P~O– postoperative
PPD– purified protein derivative (tuberculosis test)
p.r.n.– as required (*pro re nata*)
PVC– premature ventricular contraction
PVD– peripheral vascular disease
q.– every/each
q.am– every morning

q.d.– everyday
q.i.d.– four times daily
q.n.s.– quantity not sufficient
q.o.d.– every other day
q.pm– every evening
R/O– rule out
Rx:– prescription
s̄– without
SOB– shortness of breath

SP– status post
SVC– superior vena cava
TIA– transient ischemic attack
t.i.d.– three times a day
Tx:– treatment of . . .
VSD– ventricular septal defect
Wt.– weight
y/o– years old

PERIODIC TABLE OF THE ELEMENTS

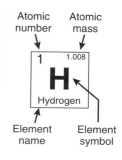

Atomic number   Atomic mass

Element name   Element symbol

Outer Electrons located in	Period	Group I	Group II	Group III	Group IV	Group V	Group VI	Group VII	Group VIII	
K shell	1	1 1.008 **H** Hydrogen							2 4.00 **He** Helium	
L shell	2	3 6.94 **Li** Lithium	4 9.02 **Be** Beryllium	5 10.82 **B** Boron	6 12.01 **C** Carbon	7 14.09 **N** Nitrogen	8 16.00 **O** Oxygen	9 19.00 **F** Fluorine	10 20.18 **Ne** Neon	
M shell	3	11 23.0 **Na** Sodium	12 24.32 **Mg** Magnesium	13 26.97 **Al** Aluminum	14 28.06 **Si** Silicon	15 30.98 **P** Phosphorus	16 32.06 **S** Sulfur	17 35.46 **Cl** Chlorine	18 39.99 **A** Argon	
N shell	4	19 39.096 **K** Potassium	20 40.08 **Ca** Calcium	21 45.10 **Sc** Scandium	22 47.90 **Ti** Titanium	23 50.95 **V** Vanadium	24 52.01 **Cr** Chromium	25 54.93 **Mn** Manganese	26 55.85 **Fe** Iron	27 58.94 **Co** Cobalt / 28 58.69 **Ni** Nickel
		29 63.57 **Cu** Copper	30 65.38 **Zn** Zinc	31 69.72 **Ga** Gallium	32 72.60 **Ge** Germanium	33 74.91 **As** Arsenic	34 79.00 **Se** Selenium	35 79.92 **Br** Bromine	36 83.7 **Kr** Krypton	
O shell	5	37 85.48 **Rb** Rubidium	38 87.63 **Sr** Strontium	39 88.92 **Y** Yttrium	40 91.22 **Zr** Zirconium	41 92.91 **Cb** Columbium	42 96.0 **Mo** Molybdenum	43 99 **Tc** Technetium	44 101.7 **Ru** Ruthenium / 45 102.8 **Rh** Rhodium / 46 106.7 **Pd** Palladium	
		47 107.88 **Ag** Silver	48 112.41 **Cd** Cadmium	49 118.70 **In** Indium	50 121.77 **Sn** Tin	51 127.6 **Sb** Antimony	52 126.93 **Te** Tellurium	53 126.92 **I** Iodine	54 131.3 **Xe** Xenon	
P shell	6	55 132.9 **Cs** Cesium	56 137.4 **Ba** Barium	Rare Earths 57—71	72 178.6 **Hf** Hafnium	73 180.9 **Ta** Tantalum	74 183.9 **W** Tungsten	75 186.3 **Re** Rhenium	76 190.2 **Os** Osmium / 77 193.1 **Ir** Iridium / 78 195.2 **Pt** Platinum	
		79 197.2 **Au** Gold	80 200.6 **Hg** Mercury	81 204.4 **Tl** Thallium	82 207.2 **Pb** Lead	83 209.0 **Bi** Bismuth	84 210 **Po** Polonium	85 211 **At** Astatine	86 222 **Rn** Radon	
Q shell	7	87 224 **Vl** Virginium	88 226.05 **Ra** Radium	Actinide Series 89—103						

Rare Earths Series	57 138.91 **La** Lanthanium	58 140.12 **Ce** Cerium	59 140.91 **Pr** Proseodymium	60 144.24 **Nd** Neodymium	61 147 **Pm** Promethium	62 150.35 **Sm** Samarium	63 151.96 **Eu** Europium	64 157.25 **Gd** Gadolinium	65 158.92 **Tb** Terbium	66 162.50 **Dy** Dysprosium	67 164.93 **Ho** Holmium	68 167.26 **Er** Erbium	69 168.93 **Tm** Thulium	70 173.04 **Yb** Ytterbium	71 174.97 **Lu** Lutetium
Actinide Series	89 227 **Ac** Actinium	90 232.04 **Th** Thorium	91 231 **Pa** Protactinium	92 238.03 **U** Uranium	93 237 **Np** Neptunium	94 242 **Pu** Plutonium	95 243 **Am** Americium	96 245 **Cm** Curium	97 249 **Bk** Berkelium	98 251 **Cf** Californium	99 254 **Es** Einsteinium	100 255 **Fm** Fermium	101 256 **Md** Mendelevium	102 254 **No** Nobelium	103 257 **Lr** Lawrencium

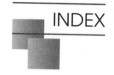

INDEX

Note: Page numbers in *italics* refer to illustrations; page numbers followed by c refer to charts, and those followed by t refer to tables.